Stone Therapy
in Urology

Stone Therapy in Urology

Edited by F. Eisenberger, K. Miller, and J. Rassweiler

with contributions by
T. Bräuner
F. Brümmer
F. Eisenberger
W. Eisenmenger
G. J. Fuchs
R. Gumpinger
D. F. Hülser
K. Miller
J. Rassweiler
J. Staudenraus
H. M. Weber

Foreword by Donald P. Griffith

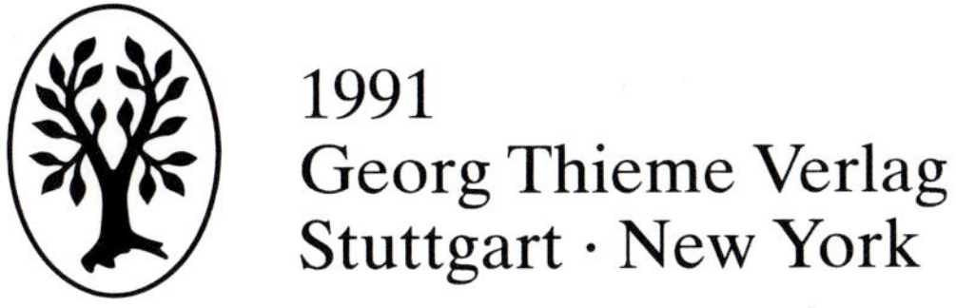

1991
Georg Thieme Verlag
Stuttgart · New York

Thieme Medical Publishers, Inc.
New York

IV

Translated by
Mario Kuntze, M.D.
Resident Urology Clinic
St. Mark's Hospital
Frankfurt University Medical School
Wilhelm-Epstein-Strasse 2
6000 Frankfurt on Main 50
Germany

With the assistance of
Sigrid Strobel
Hainer Trift 53
6072 Dreieich-Buchschlag
Germany

Library of Congress Cataloging-in-Publication Data

Urologische Steintherapie. English.
    Stone Therapy in Urology / edited by F. Eisen-
  berger, K. Miller, and J. Rassweiler.
      p.   cm.
    Translation of: Urologische Steintherapie.
    Includes bibliographical references.
    Includes index.
    1. Urinary organs -- Calculi -- Treatment.
  2. Urinary   organs -- Calculi -- Surgery.
  3. Ultrasonic lithotripsy.   I. Eisenberger, F.
  (Ferdinand)   II. Miller, K. (Kurt)   III. Rassweiler,
  J. (Jens)   IV. Title.
    [DNLM   1. Endoscopy -- methods.
  2. Lithotripsy.
  3. Urinary Calculi -- therapy.   WJ 166 U78]
  RC916.U77B13   1990
  616.6'2206 -- dc20
  DNLM/DLC   90−11328

1st German edition 1987
1st Italian edition 1988

This book is an authorized and completely revised translation from the 1st German edition, published and copyrighted 1987 by Georg Thieme Verlag, Stuttgart, Germany. Title of the German edition: Urologische Steintherapie. ESWL und Endourologie.

© 1991 Georg Thieme Verlag, Rüdigerstrasse 14, D-7000 Stuttgart 30, Germany
Thieme Medical Publishers, Inc., 381 Park Avenue South, New York, N.Y. 10016
Typesetting and Printed by Druckhaus Götz KG, D-7140 Ludwigsburg
Printed in Germany

ISBN 3-13-713301-7
(Georg Thieme Verlag, Stuttgart)
ISBN 0-86577-287-8
(Thieme Medical Publishers, Inc., New York)
                                        1 2 3 4 5 6

Foreword

Urinary stones have tormented and vexed mankind since the dawn of time. Ancient, medieval and Renaissance writings abundantly chronicle the misery and suffering they caused. Hippocrates—the father of Western medicine—counseled his followers and his patients about the effects of urinary stones and the treatments then available (ca. 400 BC).

Perhaps no other pathological condition better exemplifies the triumph of technology over misery and suffering.

Classical surgery for stones (e. g., elective nephrectomy), which was first performed by Gustav Simon of Heidelberg in 1869, ushered in the technological era. Between 1870 and the late 1970s, major technological advances evolved in surgical lithotomy and support technologies (such as anesthesia, antimicrobial treatment, and blood transfusions). These changes enhanced the success of classical surgery. Treatment was furthered by epidemiological and etiological investigations and by development of dietary and pharmacological treatments to retard or prevent stone growth or recurrence.

In the 1980s, technological developments resulted in quantum leaps in the elimination of problematic stones. Evolution of endourological instruments and techniques, and the union of fluoroscopy, ultrasonography and ancillary technologies with endoscopy, reduced surgical morbidity and improved treatment efficacy. Investigations of other forms of energy—notably shockwaves—both enhanced and competed with the evolving endourological technologies.

After approximately 100 years, the classical surgical treatment of urinary stones is now obsolete in all but a few carefully-selected patients. Advancing technology has made the minimally invasive or noninvasive elimination of stones commonplace and routine.

This textbook is written by a group of young, innovative clinical investigators, all of whom have contributed mightily to the advancements that have established the new standards. The text is a classic inasmuch as the authors themselves are the innovators and their work is already established as authoritative.

Reading this text, a perceptive reader will gain insight into the process of innovation. It is likely that similar innovations will replace the classical surgical procedures for other pathological processes as well. The reader will therefore also be learning about technologies that are likely to be applicable to other diseases.

In summary, this is an authoritative, innovative, highly readable, state-of-the-art textbook.

September, 1990

Donald P. Griffith, M. D.
Dept. of Urology
Baylor College of Medicine
Texas Medical Center
Houston, Texas

Preface

It is now twenty years since the idea was first developed of shattering calculi using shock waves that could be introduced into the body without injury. This daring research project, promoted by physicists and physicians, was both revolutionary and at the same time somewhat illusory. Scientists viewed it with disbelief and skepticism. But the project was the beginning of an incomparably productive and mutually stimulating phase of cooperation between medicine and technology that has today already become indispensable. It culminated, after ten years of intensive research, including many failures, in the first successful clinical application of extracorporeal shock-wave lithotripsy (ESWL) in 1980.

There can be no doubt that ESWL has today passed the test of time. It has transformed therapeutic approaches to urolithiasis and marginalized surgical procedures to an indication level of a mere 2%. ESWL is today the initial noninvasive treatment of choice for urolithiasis.

Our concern has been to present ESWL applications in the context of indications, together with the "tricks of the trade," at the same time listing technical variations and related treatment data, including anesthesia, auxiliary measures, and success rates. The present work is therefore not a textbook in the usual sense, but rather a user's guide corresponding to the clinical realities of nephrolithiasis in each "stone situation."

Of course, alternative endourologic procedures competing with ESWL and complementing it are also included in the book.

Contributions by physicists and biologists on the technology of shock waves and their effects on cells bring us back to the basic research that was carried out during the 1970s. This branch of research was overtaken at the time by the sudden clinical successes of ESWL, but in a period in which "minimal invasiveness" is at the center of every area of surgery, it is regaining its importance and being carried forward once again, with the aim of exploring fresh ways of applying shock waves in the future.

October, 1990   *The Editors*

Acknowledgments

The various topics dealt with in the book were written by the following authors:
Conservative stone therapy: K. Miller
Indications for interventional stone therapy: K. Miller, J. Rassweiler, F. Eisenberger
Biological side effects of shock waves: T. Bräuner, F. Brümmer, D. F. Hülser, J. Rassweiler
Shock wave physics: W. Eisenmenger, J. Staudenraus
Clinical aspects of shock-wave lithotripsy: J. Rassweiler, F. Eisenberger, G. J. Fuchs
Ureteroscopy: K. Miller, R. Gumpinger
Percutaneous and open surgery: K. Miller, R. Gumpinger, F. Eisenberger
Comparison of lithotriptors: J. Rassweiler, F. Eisenberger
Future aspects of stone therapy: J. Rassweiler, K. Miller, H. M. Weber

We should like to thank all contributors for their commitment to the field of urinary stone therapy and for their continuous work for this book. We also acknowledge the contribution of Detlef and Ulrike Rahe on the fourth generation lithotriptor, graphic support by F. Hartmann, and numerous hints for "practical ESWL" by our technician, James Göbel.

Contributors

Thomas Bräuner, Ph. D.
Dept. of Biophysics
Biological Institute
University of Stuttgart
Pfaffenwaldring 57
7000 Stuttgart 80
Germany

Franz Brümmer, Ph. D.
Dept. of Biophysics
Biological Institute
University of Stuttgart
Pfaffenwaldring 57
7000 Stuttgart 80
Germany

Prof. Ferdinand Eisenberger, M. D.
Director
School of Medicine
University of Tübingen;
Dept. of Urology
Katharinenhospital
Kriegsbergstrasse 60
7000 Stuttgart 1
Germany

Prof. Wolfgang Eisenmenger, Ph. D.
Director
Institute of Physics
University of Stuttgart
Pfaffenwaldring 57
7000 Stuttgart 80
Germany

Gerhard J. Fuchs, M. D.
Dept. of Urology
Center for Health Sciences
School of Medicine
University of California
10833 Le Conte Avenue
Los Angeles, CA 90024
USA

Rudolf Gumpinger, M. D.
Head
Dept. of Urology
District Hospital
Memminger Strasse 50–52
8960 Kempten
Germany

Prof. Dieter F. Hülser, Ph. D.
Director
Biological Institute
University of Stuttgart
Pfaffenwaldring 57
7000 Stuttgart 80
Germany

Kurt Miller, M. D.
Dept. of Urology
University of Ulm
Prittwitzstrasse 43
7900 Ulm
Germany

Jens Rassweiler, M. D.
Dept. of Urology
City of Mannheim Hospital;
School of Medicine
University of Heidelberg
Theodor-Kutzer-Ufer
6500 Mannheim
Germany

Joachim Staudenraus, Ph. D.
Institute of Physics
University of Stuttgart
Pfaffenwaldring 57
7000 Stuttgart 80
Germany

Hans M. Weber, M. D.
Dept. of Urology
University of Ulm Hospital
Prittwitzstrasse 43
7900 Ulm
Germany

Contents

1 Epidemiology, Etiology and Pathogenesis, Drug Treatment, Litholysis, and Metaphylaxis

The pathophysiology of urinary stone disease has been the subject of intensive research for many years. During this period understanding of the stone "syndrome" has considerably improved; however, a real breakthrough has never been achieved. The revolution of interventional stone therapy, mainly caused by the development of extracorporeal shock wave lithotripsy (ESWL), has had its effects both on the motivation of stone patients and stone researchers:

- Nowadays, the patient encounters calculus treatment as a noninvasive, nearly pain-free, and fairly efficient therapy. As a consequence, the patient usually prefers to occasionally undergo this therapy than to adhere to endless drug regimens or strict diet schedules.
- The decreasing attractiveness of practical metaphylaxis seems to subsequently make "conventional" stone research more and more unattractive. Hopefully, completely new points of view, such as the role of oxalobacter formigenes in the pathogenesis of calcium oxalate urolithiasis, will provide a new impact on basic stone research. The final goal, that is, preventing urinary stone disease rather than treating it, should not be forgotten.

This chapter provides a short review of the current theories of stone pathogenesis and etiology, as well as a survey of the principle possibilities of metaphylaxis. The aim is to briefly outline the present situation in this field and to emphasize the important role of the new forms of interventional stone therapy.

1.1 Epidemiology

In central Europeans, urolithiasis manifests itself mainly in the kidney and ureters (97%). Calculi in the lower urinary tract are rare and almost always represent a symptom of micturi-tion disturbances. Prevalence and incidence of urolithiasis stress the importance of adequate treatment. 2%−3% of the West German population experience an episode of lithiasis once in their lifetime. The annual rate of primary disease is 0,1% (Vahlensieck 1980, 1982). In the Federal Republic of Germany (FRG), about 320000 people develop urinary calculi every year (primary diseases and recurrences). About 40000 people underwent kidney and ureter surgery in the FRG in 1979 (Schneider, 1986).

Men are affected by urolithiasis more frequently than women; the ratio in Europe is 2:1. Most of the patients develop nephrolithiasis between 30 and 50 years of age (Vahlensieck, 1982). The recurrence rate of untreated urolithiasis is reported to range between 50% and 70%. In the FRG, about 5% of all diseases requiring dialysis are caused by urolithiasis (Schneider, 1983).

1.2 Etiology and Pathogenesis

Etiologically, urolithiasis (Table 1.**1**) can be classified into three groups:

1. Defined clinical pictures (e.g., hyperparathyroidism);
2. Pathological laboratory values (e.g., hypercalciuria) that cannot be attributed to a defined clinical picture;
3. Idiopathic urolithiasis in which differences between healthy subjects and patients developing urinary calculi cannot be established by current laboratory methods.

Even in the case of well-defined clinical syndromes, the term "etiology" is a bit exaggerated. For example, only 65% of all patients suffering from primary hyperparathyroidism actually develop urinary calculi (Hautmann, 1986). In urolithiasis, as in other medical conditions, risk factors must serve as a general

Table 1.1 **Etiological classification of nephrolithiasis in 1,936 patients** (after Rapado)

Known Cause	n	%
Uric acid	260	13.0
Hypercalciuria	213	11.1
Urinary tract infection (UTI)	191	9.9
Malformation of the urinary tract	87	4.4
Increased alkali intake	57	2.9
Hyperparathyroidism	54	2.7
Cystinuria	21	1.1
Bone metaplasia	19	1.0
Hyperoxaluria	8	0.4
Tubular acidosis	6	0.3
Xanthinuria	1	–
Idiopathic lithiasis	1029	53.2

guide until the exact etiological correlations have been established. As per definition, it can be said that such risk factors provide possible but not imperative preconditions for the development of, for example, calcium oxalate stones. In general, distinctions can be made between prerenal, urinary, and chemical risk factors (Fig. 1.**1**).

In the pathogenesis of urolithasis (Fig. 1.**2**), substantiated theories and open questions balance each other.

– Although urinary supersaturation with the lithogenous substance is regarded as a "conditio sine qua non" for stone formation, not all patients meeting this condition actually develop urinary calculi.
– The starting point for stone formation is the so-called nucleus. However, it has not yet been fully elucidated whether this nucleus represents a crystal aggregation of the lithogenous substance itself (homogeneous nucleation) or particles of other substances (heterogeneous nucleation). The site of primary nucleation is also unclear.
– Aggregation and crystal growth ultimately lead to stone formation. It is unknown why the crystal aggregations are not discharged with the urine, or where and how they are temporarily retained in the urinary tract.
– Although the existence of so-called antilithic substances (such as the glycosaminoglycans in the urine) has been established, their exact mode and site of action in the patho-

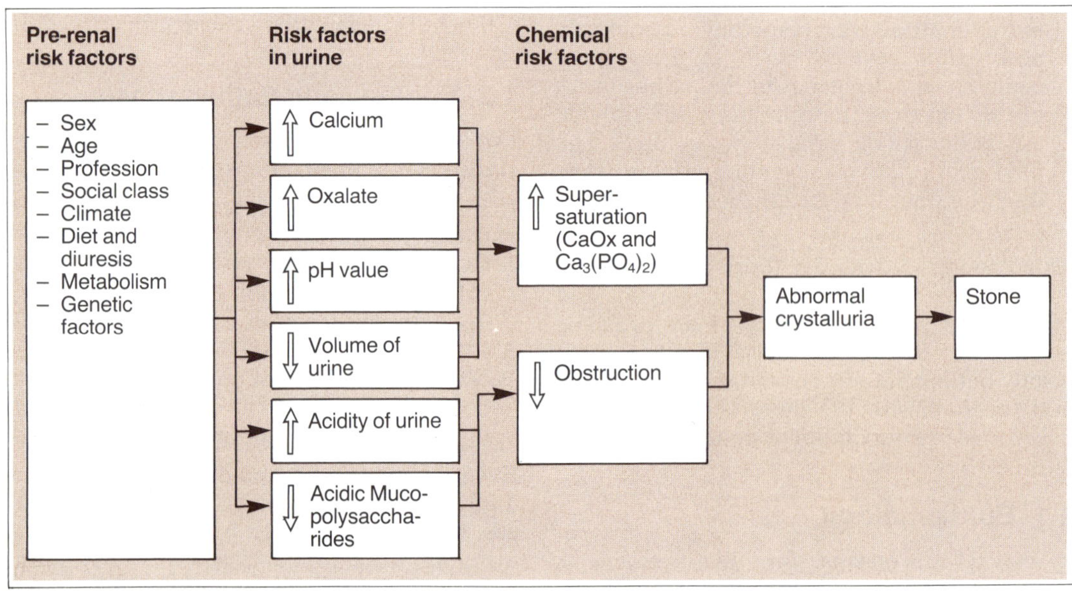

Fig. 1.1 **Risk factor model of calcium oxalate stone formation** (after Robertson)

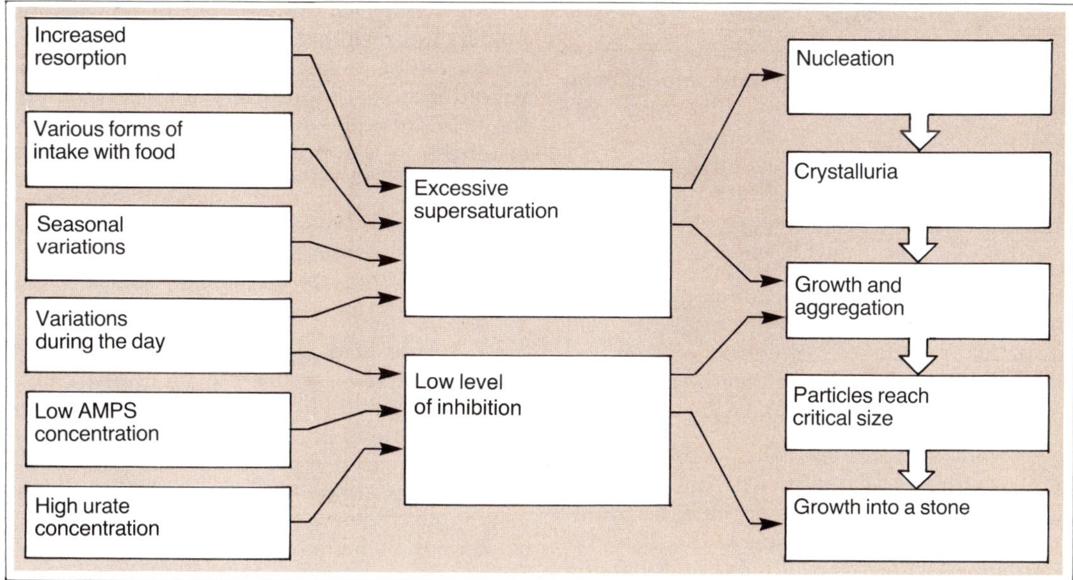

Fig. 1.**2 Pathogenesis and phases of calcium stone formation.** AMPS = acid mucopolysaccharides (after Robertson)

genesis of stone formation still remains unclear.

1.3 Drug treatment and Metaphylaxis

The ideal situation of stone dissolution by drugs has so far only materialized in the case of uric acid stones. Although in vitro dissolution of cystine stones is possible, the clinical experience gained to date with this method is rare and controversial (Hautmann, 1983).

The measures to prevent recurrent stone formation (metaphylaxis) can be classified into two groups:

1. unspecific measures not dependent upon the composition of the stone;
2. specific treatments especially attuned to the stone composition and the patient's metabolic situation.

1.3.1 General Metaphylaxis

The most important general preventive measure to be observed by all stone patients is a sufficient daily fluid intake to effect urinary dilution (specific gravity <1.012, determined

by a urometer). This has a favorable influence on all phases of stone formation (see Fig. 1.**2**):

– As a result of urinary dilution, the concentration of all dissolved substances is reduced, and thereby supersaturation is prevented.
– The increased flow rate of the urine effects better elimination of already formed crystals and aggregates, and prevents their fixation in the urinary system.

The most important difficulty that has to be faced with regard to urinary dilution is the steady fluid intake over a period of 24 hours. Concentration peaks occurring, for example, as a result of nocturnal fluid restriction are difficult to avoid as it is often impossible for the patient to meet the requirement of uniform fluid distribution over day and night.

Additional general preventive measures to be observed by stone patients are

– avoid intensive sweating (urinary concentration);
– avoid exposure to intensive sunlight (elevated vitamin D activity, mobilization of calcium, hypercalciuria);
– reduce body weight in the case of adiposity.

1.3.2 Specific Metaphylaxis

1.3.2.1 **Calcium-containing stones.** Calcium stones, such as calcium oxalate and calcium phosphate, cannot be dissolved by drugs. After the primary stone episode, treatment may be restricted to general preventive measures. Specific metaphylaxis is indicated in the case of patients suffering from recurrent episodes.

First of all, a possible underlying disease (hyperparathyroidism, renal tubular acidosis) should be excluded by laboratory tests, and the patient's metabolic situation established. A specific metaphylaxis can then be attempted according to the results obtained.

A generally accepted measure to prevent calcium urolithiasis is treatment with thiazides. These substances effect hypocalciuria by increasing calcium reabsorption at the distal renal tubule. A controversial point of discussion is whether this treatment is also indicated in cases of absorptive and renal hypercalciuria, as well as in patients exhibiting normal calcium values (Yendt, 1983; Pak, 1982). On the basis of the favorable results (reduction of the recurrence rate to about 10%), the application of thiazides appears to be justified in patients suffering from recurrent calcium stones without extensive laboratory testing prior to treatment. The main problem, and hence the primary cause of treatment failure, appears to be the noncompliance of patients regarding the regular intake of medication.

Further specific metaphylactic measures are as follows:

– Calcium stone patients exhibiting an additional disturbance of uric acid metabolism (about 27% of all patients with calcium oxalate stones suffer from hyperuricemia) should be treated with allopurinol.
– Dietary restriction of calcium-containing food (e.g., dairy products) is reasonable in the case of the absorptive hypercalciuria.

1.3.2.2   **Magnesium-ammonium-phosphate stones.** These stones are mainly found in connection with urinary tract infections (UTI). The urease activity of various bacteria (Proteus, Pseudomonas, Klebsiellae, Staphylococci) splits urinary urea into ammonia and CO_2. The result is an increase in the ammonium and bicarbonate concentrations leading to an alkalization of the urine to pH 8 or 9. As phosphate is only slightly soluble in an alkaline milieu, the resultant supersaturation leads to the formation of calculi. After complete removal of the stone, appropriate drug treatment of the UTI, possibly in combination with urinary acidification, can prevent about 80% of recurrences (Griffith, 1979).

Instrumental litholysis (direct irrigation) of infectious stones with Renacidin via a percutaneous nephrostomy is possible in special cases (see Chapter 4).

1.3.2.3 **Uric acid stones.** The dissolution of uric acid stones by the use of drugs is also applied as a metaphylactic measure. The solubility of uric acid depends on the pH value; it is greatly decreased at pH values of less than 5.8. Treatment is aimed both at dissolving already crystalline concretions and at preventing recrystallization by increasing the urinary pH value. By administration of a citrate acid mixture and under daily monitoring, the urinary pH value is maintained within a range of 6.2 to 6.8 (stronger alkalization would encourage phosphate precipitation).

As the dissolution of uric acid stones with drugs is rather time consuming, instrumental litholysis as a "semi-invasive" method is preferable in the presence of stone-related obstruction. After installation of a percutaneous nephrostomy, the urinary tract is irrigated with 1.6% sodium bicarbonate solution (see Chapter 4).

Patients exhibiting hyperuricemia in addition to uric acid stones should be treated with allopurinol.

1.3.2.4 **Cystine stones.** Cystine stones develop as a result of a congenital tubular transport disorder associated with an excessive excretion of cystine, lysine, arginine, and ornithine. Owing to the poor solubility of cystine, the disease manifests itself in the formation of cystine concrements in about 50% of all patients with homozygote cystinuria. In adult cystinurics, the excretion of cystine is between 600 and 2000 mg/day. The aim of drug treatment is to achieve a reduction to values of < 100 mg/day.

The current treatment of choice (Table 1.**2**) is therapy with alpha-mercapto-propionylglycine (alpha-MPG), which should be preferred to penicillamine for its fewer side effects. Alpha-

Table 1.**2** **Therapeutic principles with cystine stones** (after Hautmann)

Pathophysiological principle	Therapeutic measure	Problems
Reduced cystine excretion	Low-protein diet	Children in growth age
Increase of urine output	Daily fluid intake of 4−7 liters	Hypertension, cardiovascular disease, renal insufficiency
Increase of cystine solubility	Urinary alkalization (pH 7.5)	Phosphate precipitation, hypercalcemia, edema, alkalosis
Conversion of cystine into substances of better solubility	α-mercapto propionyl glycine (α-MPG), D-penicillamine, vitamin C, N-acetyl cysteine	Side effects, loss of activity with long-term use

MPG effects a conversion of cystine into substances of better solubility (cysteine). A disadvantage of alpha-MPG treatment is a loss of therapeutic activity on long-term administration (up to 10 years) (Hautmann, 1983). A reduction of the alpha-MPG dose or a compensation of the loss of efficacy can be achieved by the additional administration of vitamin C.

Additional measures to be observed in the case of cystinuria are excessive fluid intake over 24 hours (4 liters minimum, preferably 5−7 liters) and a urinary alkalization to pH 7 (better solubility of cystine) by a substance such as Uralyt-U. In special cases, instrumental litholysis can also be performed in patients with cystine stones by irrigating the urinary tract with N-acetyl cysteine.

2 Indications for Multimodal Stone Therapy

2.1 General Therapeutic Guidelines

The introduction of ESWL and endoscopic methods (percutaneous nephrolithotomy [PCNL]; ureteroscopy [URS]) should not, at least theoretically, have changed the current indications for interventional stone therapy. Even with all the enthusiasm over the new techniques, it should not be forgotten that

– application of appropriate adjuvant measures effects spontaneous stone passage in about 80% of cases. Various methods are available for conservative treatment of stone-related symptoms (Table 2.**1**);
– asymptomatic calyx stones without growth do not require treatment per se (Fig. 2.**1**). Special indications must be considered in the case of professional demands (professional pilot).

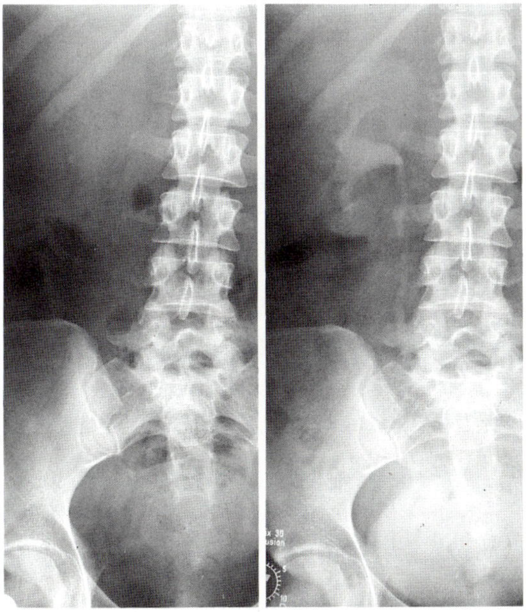

Fig. 2.1 **Lower calyx stone in the right kidney without symptoms** (no pain, no UTI, no incrase in size); no indication for treatment. Controls in 6- to 12-month intervals

Table 2.1 **Conservative Stone Therapy**

General measures	Abundant fluid intake Much physical exercise
Drug treatment	Prevention of ureter colic: papaverine preparations (e. g., papaverine HCl) Therapy of ureter colic: Spasmoanalgesics (e. g., combination of metamizol + pitofenone HCl + fenpiverinium bromide; propyphenazone + drofenine HCl + codeine phosphate) as suppositories or drops or by intravenous administration Spasmoanalgesics as infusion (e. g., 2 ampullae of metamizol + pitofenone HCl + fenpiverinium bromide, n-butyl scopolamine bromide/metamizol Na in 500 ml saline solution) Morphine derivatives + parasympatholytics (e. g., hydromorphine HCl + atropine sulphate)
Adjuvant measures	Physiotherapy (hot bath) Laxatives, clysma, antiemetics

On the other hand, an increasing tendency can be observed (at least in the FRG) towards treating asymptomatic caliceal stones. The rationale for this approach is that an asymptomatic caliceal stone is a potential symptomatic ureteral stone. In other words, to treat an asymptomatic caliceal stone with ESWL is actually inducing a planned passage of the calculus (in the form of fragments) rather than waiting for this event to take place by chance.

This approach is naturally endorsed by the evidence that ESWL has added a completely new dimension to renal stone therapy. This is especially true when compared with surgical nephrolithotomy, which was the only method available for the removal of caliceal stones in the pre-ESWL era.

While the indications for the treatment of caliceal stones and small ureteral calculi (which may pass spontaneously) may still be debatable, indications for interventional stone treatment in general have remained clearly defined.

- Stone size exceeding 8–10 mm in diameter:
  normal passage unlikely.
- Recurrent pain or continuous colics:
  control by drug treatment impossible.
- Prolonged urinary obstruction:
  risk of renal dysfunction.
- Urinary obstruction and UTI:
  risk of pyonephrosis and septicemia.

2.2 Current Role of Endourological Techniques

When open surgery represented the only therapeutic modality for renal and ureteral calculi, the attending urologist had no difficulty in making a treatment decision. The introduction of new techniques with minimal invasiveness, however, at first entailed considerable difficulties in finding the optimum treatment for the variety of stone modifications.

Currently, about 90% of all stone bearers can be treated by ESWL. This widening of the ESWL indications (compared with the situation of about three years ago) is due to three recent advancements:

1. The use of Double-J stents prior to ESWL has significantly reduced the problems connected with the treatment of large stones (Lingeman, 1987; Libby, 1988);

2. Lithotriptors, featuring ultrasound localization system allow noninvasive treatment of nonopaque stones (see Chapter 3; Rassweiler, 1988; Zwergel, 1987);

3. The introduction of piezoelectric shock wave sources (Wolf, Edap) was the starting point for the era of ESWL without major forms of anesthesia (Ziegler, 1986; Zwergel, 1987). Other technologies, such as the sparkgap and the electromagnetic shock wave source, have been modified accordingly. Anesthesia-free ESWL is currently the standard in the FRG and in Europe. It has certainly added to the attraction of ESWL, on the one hand; on the other hand, the efficiency of anesthesia-free lithotriptors seems somewhat reduced. Repeated treatment sessions in 20%–50% of patients have to be taken into account (Zwergel, 1987; Graff, 1987).

As a consequence of the aforementioned advancements of ESWL indications for PCNL and URS have continuously decreased, with only about 10%–15% of the patients currently requiring endoscopic stone removal. Moreover, there are still two groups of "problem" stones that are reason for ongoing discussions regarding the treatment of choice. These are large calculi (>2 cm, partial and complete staghorn stones) and ureteral calculi.

2.2.1 Treatment of Large Stones

Placement of a Double-J ureteral catheter prior to ESWL provides drainage of the kidney during the period of stone passage. Symptoms linked with a persistent, acute obstruction of the kidney can thereby be significantly reduced. The search for the limits of this treatment modality in terms of stone size has not yet been completed, as various groups have presented contradictory results (Eisenberger, 1987; Lingeman, 1987; Alken, 1987; Abomelha, 1987; Groenveld, 1987; Zwergel, 1987; Tiselius, 1988; Miller, 1988, 1989).

Nevertheless, some facts have been repeatedly confirmed.

- The outcome of the treatment does not only depend on the stone size but also on the grade of deformation or dilatation of the renal collecting system (RCS), since the integrity of the RCS seems to be an important factor in the sufficient elimination of stone

fragments after ESWL (Lingeman, 1987).
- The chemical composition and physical properties of the stone (i.e., stone hardness) have significant influence on the results after contact-free lithotripsy (Dretler, 1988; Miller, 1989).

The role and the fate of residual stones are also not yet clearly defined. Some reports (Rassweiler, 1987; Michaels, 1988) suggest that residual fragments from infected stones do not necessarily cause persistent UTIs, but may be asymptomatic. The explanations for this is that enclosed or adherent bacteria can be efficiently eliminated by antibiotics once the infected stone is broken into small fragments.

The final definition of reasonable indications for ESWL therapy with ureteral stenting must obviously influence the "residual" indications for percutaneous stone operations. There is no doubt that, along with the greater invasiveness of PCNL, a higher risk for periprocedural complications must be taken into account. Accordingly, PCNL is only indicated in those stones (which are still to be exactly defined) in which the higher risk is outweighed by significantly better results.

2.2.2 Treatment of Ureteral Stones

Lithotriptors with a fluoroscopic localization system generally bring about in situ ESWL of all ureteral calculi, no matter what the site. This flexibility has been achieved by varying and improving the positioning techniques (Puppo, 1987; Miller, 1987, 1988). Independent from these advancements, the truth remains that the disintegration rate for ureteral calculi is only 60% to 80% (Miller, 1989). Hence, treatment of ureteral calculi is still under discussion.

- Should upper ureteral calculi routinely be mobilized or bypassed with a ureteral stent to improve treatment results, or should they primarily be treated in situ?
- Should distal ureteral calculi be treated by ureteroscopy, or is ESWL preferable as the primary approach?

Various algorithms for the management of ureteral calculi have been presented by various authors (Dretler 1986, 1988; Lingeman 1986, 1987; Fuchs, 1988; Miller, 1989). It is obvious that the preference for either treatment depends on many factors, such as personal experience of the operator, availability of a lithotriptor, type of the lithotriptor, cost considerations, and inpatient or outpatient philosophy. Since there is a rapid development of new technologies in this field, further improvements of anesthesia-free ESWL on the one hand, as well as advancements with laser lithotripsy on the other hand, may provide new arguments for both sides. Thus, an approach that is based on the technical possibilities of August 1990 may be outdated at the end of the same year.

2.2.3 Intercontinental Differences

The therapeutic concepts presented in this book for the application of ESWL, PCNL, and URS are based on experiences with all three methods since 1983. They have been well accepted, with minor modifications, in many centers in Central Europe.

Naturally, these concepts are also based on the "social" health systems in these countries, giving minimal invasiveness a chance without the imperative need for immediate success. Repeated treatment sessions and a reasonable extension of the hospitalization period are well tolerated both by the patient and the insurance companies.

In the USA, on the contrary, it is the primary success of treatment, being carried out mainly in outpatient clinics, that is under main focus today. This philosophy has its roots in the politics of the insurance companies, which above all emphasize the costs of the treatment. The result is an increased rate of adjuvante procedures prior to ESWL, such as retrograde mobilization of ureteral calculi and generous placement of Double-J stents, which in turn is associated with a higher level of invasiveness and morbidity.

In Asia, despite comparable cost impact, ESWL is primarily applied as monotherapy. This is mainly due to the patients' fear of invasive methods, including PCNL, and to the education process now under way in association with the use of endourological methods.

2.2.4 Lithotriptor System Differences

With the introduction of second generation lithotriptors in 1986, the Dornier HM3 monopoly has come to an end. Technical details, advantages, and drawbacks of the different lithotriptor systems are described in detail in Chapter 3. Since the indications are influenced to some extent by the technical features of the lithotriptor, some general considerations are necessary at this point.

– Localization system:

The lithotriptors currently available are equipped with either a fluoroscopic or a ultrasonic localization system or, most recently a combination of both.

Examples of fluoroscopically guided devices are the Dornier HM3, HM3+, HM4, and MFL 5000; the Siemens Lithostar; and the Medstone 1050.

Ultrasound-based machines are represented by the Wolf Piezolith 2300, the Edap LT01, and the Technomed Sonolith 3000.

Systems providing both fluoroscopy and ultrasound are the Dornier MPL-X, the Storz Modulith and the Wolf Piezolith 2500 (see Chapter 3 for details).

The obvious drawback of the ultrasound-guided machines is that ureteral calculi cannot be routinely localized, except immediately below the ureteropelvic junction and in the intramural part of the distal ureter.

– Anesthesia:

Various systems are available requiring no anesthesia or only minor forms (i.e., analgosedation). There seems to still be an inverse correlation between the amount of "pain-freedom" and the efficacy of the lithotriptor system. Accordingly, centers featuring a truly pain-free machine like the Wolf 2300 must naturally tend to a "multiple-sessions philosophy". On the other side of the spectrum, a one-session approach under anesthesia (general or epidural) can be pursued when a powerful machine (Dornier HM3, Dornier MPL 9000) is available (Rassweiler, 1988).

2.3 Specific Indications

2.3.1 Radiopaque Kidney Stones (renal pelvis, calyx)

Stone	**Collecting system**	**Stone**	**Collecting system**
Diameter < 2 cm. Multiple stones of corresponding volume (< 5 cm^3).	No urinary obstruction.	Diameter < 2 cm. Multiple stones of corresponding volume (< 5 cm^3).	Narrowing of the caliceal without primary indication for surgical correction.

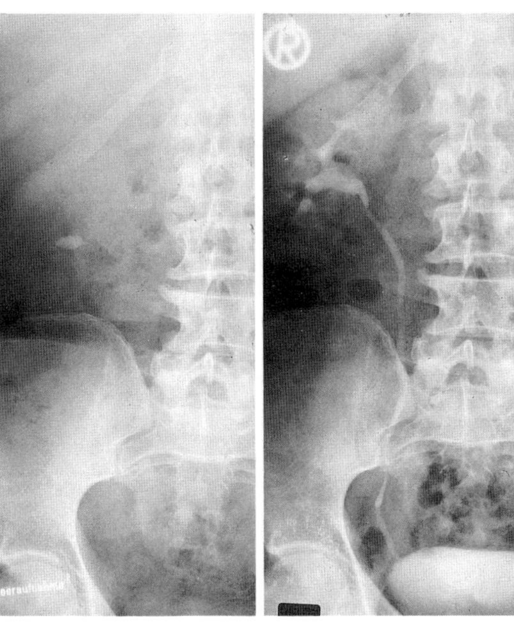

Fig. 2.**2** **"Ideal" ESWL stone:** radiopaque concrement in the renal pelvis of 1.5 cm diameter (left). No obstruction in the IVP (right)

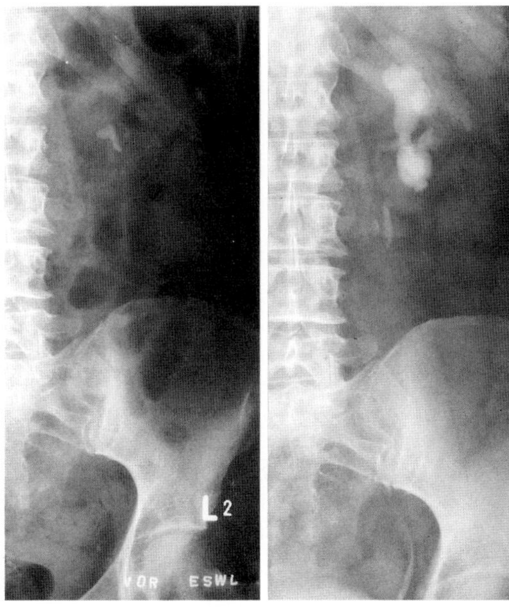

Fig. 2.**3** **Branched pelvic stone;** two small caliceal stones in the lower and middle calyx (left). Marked hydronephrosis on the IVP, probably stone related (right)

Therapy:	ESWL	**Therapy:**	"diagnostic" ESWL
Reasons:	Noninvasive method, lowest possible complication rate, lowest morbidity.	**Reasons:**	Lack of invasiveness justifies probatory ESWL. If stone fragments do not pass, percutaneous stone extraction should be made.

Indications are not dependent on the localization system of the lithotriptor

Stone	**Collecting system**	**Stone**	**Collecting system**
2–3 cm in diameter.	No urinary obstruction.	Multiple stones in various calyces. Stone volume > 5 cm^3	No urinary obstruction. Narrow dendritic collecting system.

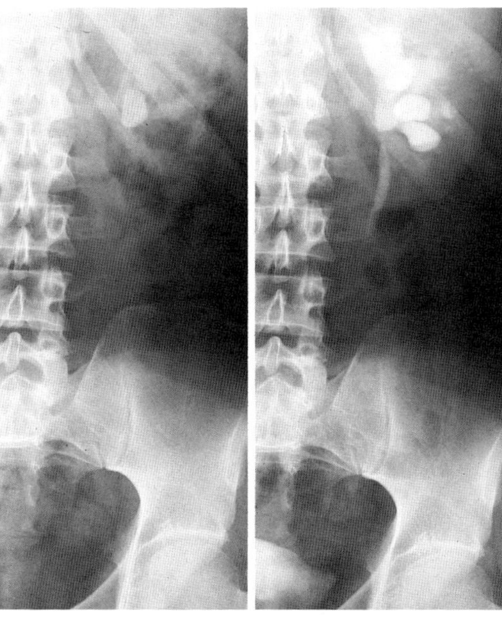

Fig. 2.4 **Large pelvic stone** (>2 cm in diameter) **causing marked hydronephrosis;** medium "central" stone burden

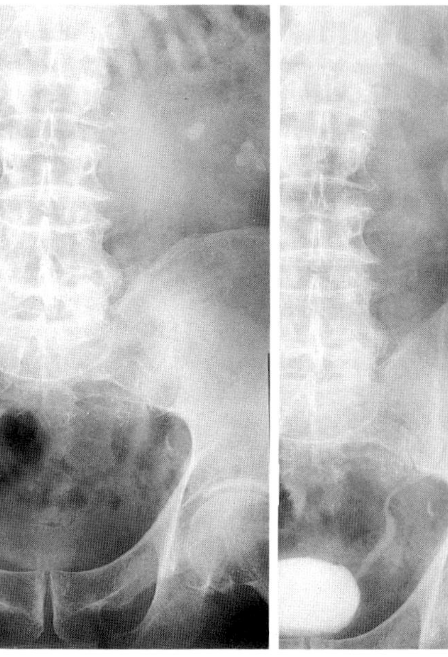

Fig. 2.5 **Three caliceal stones in different calices;** narrow, dendritic RCS, "peripheral" stone burden

Therapy:
1. ESWL with preceding insertion of a Double-J ureteral stent
2. PCNL is a valid alternative in solitary stones of the lower calyx or the renal pelvis (= central stone burden)

Reasons:
1. Double-J prior to ESWL significantly reduces the postprocedural morbidity
2. The morbidity after ESWL is favorably influenced by the Double-J stent, yet the results in terms of stone-freedom are not improved. This is particularly important for lower calyx stones. In the hand of the experienced operator, more than 90% of patients with lower calyx or pelvic stones can be completely rendered stone-free by percutaneous surgery. Naturally, the higher risk linked with PCNL must be taken into account.

Indications are not dependent on the localization system of the lithotriptor

Stone

Multiple stones or branched stones up to complete staghorn stones, medium stone burden.

Collecting system

Normal RCS, no or only mild dilatation (Emmet 1), no deformation.

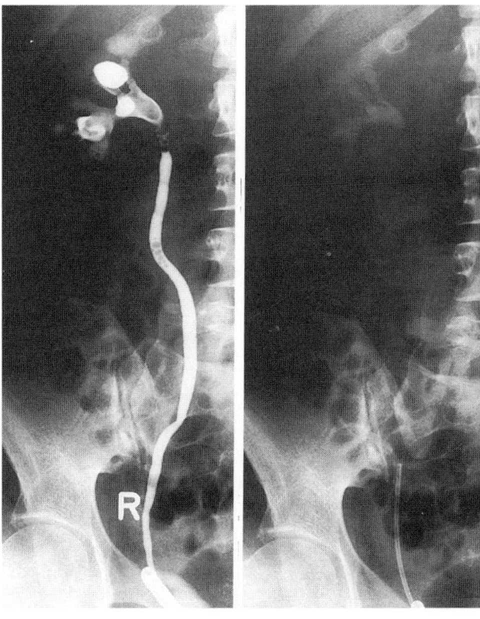

Fig. 2.**6 Complete staghorn stone in a normal RCS;** medium stone burden

Therapy: 1. ESWL + Double-J ureteral stent
2. PCNL + ESWL

Reasons: A normal RCS is the prerequisite for an efficient elimination of stone fragments after ESWL. Depending on the actual stone burden, percutaneous debulking is an option but not uniformly necessary.

Indications are not dependent on the localization system of the lithotriptor

Stone	**Collecting system**
Diameter > 3 cm large central stone burden, filling maximal 2 calices and renal pelvis.	Normal RCS, no or only mild dilatation (Emmet I), no deformation.

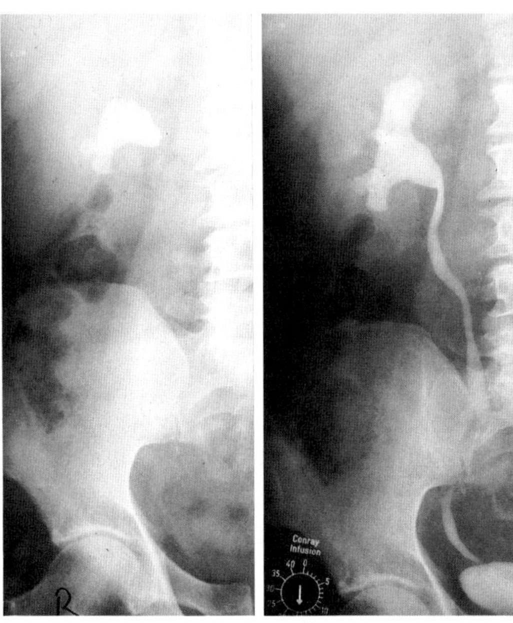

Fig. 2.**7 Partial staghorn stone casting the renal pelvis and two lower calices;** mildly dilated, wide RCS; large, central stone burden

Therapy: 1. PCNL
2. ESWL + Double-J ureteral stent

Reasons: Complete stone removal via one percutaneous tract is technically feasible in one session. The results of ESWL with a Double-J stent in terms of stone freedom are uncertain when very large stone burdens are to be dealt with.

Indications are not dependent on the localization system of the lithotriptor

Stone	**Collecting system**
Multiple stones of large volume; branched stones.	Deformated (Fig 2.**8**) or dilated (Fig. 2.**9**) RCS (Emmet II–IV).

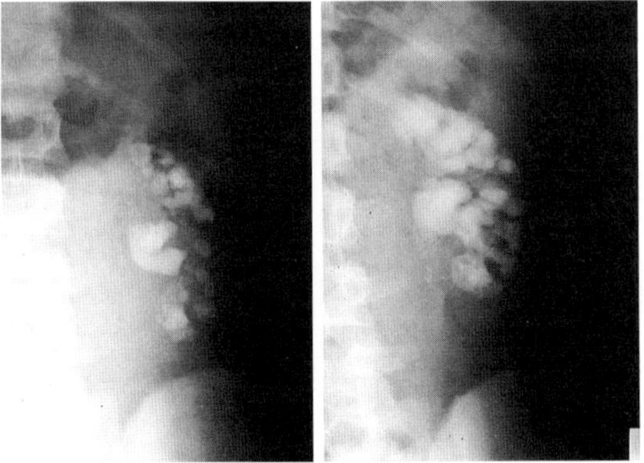

Fig. 2.**8** **Pelvic stone and multiple caliceal stones;** dysplastic RCS, large stone burden

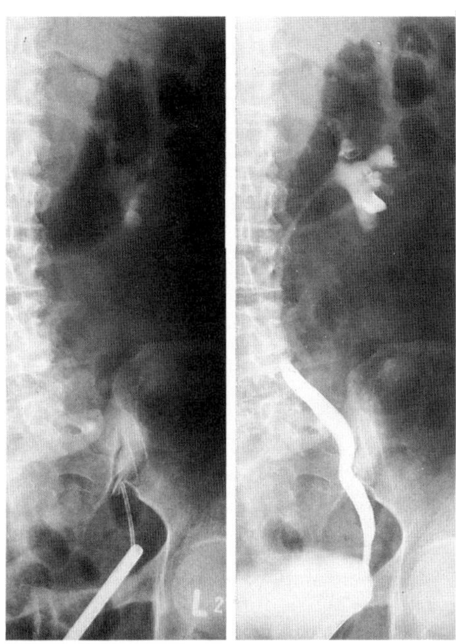

Fig. 2.**9** **Complete staghorn in a dilated RCS;** large stone burden

Therapy: 1. Combination PCNL + ESWL
2. ESWL + Double-J ureteral stent

Reasons: In substantially dilated or deformed renal collecting systems, passage of debris following ESWL is doubtful. Therefore, percutaneous stone debulking and secondary percutaneous removal of stone debris is preferable to ESWL monotherapy.

Indications are not dependent on the localization system of the lithotriptor

Stone

Multiple stones or branched concrements.

Collecting system

Narrow, dysplastic RCS. Multiple caliceal neck stenoses.

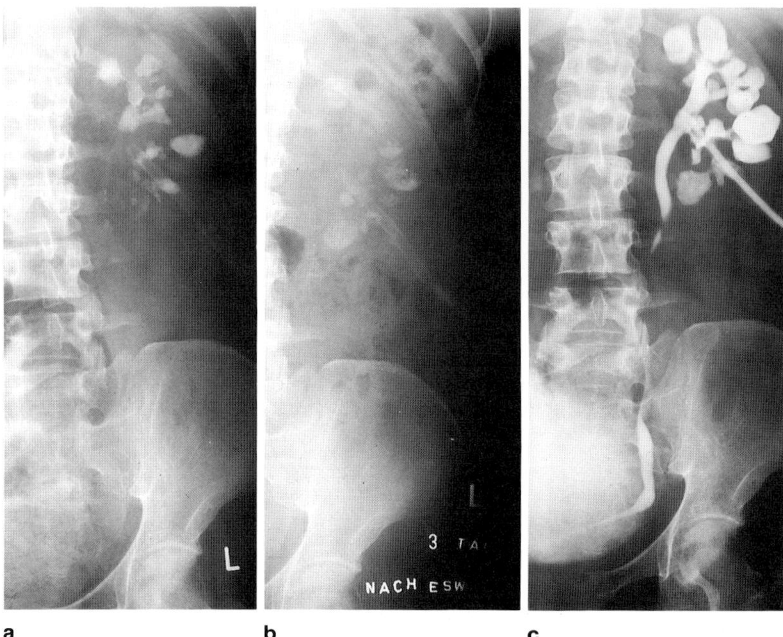

a   b   c

Fig. 2.**10 Complete staghorn stone**
a Treatment by PCNL
b Treatment by ESWL
c Stone fragments in multiple calyces without tendency to pass spontaneously

Therapy:
1. Surgical stone removal: pyelocaliectomy (Gil Vernet principle), radial nephrotomies, plastic correction of calyx neck stenoses where possible.
2. PCNL + flexible nephroscopy + electrohydraulic (in the future laser?) lithotripsy.
3. ESWL + Double-J ureteral stent.

Reasons:
1. Percutaneous manipulation in the dentritic RCS is difficult and inefficient.
2. When the patient denies an open surgical approach, a percutaneous attempt should be made. The use of a flexible nephroscope in combination with a flexible lithotripsy system is of particular advantage in these cases.
3. Passage of stone debris after ESWL is doubtful in the presence of caliceal neck stenoses and a dysplastic RCS.

Indications are not dependent on the localization system of the lithotriptor

2.3.2 Nonopaque Kidney Stones

Stone

Slightly opaque, nonopaque stone. Varying stone position. Varying volume, size, and number.

Collecting system

No urinary obstruction.

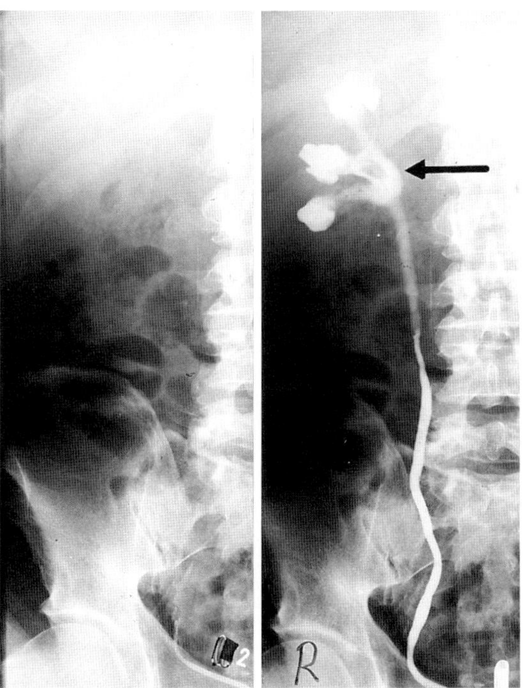

Fig. 2.**11** **Nonopaque stone, filling defect on the retrograde pyeologram**

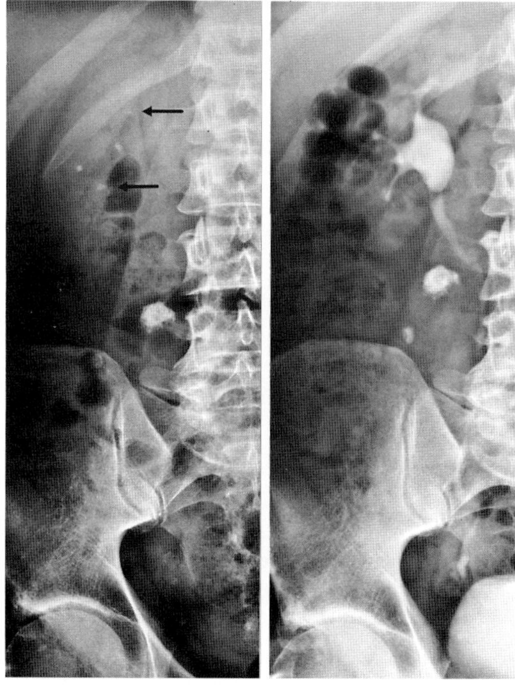

Fig. 2.**12** **Slightly opaque, small caliceal stones**

With the advent of ultrasound-equipped lithotriptors, rules for the treatment of opaque stones can now accordingly be applied to nonopaque calculi as there is no longer a localization problem. If only a fluoroscopically guided lithotriptor is available, indications for ESWL should be limited to small caliceal stones (Fig. 2.**12**) that can be localized with contrast medium. Larger stones may either be referred to a center equipped with an ultrasound location system or treated by percutaneous surgery.

2.3.3 Ureteral Calculi

To date, stones at any site of the ureter can be reached by direct application of shock waves (Fig. 2.**13**). However, stone localization depends on the lithotriptor system. Ultrasound localization can only visualize stones in the extreme upper ureter and in the intramural part of the distal ureter.

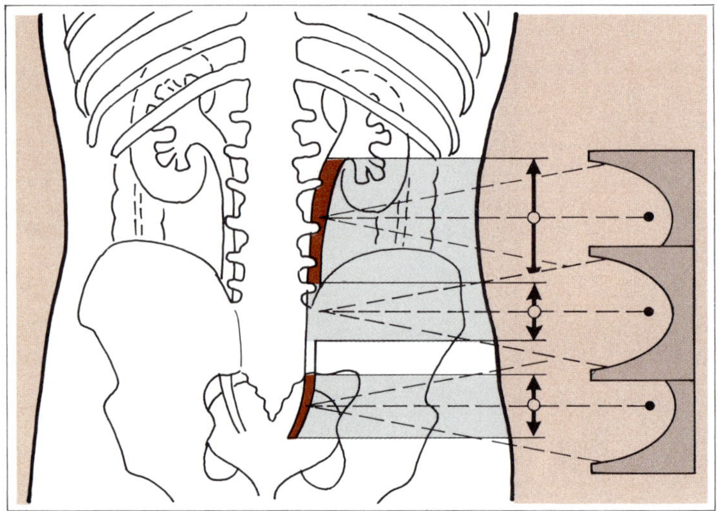

Fig. 2.**13 The use of varying positioning techniques** (see text) brings about direct shock wave exposure of all parts of the ureter

2.3.3.1 Proximal ureteral calculi
(Figs. 2.**14**–2.**15**).

Algorithm for proximal ureteral calculi positioned above the linea terminalis (Fig. 2.**16**).

1. ESWL in situ
2. Retrograde mobilization of the stone or passage with the ureteral catheter. Option: Retrograde mobilization by ureteroscopy (see Chapter 5)
3. Retrograde and antegrade ureteroscopy
4. Ureterolithotomy

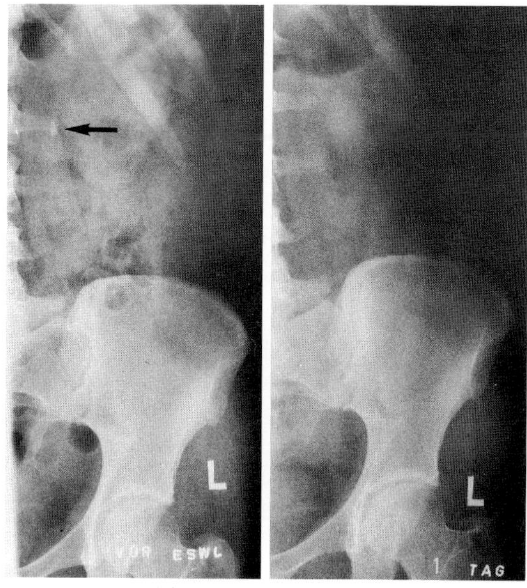

Fig. 2.14 Proximal ureteral stone, no obstruction in the IVP (not displayed). Complete discharge of stone debris one day after in situ ESWL

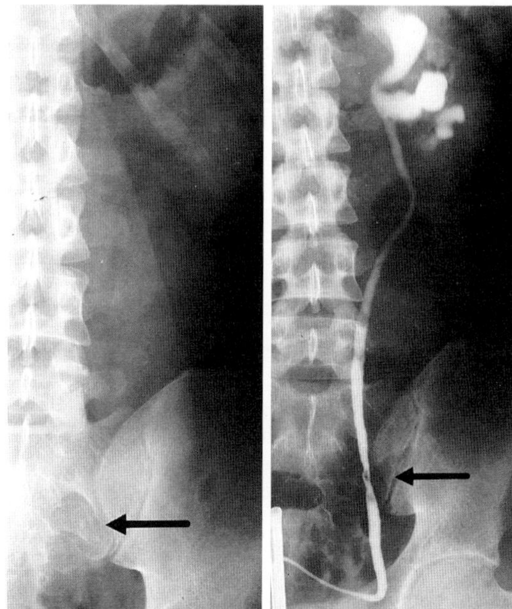

Fig. 2.15 Stone in projection over the bony pelvis. For in situ ESWL in the prone position, intravenous dye is used for stone localization

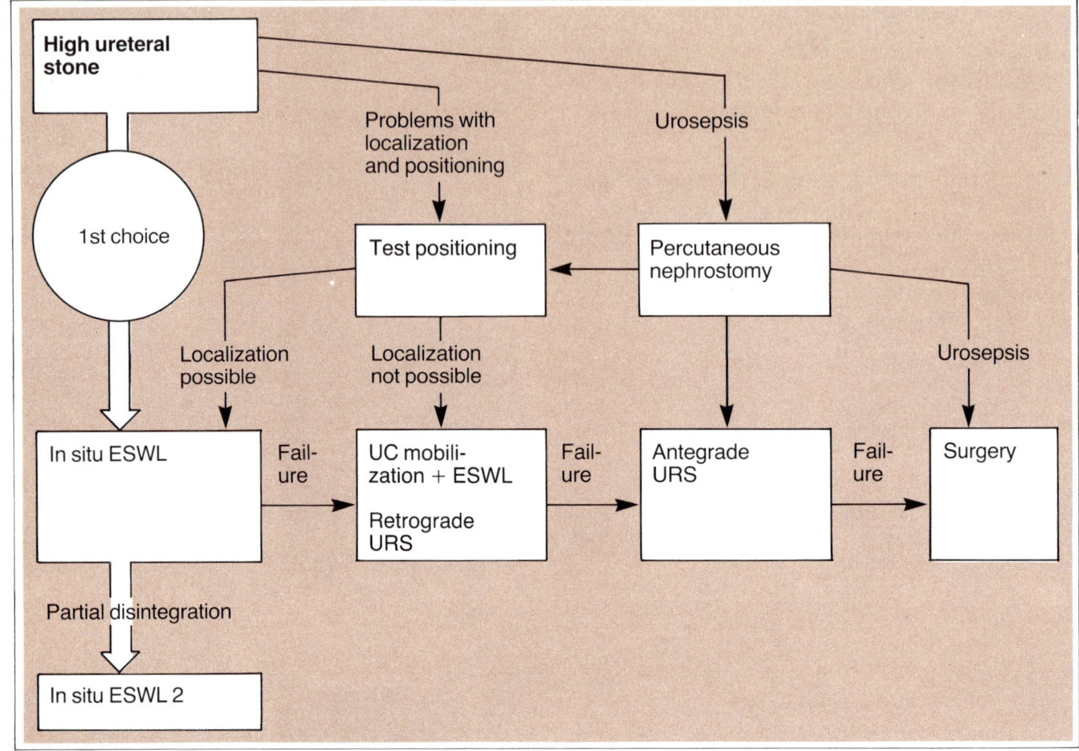

Fig. 2.16 Algorithm for the treatment of ureteral calculi above the linea terminalis

Reasons:

1. The success rate of in situ ESWL ranges between 60% and 80%. This justifies the application of primary in situ ESWL as a noninvasive method, particularly if anesthesia-free lithotripsy is available. For stones in projection over the bony pelvis (Fig. 2.**15**), ventral shock wave exposure must be used to avoid damping of the shock waves by the bone.

   When a partial stone disintegration is achieved, a second and, likewise, a third in situ ESWL is indicated.

2. Indications for retrograde mobilization (ureteral catheter) are (Fig. 2.**17**)
   - unsuccessful in situ ESWL;
   - localization of stone impossible (gross adiposity, skeletal anomalies);
   - only lithotriptor with ultrasonic localization system available.

   Once the stone is flushed back into the RCS, subsequent disintegration is successful in more than 95%. When mobilization of the calculus fails, irrigation with saline through the ureteral catheter may be useful to produce an "expansion chamber" for the stone.

3. Impacted stones that can neither be mobilized nor passed with the ureteral catheter should be approached ureteroscopically. As URS is mostly preceded by an attempt of retrograde mobilization, the transurethral route should be tried first. If the stone cannot be managed this way, antegrade URS via a percutaneous track is the next step.

4. If any of the aforementioned attempts have failed, ureterolithotomy is the last option. Depending on the consent of the patient, open surgery can be performed in the same session as the endourological approach.

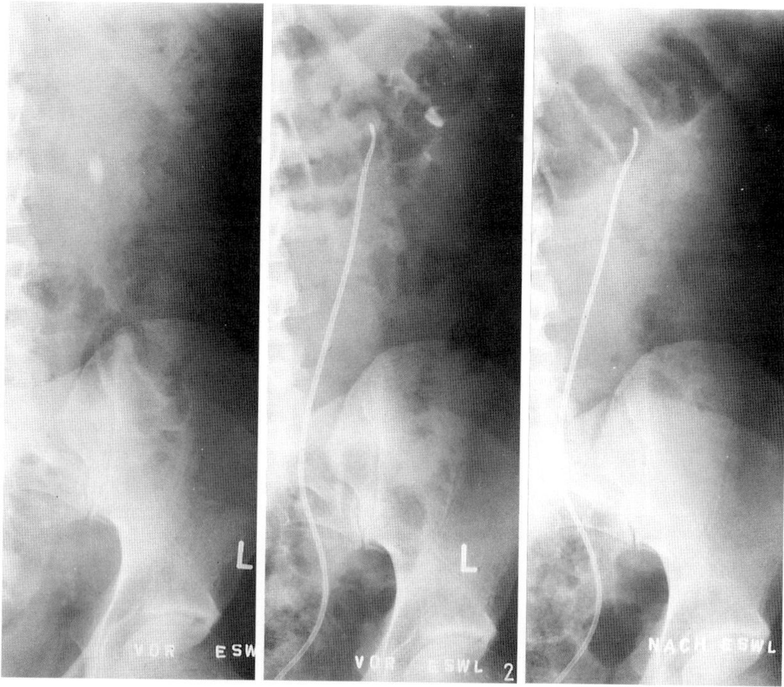

Fig. 2.**17 Obstructive ureteral stone** on left side
successfully mobilized with ureteral catheter (middle)
for consecutive ESWL. Right picture shows situation
after shock wave treatment

2.3.3.2 Distal ureteral calculi
(Fig. 2.**18**).

The algorithm (Fig. 2.**19**) for distal ureteral calculi (positioned below the linea terminalis) parallels that for proximal ureteral calculi.

1. ESWL in situ
2. Retrograde URS
3. Ureterolithotomy

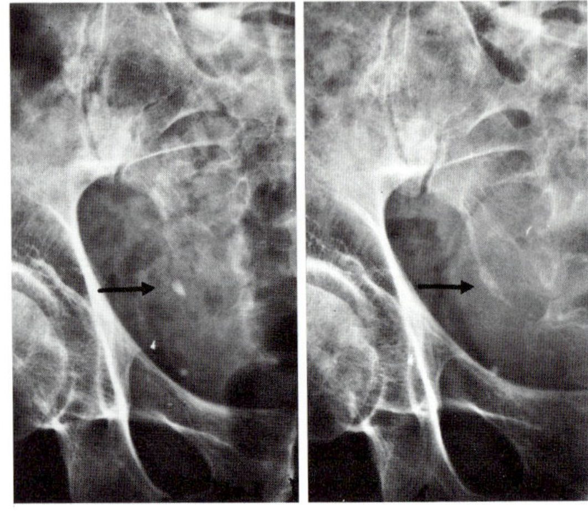

Fig. 2.**18**   Distal ureteral stone before (left) and after (right) in situ ESWL

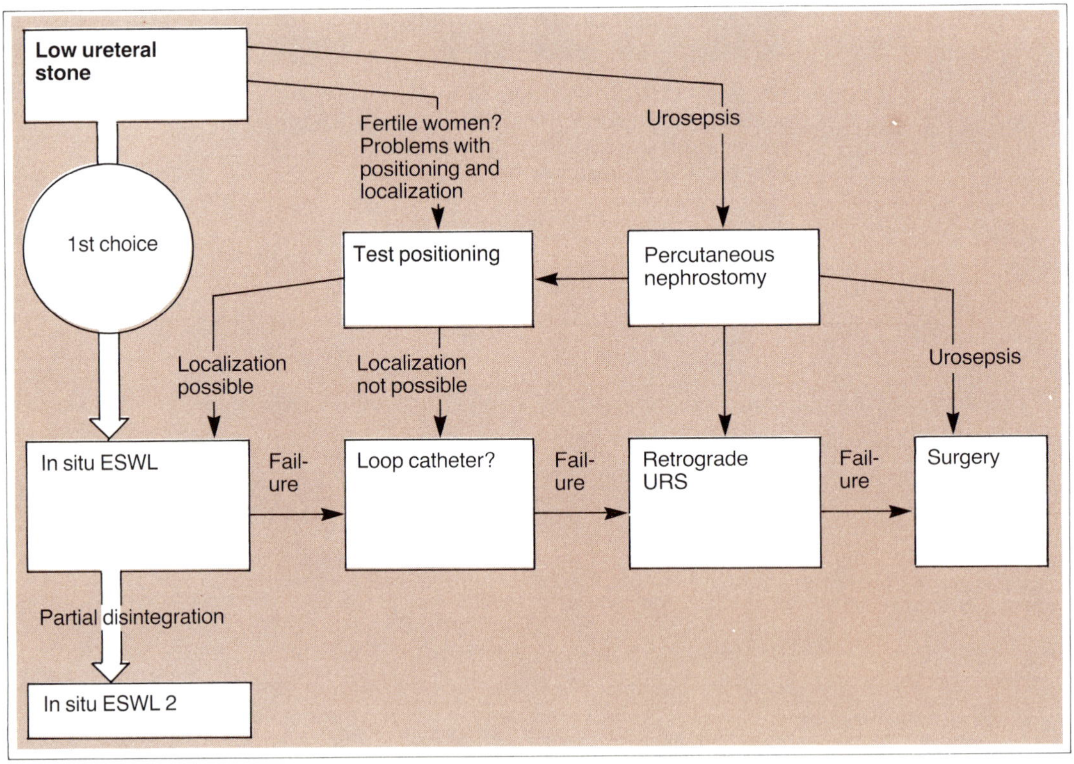

Fig. 2.**19**   Algorithm for the treatment of distal ureteral calculi

Reasons:

1. Several reports (Miller, 1988; Becht, 1988) demonstrate the efficacy of ESWL for distal ureteral calculi. Compared with ureteroscopy, there is no risk whatsoever of damaging the ureter. The treatment of fertile women is still a subject for discussions, reflecting a potential damage of the ovary by the shock waves. However, experimental data clearly suggest that the ovarian tissue is not altered by shock wave exposure (McCullough 1990).

When a partial stone disintegration is achieved, a second and, likewise, a third in situ ESWL is indicated.

2. If the calculus shows no sign of disintegration after ESWL, endoscopic stone removal is the next step. The authors see no rationale for mobilizing a distal ureteral stone and attempting to flush it all the way back up to the renal pelvis. The use of URS for stone removal in the distal ureter uniformly yields excellent therapeutic results in conjunction with a comparably low complication rate.

Depending on the experience of the operator, URS can be considered as primary treatment for distal ureteral calculi if ESWL can only be performed under anesthesia.

2.4　Indications for Special Cases

2.4.1　Compensated Renal Insufficiency

Patients suffering from compensated renal insufficiency can, in principle, be treated in accordance with the aforementioned therapeutic guidelines. The new methods afford the additional advantage that no further impairment of kidney function must be expected.

Patients with compensated renal insufficiency, a single kidney carrying multiple stones, and several previous surgeries (Fig. 2.**20**) can be treated with the combination of PCNL and ESWL. However, the number of sessions required and the final therapeutic result (reduction of retention values, elimination of UTIs, postponement of dialysis) are difficult to anticipate in each individual case. In the event of imminent dialysis, this approach can be considered as a last option and is preferable to open surgery.

Exact limits have not yet been defined as to under what clearance values ESWL can still be performed successfully. The authors consider a iodine-hippurane clearance of the stone-bearing kidney of less than 100 ml/min as contraindication for shock wave therapy, since a sufficient elimination of stone fragments is doubtful in this situation.

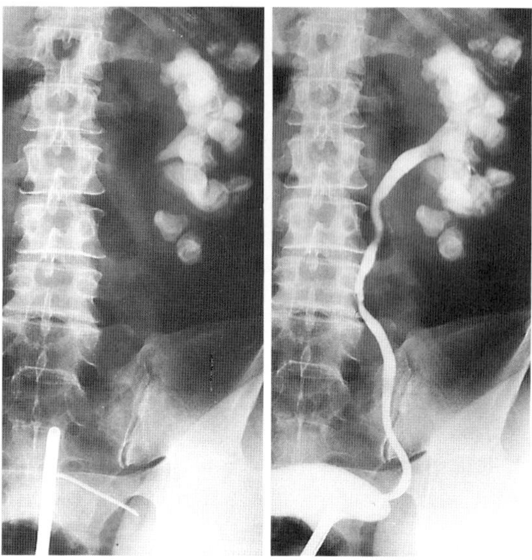

Fig. 2.**20**　**Large stone burden in a solitary left kidney.** Multiple previous operations, compensated renal insufficiency (creatinine 4.5 mg/dl)

2.4.2　Urolithiasis in Children

While only a few years ago ESWL of small children (< 100 cm) was considered to be contraindicated, recent experience has shown otherwise.

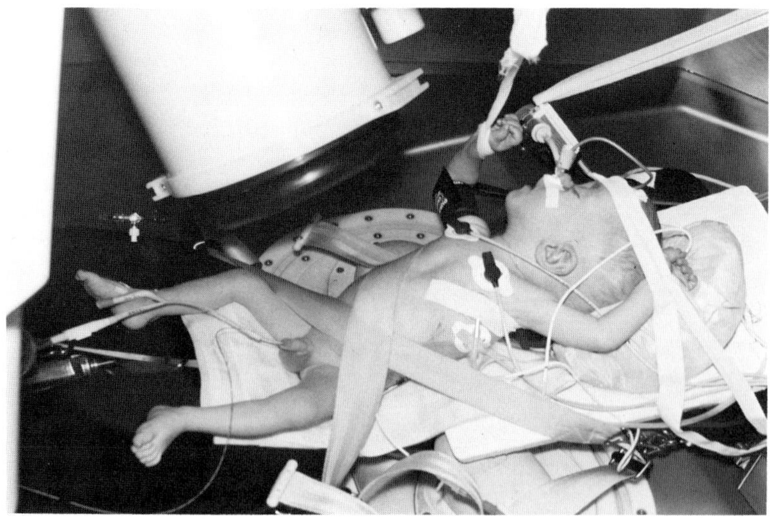

Fig. 2.**21**　**ESWL of a 6-month-old baby with a pelvic stone on the left side.**

Children as young as 6 months of age have been treated successfully without adverse side effects (Fig. 2.**21**). As a consequence, restrictions for shock wave lithotripsy with regard to size and age of children must no longer be considered. The only practical rule to adhere to with any pediatric ESWL is shielding the area of the lungs with a styrofoam sheet at the back in order to avoid shock wave exposure of the lungs. With the advent of ultrasonic-guided and dry-coupling shock wave sources that provide a small focal area (e.g. Siemens Lithostar overhead module, Dornier MPL 9000, Storz Modulith), unproblematic treatment of infants has become feasible (Köhrmann, 1990).

Percutaneous surgery in children is only restricted by the anatomical conditions of the renal collecting system. Children up to 4 years of age can generally be treated using the conventional set of instruments (24Fr or 26Fr nephroscope sheath). If small instruments seem necessary, care must be taken that the use of the auxiliary tools (i.e., ultrasonic-electrohydraulic lithotripsy probes, stone forceps) ist not compromised. In some cases, the use of a small, rigid ureteroscope (9.5Fr) via an 18Fr sheath may be helpful.

If pediatric cases with unilateral or bilateral staghorn stones are to be dealt with (Fig. 2.**22**), it must be kept in mind that each treatment session requires general anesthesia, whether PCNL or ESWL is applied. Therefore, open surgery may be preferable in some situations, since multiple sessions must be anticipated with the endourological approach.

2.4.3 Immobile Patients

Shock wave lithotripsy of patients suffering from hemiplegia or tetraplegia has shown that, despite the patients' immobilization, spontaneous discharge of the stone fragments can be achieved (Lazare, 1988). As a prerequisite, sufficient drainage of the urinary bladder must be provided.

2.4.4 Upper Urinary Tract Obstruction

Stenosis of the ureteropelvic junction (UPJ) with or without stone formation (Fig. 2.**23**) remains an indication for surgical pyeloplasty with or without simultaneous stone removal.

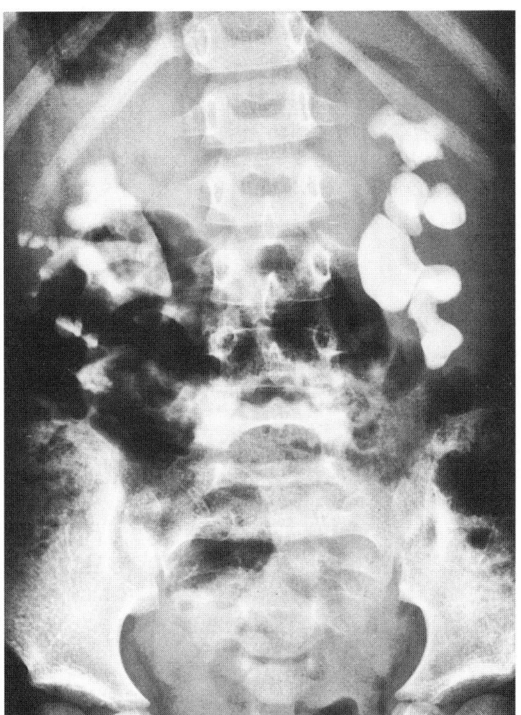

Fig. 2.**22   Bilateral nephrolithiasis in a 2-year-old child:** one of the few indications for open surgery

The results, recently presented with the percutaneous correction of a congenital UPJ-stenosis, are satisfactory (60%−80% success rate) but cannot quite match the success rates of open surgery (Karlin, 1988). In this situation, the lesser invasiveness of the percutaneous operation has to be weighed against the slightly better results of open surgery. As a consequence, an individual decision must be made according to the preference of the patient and the experience of the surgeon. However, endoscopic pyeloplasty should be preferred in any case of secondary stenosis (following previous open surgery) of the UPJ as this approach yields uniformly good results. Furthermore, open operations are more difficult in these cases.

The urodynamic effect of a caliceal neck stenosis or of a caliceal diverticulum is difficult to predict. Several reports indicate that, particularly in the case of a diverticulum stone, ESWL is less effective than a percutaneous

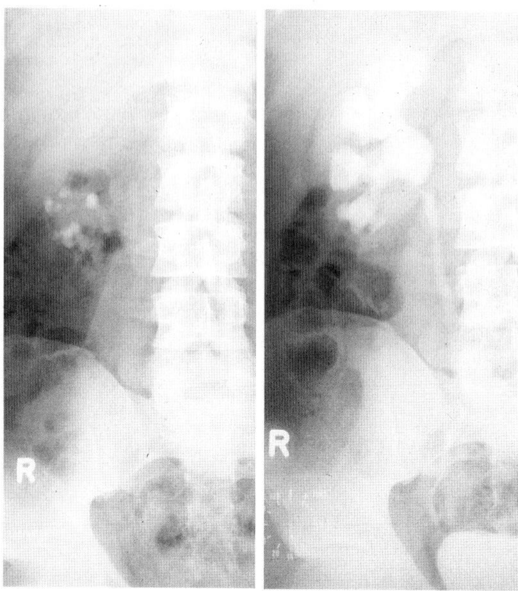

Fig. 2.**23 Several caliceal stones in conjunction with a UPJ stenosis**

approach (Lingeman, 1987; Janetschek, 1988). However, the authors maintain that in the era of anesthesia-free shock wave lithotripsy, an ESWL attempt should be made (Fig. 2.**24**). If passage of stone fragments does not occur, a percutaneous operation can be performed sec-

ondarily by directly approaching the stone-bearing calyx or diverticulum.

If stones in hydronephrotic lower calyces have to be dealt with, a primary percutaneous approach should be considered (Fig. 2.**25**) since the tendency of stone fragments passing from these calyces is poor. After recurrent stone formation, resection of the lower pole of the kidney is indicated.

2.4.5 Kidney Anomalies

Horseshoe kidneys or malrotated kidneys (Fig. 2.**26**) can be treated by ESWL or percutaneous surgery as well, depending on the stone size. ESWL may be difficult in anteriorly located calyces in a horseshoe kidney. In these cases, a prone position for shock wave lithotripsy must be utilized. If a percutaneous approach is made to a horseshoe kidney, the different anatomic situation (Janetschek, 1988) has to be taken into account.

When pelvic kidneys (Fig. 2.**27**) or transplanted kidneys are dealt with, ESWL can be applied either in a prone position (ventral shock wave exposure) or in a sitting position similar to distal ureteral calculi (perineal shock wave exposure) (Fuchs, 1988).

The authors are not aware of the existence of any reports on percutaneous approaches to congenital ectopic kidneys in the pelvis. Ho-

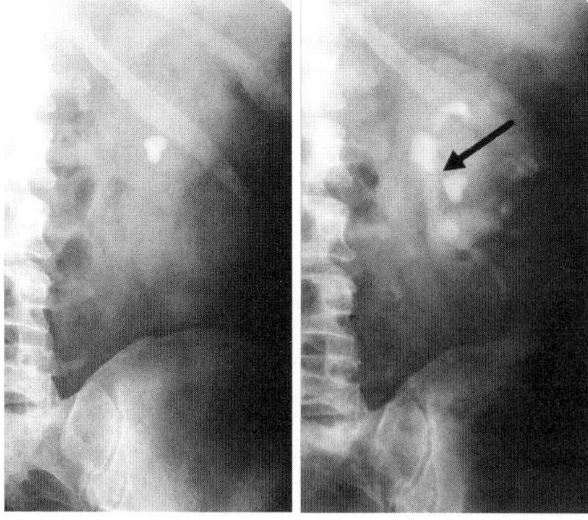

Fig. 2.**24 Stone debris after ESWL in a caliceal diverticulum.** No spontaneous passage of the fragments due to a narrow outlet of the diverticulum (arrow)

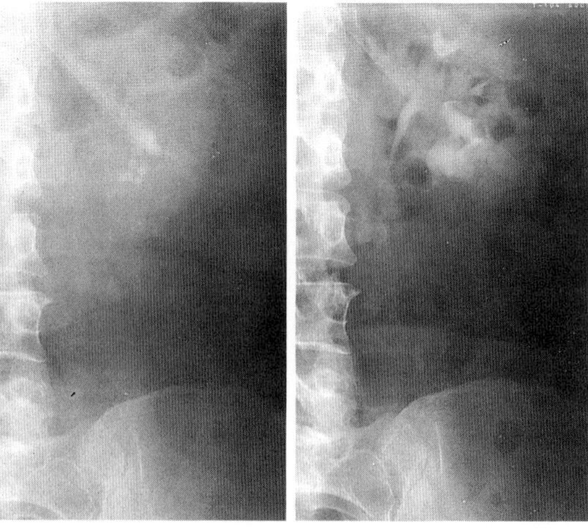

Fig. 2.**25 Caliceal stones in a dilated lower calyx** (see text)

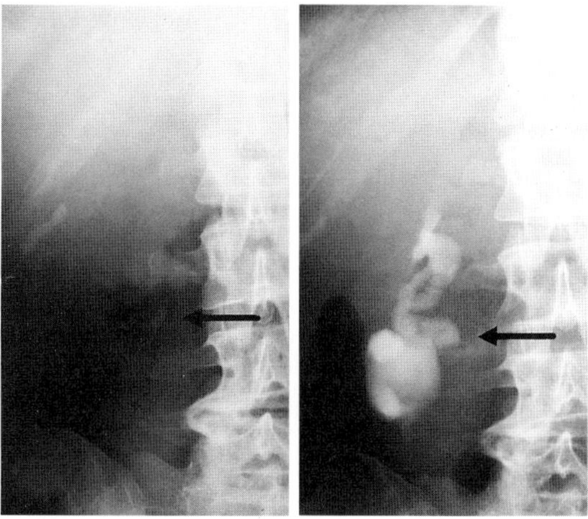

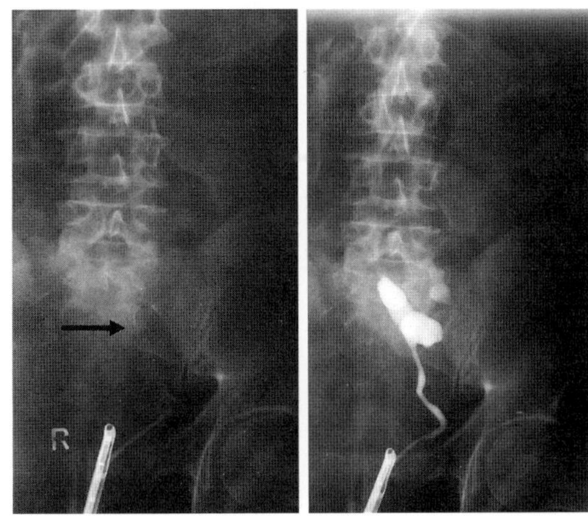

Fig. 2.**26** **Stone in middle calyx of a malrotated kidney**

Fig. 2.**27** **Pelvic stone** (arrow) **in a dystopic pelvic kidney**

wever, since percutaneous nephrostomy of transplanted kidneys is a routine procedure in the case of obstruction, percutaneous surgery in these kidneys should at least theoretically be possible.

2.4.6 Skeletal Anomalies

Patients with pronounced deformation of the spine (Fig. 2.**28**) should undergo a "test positioning" (simulation) on the shock wave device to clarify if the stone can be focused; the same holds true for percutaneous surgery. It should be clear before surgery if the patient can be positoned in a prone position and if the kidney can be reached through a percutaneous tract.

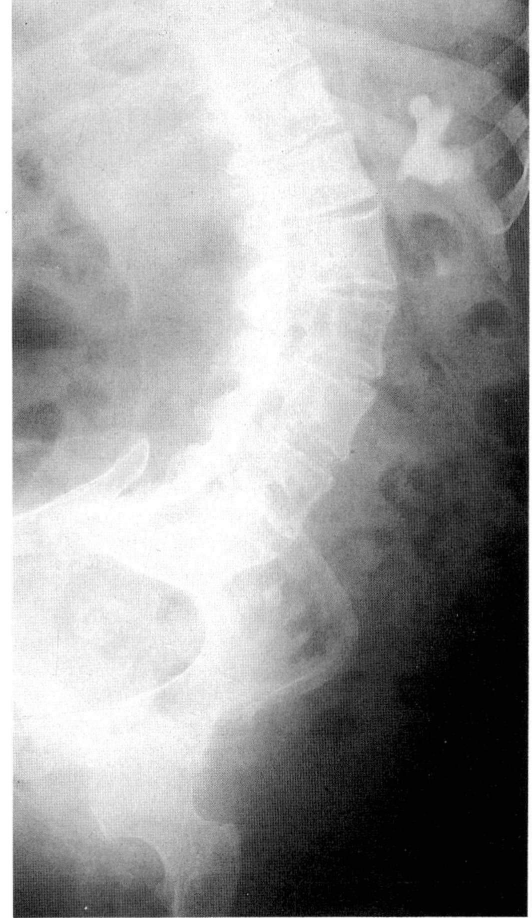

Fig. 2.**28** **Pronounced kyphoscoliosis with left-sided stone formation**

3 Extracorporeal Shock Wave Lithotripsy (ESWL)

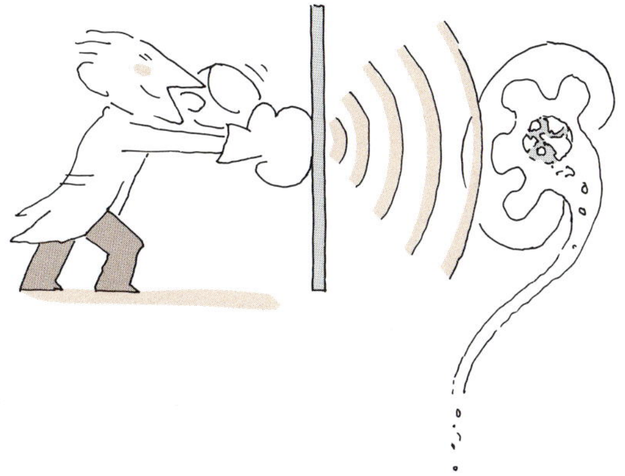

Principle

Disintegration of urinary calculi is achieved by extracorporeally induced shock waves. Penetrating the body without damaging tissue, the focused shock waves disintegrate the concrement into particles that may pass spontaneously.

3.1 Development of ESWL

The first physical classification of electromagnetically induced, unfocused shock waves was performed by Eisenmenger in 1959. However, systematic investigations on shock wave generation and its effects were carried out in the sixties within the framework of the elementary research of an aerospace company, namely, Dornier System. Typical examples of shock wave generation can be found, for instance, when a raindrop hits the surface of a supersonic aircraft; when meteorites collide with spacecraft; or in the blast effect associated with explosions. It was shown that shock waves are reflectable and, therefore, can be focused.

In the early seventies, the damaging effects and thresholds of shock wave application to biological tissue were studied in order to assess the risk that tank crews face on exposure to shock waves. At the same time, the medical utilization of focused shock wave energy was considered. The following application fields appeared to be interest:

- disintegration of urinary and biliary calculi;
- mechanical stimulation of the heart in the case of asystolia

ESWL for urinary calculi. *In 1971,* the first in vitro disintegration of kidney stones by shock waves was achieved by Häussler with the Dornier System shock wave gun. In the initial test phase, the generation of only four shock waves took an entire day and produced only a network of cracks in a kidney stone.

From 1972 to 1974, laboratory tests on the disintegration of kidney stones by focused shock waves were carried out. These experiments were subjected to the following criteria:

- reproducible generation of shock waves
- adequate focusing of shock wave energy
- acoustic coupling to guarantee energy transfer
- localization of the stone
- determination of optimal stone-disintegrating energy

In vitro and in vivo studies on the action of focused shock waves on biological tissue followed from *1974 to 1978*. The clinical application of ESWL was demonstrated on a canine kidney stone model.

On February 7, 1980, the first patient suffering from a kidney stone was successfully treated with ESWL at the Department of Urology of the University of Munich.

Table 3.1   History of ESWL

1959	Physical characterization of electro-magnetically induced shock waves (Eisenmenger)
1966	First observation of the transmission of shock waves through human body (Dornier System)
1969	First animal experiments to study the effect of focused shock waves on biological tissue (Dornier System)
1971	First in vitro destruction of urinary stones by a multistage shock-wave gun (Häussler)
1972–1978	Systematic in vitro and in vivo experiments with focused shock waves (Eisenberger, Chaussy, Schmiedt, Brendel)
Feb 7, 1980	First clinical application at Dept of Urology, University of Munich (Chaussy)
1982	Installation of the first ESWL center at Dept of Urology, University of Munich (Chaussy, Schmiedt)
Oct 1983	Installation of the second ESWL center worldwide at Katharinen Hospital, Stuttgart (Eisenberger)
1980–1984	Experimental in vitro and in vivo investigations with ESWL for gallstones (Sauerbruch, Delius, Brendel, Paumgartner)
1985	First clinical gallstone ESWL at the Dept of Gastroenterology, University of Munich (Sauerbruch)
1985–1990	Development and clinical introduction of more than 20 different 2nd and 3rd generation lithotriptors.

Two years later, the first ESWL center was inaugurated at the Grosshadern Urologic Clinic of Munich University. This was followed by the installation of the second center in 1983 at the Urologic Clinic of the Katharinen Hospital in Stuttgart. The first series model (Dornier HM3) was installed there.

To date, more than 800 centers have been established worldwide, where more than 2,000,000 patients have been successfully treated.

ESWL for biliary calculi. *From 1980 to 1984*, in vitro and in vivo studies were carried out on the application of ESWL to human gallstones. These studies were performed at the Department of Gastroenterology at Munich University. Using a canine model, it was shown that human radiolucent calculi can be fragmented by ESWL and may pass spontaneously via the bile duct into the duodenum.

In 1985, a patient suffering from a gallstone was the first to be treated with a modified Dornier HM3 lithotriptor. The treatment concept of biliary ESWL, however, included oral chemolysis. To date, more than 10,000 patients have been treated in the FRG.

New lithotriptors and further indications. *Since 1985*, an increasing number of new lithotriptors, the so-called second generation lithotriptors, have been developed and introduced for clinical application. These devices employ different principles of shock wave generation, focusing, acoustic coupling, and stone localization. In general, the lithotripors became smaller, cheaper, multifunctional, or a combination thereof. The interdisciplinary use of ESWL has lead to the installation of stone centers with two machines (Table 3.**1**).

Further indications for ESWL may be pancreatic duct calculi and parotid gland concrements.

3.2 Physical Background

Ultrasound waves are characterized by alternate compression and rarefaction. For low-amplitude disturbances, a *linear* correspondence exists between pressure and density in the carrying medium (Fig. 3.**1**).

As a result of the high attenuation when passing through tissue, and hence, low depth of penetration, the application of ultrasound

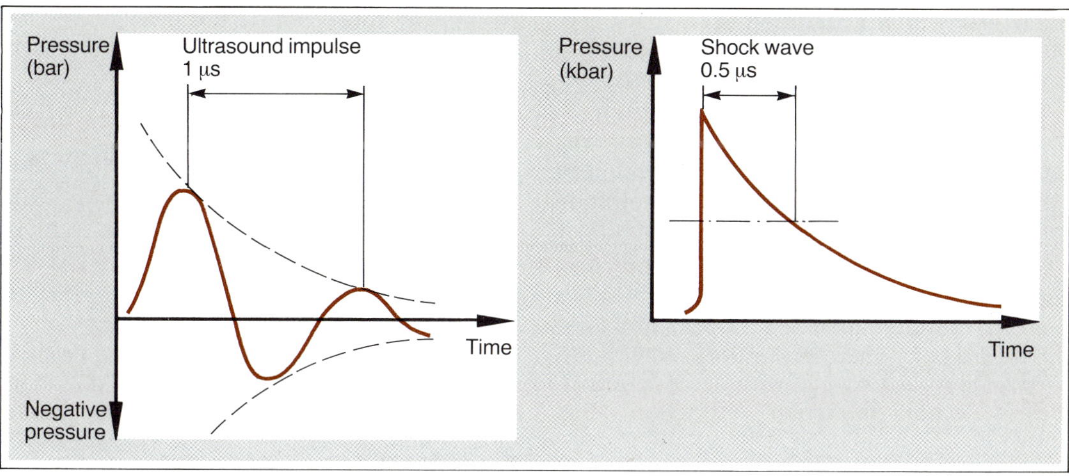

Fig. 3.**1** **Pressure wave form of ultrasound waves and shock waves**

waves for contact-free disintegration of stones is problematic in the energy range that can be utilized for medical purposes. Another disadvantage of ultrasound wave application is the risk of thermal tissue damage.

On the other hand, a *shock wave* consists of a *nonlinear* high pressure impulse with a rapid rise forming the shock front and a gradual decline (Fig. 3.**1**). It includes a wide continual spectrum of frequencies ranging from a few hundred kHz to a few hundred MHz.

Principally, each high-pressure impulse, if high enough, may become a shock wave on transmission. The main reason for this is caused by the nonlinear acoustic behavior of such waves. Large amplitude compression pulses will be distorted as they travel through a medium. Consider a plane wave front where pressure continuously increases and then falls. High-pressure parts of the wave commence after the low-pressure components. However they travel faster, pushing forward to increase the pressure at the wave front. As the wave continues through the medium, a steep shock front is formed — a travelling discontinuity where there is a sudden rise in pressure and density (Fig. 3.**2**).

Shock fronts have definite width and amplitude. They can be characterized by their peak pressure and rise time (~1 ns). Depending on the energy source, shock fronts are formed

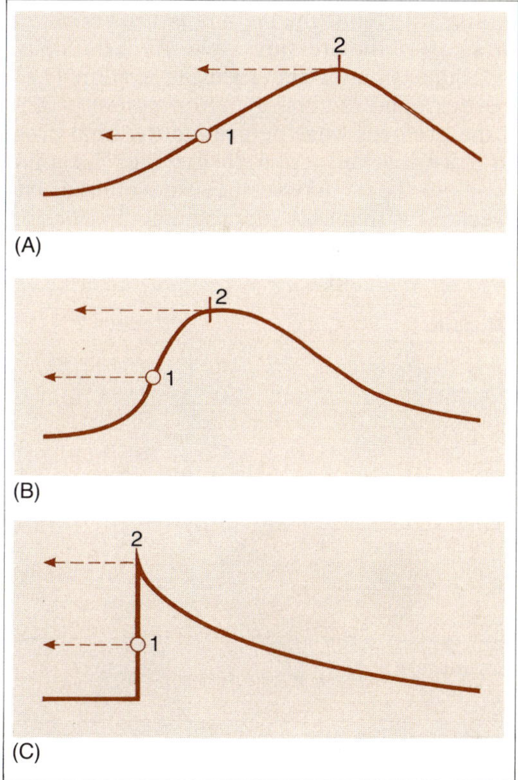

Fig. 3.**2** **The formation (= steepening) of a shock front.** High pressure parts (2) of the wave start out later than the lower pressure ones (1) but travel faster, pushing forward to increase the rate of pressure rise at the wave front

immediately after generation (i.e., spark gap, pulsed laser, microexplosion) or develop when travelling through the medium (i.e., piezoelectric elements, electromagnetic membrane).

When passing through biological tissue the attenuation of shock waves is minimal ($10\% - 20\%/10$ cm), enabling deep penetration into the body.

Even though shock waves are faster than sound waves, the increase of velocity is less than 5% in water and tissue for peak pressures up to 1 kbar. Therefore, shock waves still propagate in accordance with acoustic principles (reflection, refraction, diffraction) (Fig. 3.3).

This is the main reason why shock wave energy can be focused, which is one of the essentials for shock wave lithotripsy. However, with respect to physical classification, the situation becomes more complicated. As a pressure wave converges towards its geometrical focus, nonlinearity limits the peak pressure and alters the shape of the pressure wave. Both the shape and dimension of the focusing system (i.e., aperture) and the energy and pressure profile of the prefocus wave determine the final pressure distribution at the focus (Fig. 3.4). No complete theory has yet been developed, but direct measurements of pressure distribution around the focus can be taken as a basis for comparing lithotriptors and developing their design (see Chapter 7).

3.3 Measurements of Shock Waves

A detailed characterization of the acoustic field generated during ESWL may be useful in understanding the parameters that affect the performance of the equipment and safety of the treatment.

Measurement of shock wave pressure necessitates a probe size of less than 1 mm, due to its high resolution. Therefore, the hydrophones most commonly used for shock wave measurement consist of the piezoelectric material, polyvinyliden fluoride (PVDF). The membrane hydrophones of PVDF are elastic and thus less sensitive to shock wave-induced fractioning than the piezoceramic probes used previously. in such hydrophones, the voltage wave form is displayed on a digital oscilloscope. The measured voltage is calibrated to the level of shock wave pressure (in degassed, deionized water at $20\,°C$ at pressures below 0.5 MPa).

A PVDF needle hydrophone (Fig. 3.5) consists of an inner electrode shielded with PVDF. The outer electrode represents a silver covering of the PVDF layer. The PVDF needle hydro-

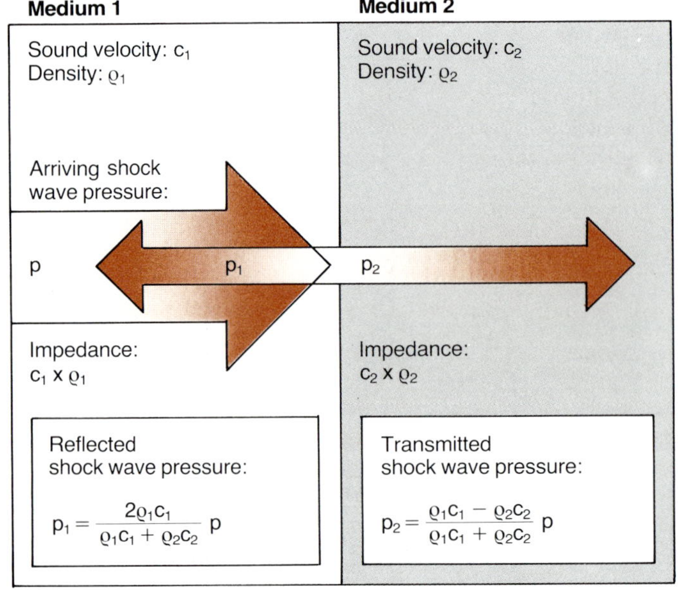

$$p_1 = \frac{2\varrho_1 c_1}{\varrho_1 c_1 + \varrho_2 c_2}\, p$$

$$p_2 = \frac{\varrho_1 c_1 - \varrho_2 c_2}{\varrho_1 c_1 + \varrho_2 c_2}\, p$$

Fig. 3.3 **Physical characteristics when shock waves meet acoustic interphases**

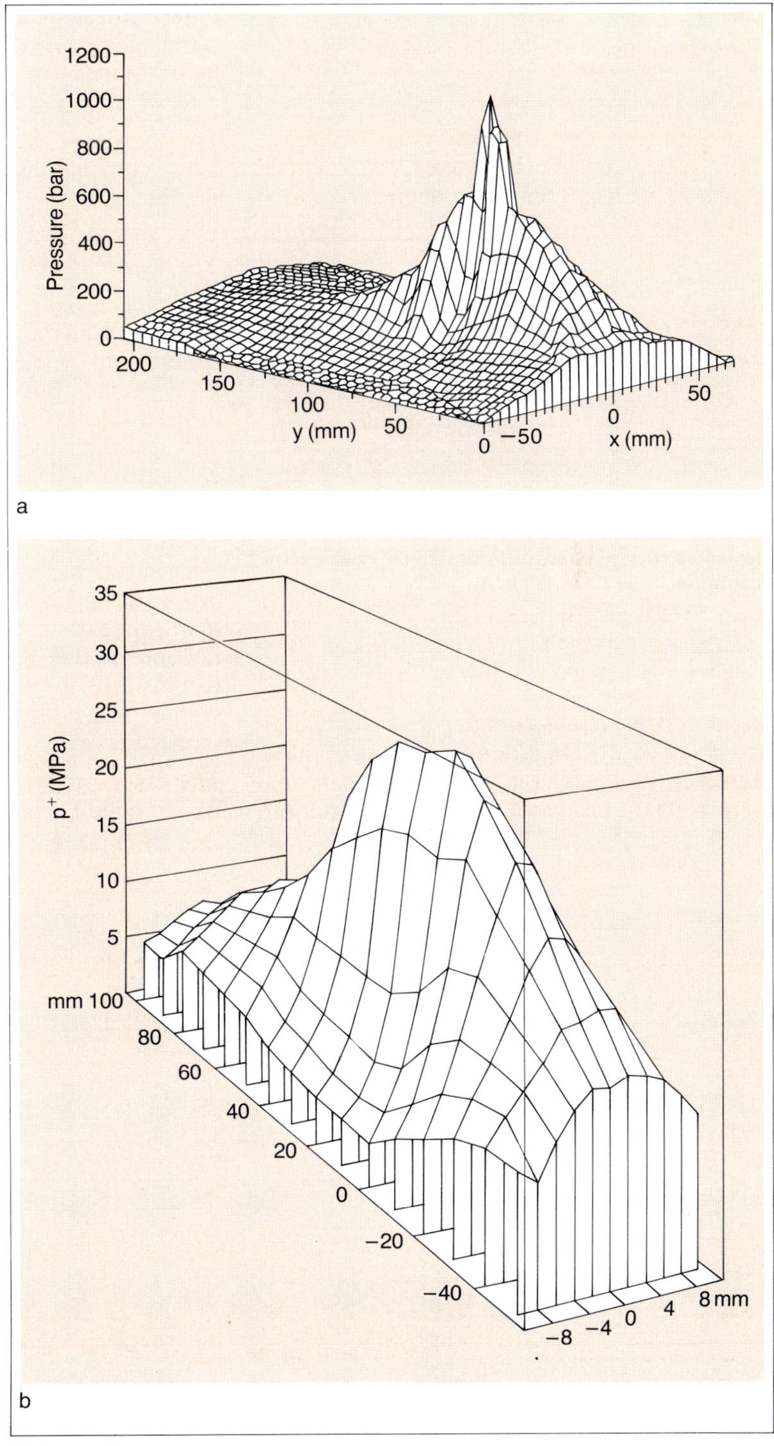

Fig. 3.4 **Pressure distribution within the focal area of two different lithotriptors**
  a Dornier HM3 (measured with PCB-transducer)
  b Siemens Lithostar (measured with PVDF-probe)

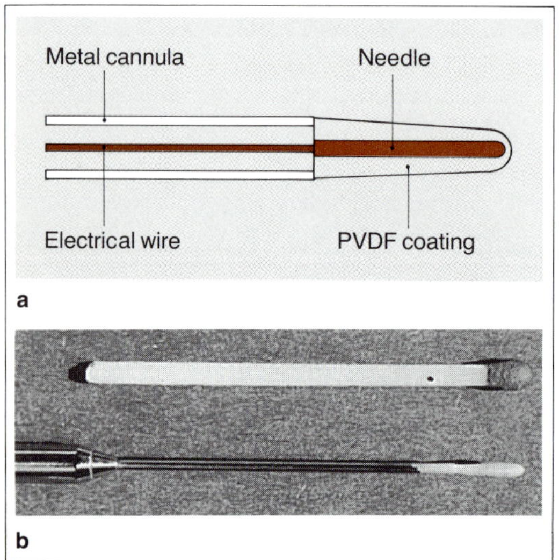

Fig. 3.5 Polyvinyliden fluoride (PVDF) needle hydrophone
a Schematic drawing
b Original probe

phone is considerably smaller than the bilaminar shielded PVDF membrane hydrophone. However, its lifespan is restricted to approximately 100 measurements due to cavitation-induced destruction of the silver covering (= outer electrode). Therefore, PCB membrane hydrophones are still used by the manufacturers for routine measurements.

Two newly developed hydrophone principles may overcome the disadvantages of the PVDF probes:

1. a capacitive probe hydrophone;
2. a laser hydrophone.

The *capacitive probe hydrophone* measures the movement at the surface of the liquid during shock wave propagation. For this purpose, the level of the fluid has to be adjusted to the desired distance from the generator. The advantage of this system is the easy mechanical calibration and long lifespan, since the membrane of the capacitive probe is not damaged by cavitation (Fig. 3.**6**).

For routine measurements, however, the *laser probe,* using a quartz fiber with an Argon laser light, appears to be more interesting. The reflection of the laser light at the shock wave front can be measured photoelectrically at the voltage wave form displayed on an oscilloscope (Fig. 3.**7**).

The laser probe is certainly as good as the PVDF needle hydrophone (Fig. 3.**8**), whereby

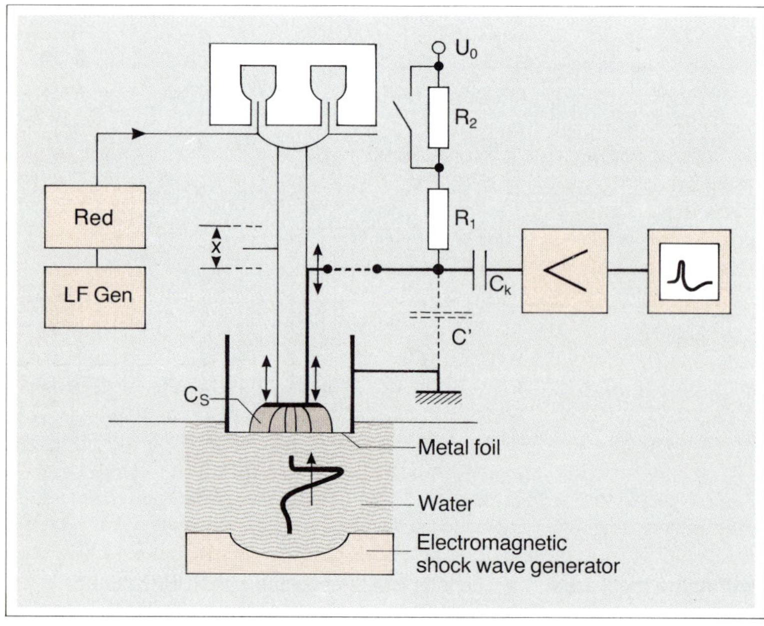

Fig. 3.6 Capacitive probe hydrophone. Shock wave-induced change of the probe capacitor (C_s) is transmitted into an oscillogram of the shock wave pressure

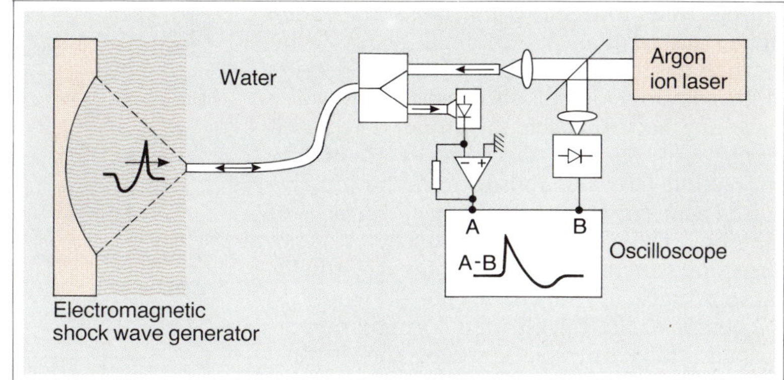

Fig. 3.7 Laser hydro-phone. Shock wave-induced changes of the Argon laser light are transformed into the oscillogram of the shock wave pressure

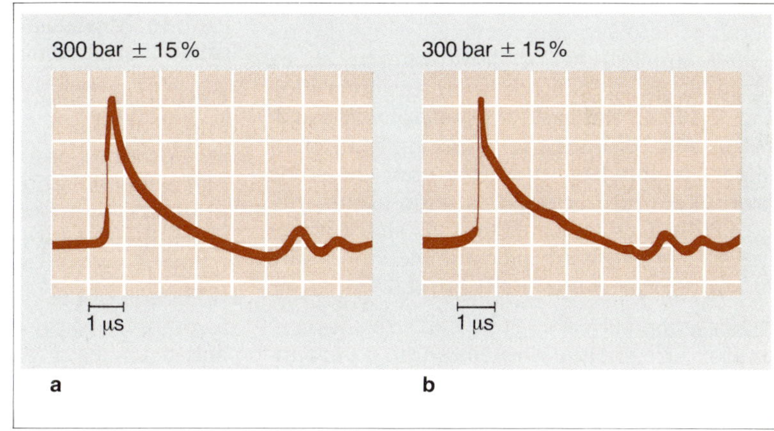

Fig. 3.**8 Comparison
of the signals (pressure
wave form) of two different
hydrophones**
a   PVDF needle hydrophone
b   Laser hydrophone

the quartz fiber seems to last considerably longer. Moreover, repair or replacement, or both, of the quartz fiber is much easier and less expensive. Furthermore, the small size of the quartz fiber (600 µm) enables *in vivo measurement of shock wave fronts* via an ureteral catheter or a nephrostomy tube.

3.4 The Principle of Stone Disintegration

The amount of transmission and reflection of the shock wave when travelling through the body depends on the acoustic impedance of the different tissues (Fig. 3.3). Acoustic impedance is a characteristic of any medium and is equal to the product of density and sound velocity (Table 3.2). Water has a similar acoustic impedance to tissue, and this is the reason it can be used as a transmission medium for shock waves from the generator into the tissue. Air has a very different impedance to tissue and, therefore, all lithotriptors operate with degased water to avoid attenuation of shock wave energy by released airbubbles (nondissolved gas).

Tear and stress forces. Due to the similar acoustic impedances of water and tissue, shock waves travel through the body with minimal reflection and refraction. Therefore, the location of the focal zone in vivo is nearly identical to that in vitro. In contrast to this, the acoustic impedance of urinary calculi is 5 to 10 times higher than that of tissue. When a shock wave hits the surface of a stone, some of the energy is reflected and thereby creates a compressive force on the front surface of the stone (Fig. 3.3). A compression pulse will then travel through the stone, stressing the sides of the stone, faster than its original shock front through tissue. On its back surface, reflection of the compression pulse creates a tensile pulse travelling back through the stone. The maximum tensile stress is theoretically created by interaction between tensile and compressive pulses near the front and the back surfaces of the stone. Depending on the often heterogeneous stone structure, these complex stress fields cause a crack network from the periphery to the center of the calculi, thus forming numerous additional interfaces where shock wave energy is released (Fig. 3.9).

Preliminary studies have shown that single, high-energy shock wave applications shatter the stone into big concrements, while the repeated application of lower-energy shock waves leads to a much finer disintegration (Fig. 3.10). In this case, the concrement usually starts to disintegrate after application of numerous impulses; therefore once the stone has broken, further fragmentation occurs more rapidly. This indicates that the shock waves first shatter the weak parts of the stone until the stronger parts are finally broken.

The described effect of "tear and stress forces" for stone fragmentation necessitate a very rapid rise of pressure. In contrast, a pressure wave with a lower rising time would never be capable of disintegrating a stone.

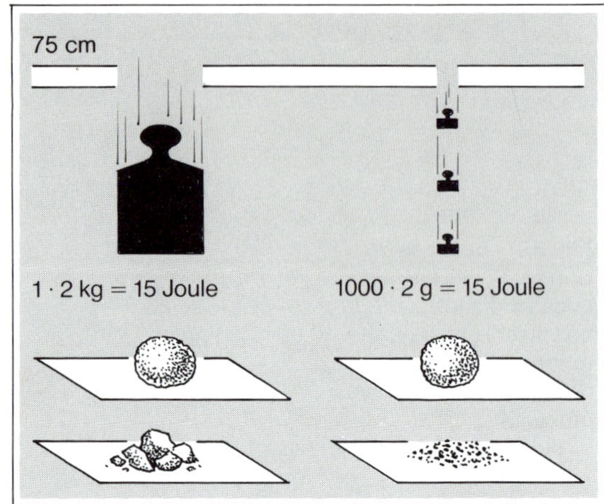

Fig. 3.**10** **Effective lithotripsy by repetitive application of small amounts of shock wave energy**

Cavitation. Besides the direct disintegrative effect of shock waves, stone fragmentation may occur secondarily due to the phenomenon of *cavitation* around the stone. Cavitation is produced by negative pressure that immediately follows the shock wave front. On the other hand, negative pressure may be produced by reflection of the shock front at interfaces when a compressive pressure pulse changes its action and becomes a *tensile pulse*. If tensile forces are strong enough, they may locally exceed the strength of a medium. This causes cavitation in liquids (water, blood, urine, bile), where the

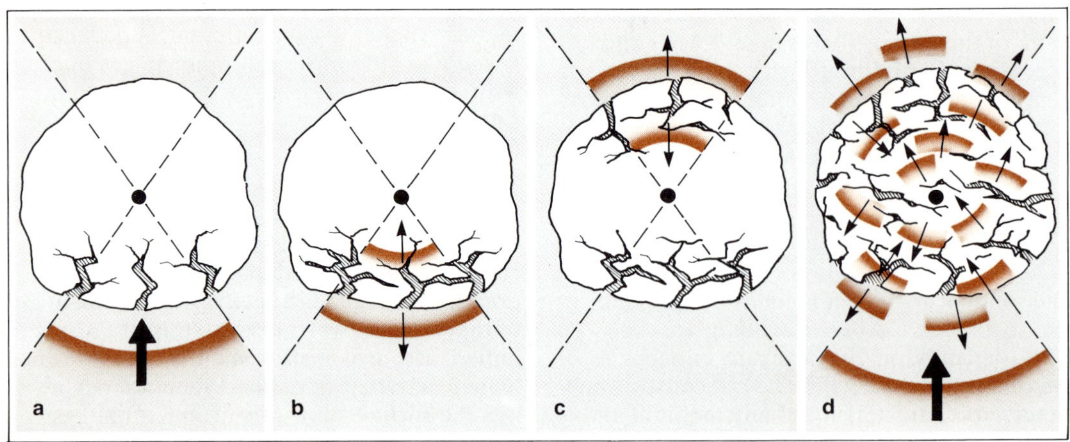

Fig. 3.**9** **Schematic drawing of the stone disintegration by shock waves**

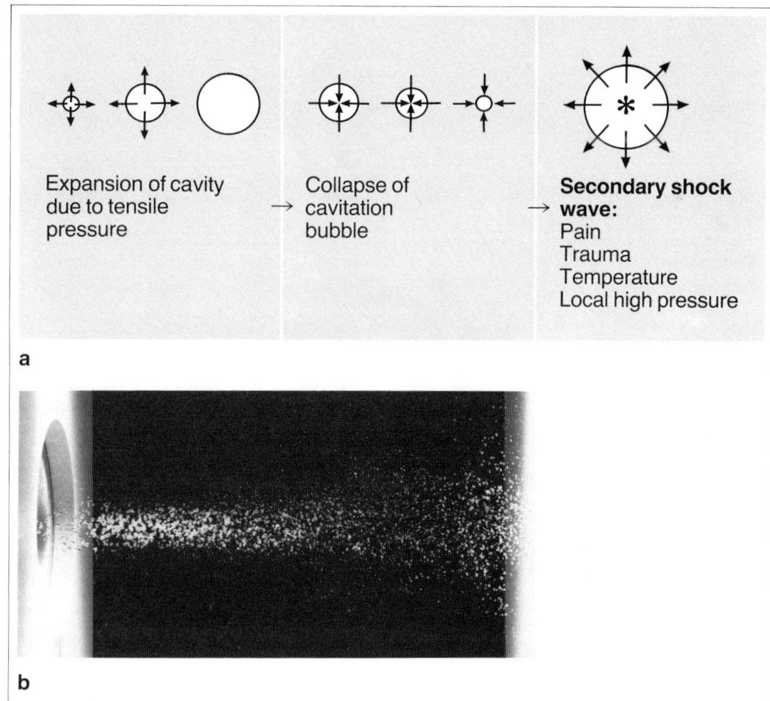

Fig. 3.**11** **The generation of cavitation bubbles by tensile and negative shock wave pressures**
a The collapsing cavitation bubble leads to a secondary shock wave
b Cavitation along the z-axis of an electromagnetic self-focusing shock wave generator

liquid is pulled apart to create a small bubble. These bubbles form around nuclei, such as dust particles and stone crystals, and collapse immediately once the shock front has passed (Fig. 3.**11**). This collapse leads to high pressures locally that may produce secondary shock waves, microscopic high-speed jets within the liquid, high temperature, and even illumination. Such collapsing cavitation bubbles found around the stone may cause erosive surface damage comparable to the cavitation-induced damage of high-speed propellors on racing boats.

Cavitation on the skin at the point where the shock front enters into the body should be minimized, since it may lead to local petechiae.

3.5 Shock Wave Generation

In principle, any physical mechanism converting energy into its acoustic form could be used for ESWL (Fig. 3.**12**). Up until the present time, only a limited number of options have been realized. These ESWL sources can be classified into two different types:

1. **Point Sources,** which always emit spherical shock waves due to sudden evaporation of the fluid. A compressive pressure pulse results from expansion of the heated gases, followed sometime later by a negative pressure pulse as the gas bubble around the energy source collapses. Point sources are the *spark gap,* a *pulsed laser,* and *microexplosive lead pellets.*

   Of these three sources, the **spark gap system** has proved to be the most reliable method of shock wave generation. Two underwater electrodes are serially connected with a capacitor that is charged to a high voltage. The discharge of the energy contained in the capacitor leads to explosive plasma formation and evaporization of the water, thus generating a spherical shock wave (Fig. 3.**13**) that is focused by means of an *ellipsoid metal reflector.* The electrodes are placed at one focus (F 1). As a result of the geometrical property, all rays emitted at F1 will

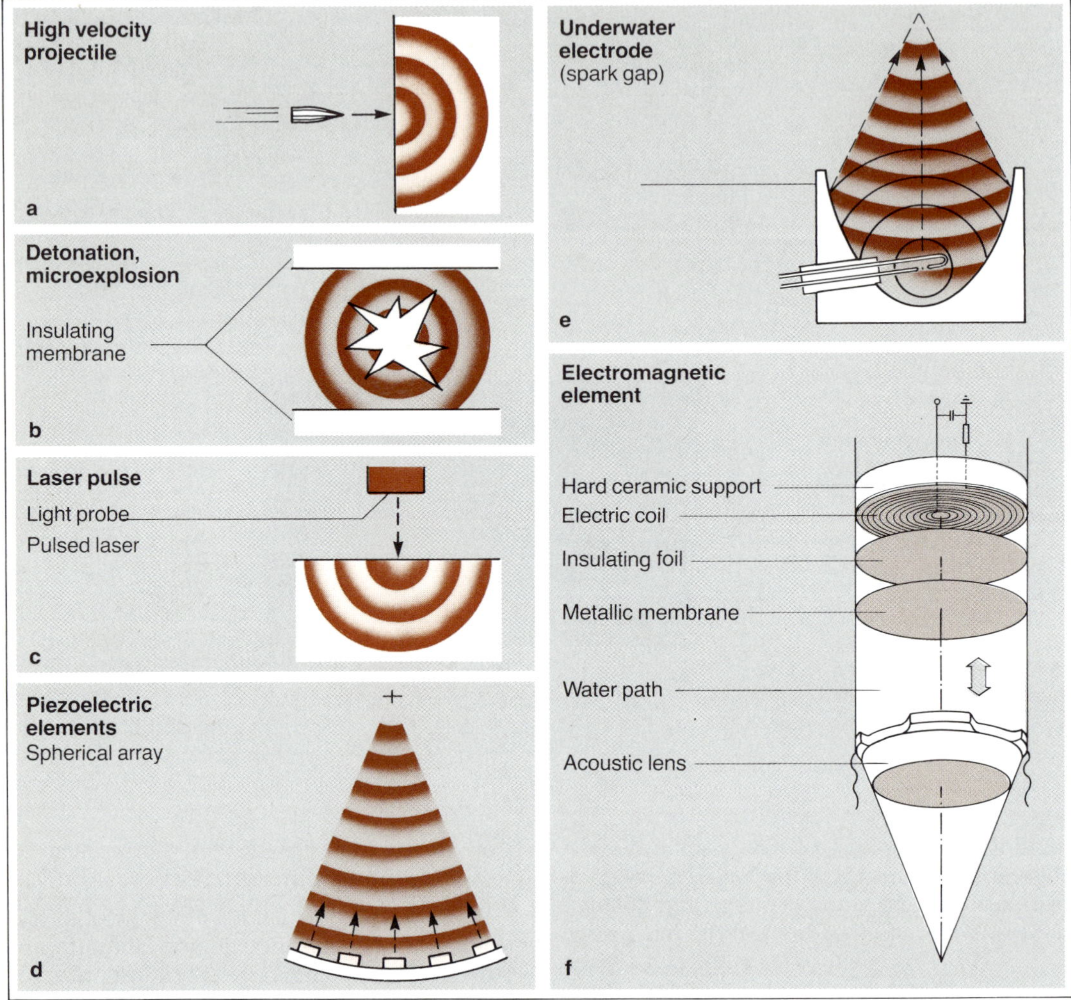

Fig. 3.12 Different principles of shock wave generation and focusing

a High-velocity projectile hits a membrane, inducing a shock wave in the adjacent medium (i.e., light gas-gun)
b Microexplosion of lead acid pellets in water
c Evaporization of water by laser-induced plasma formation
d Modified ultrasound waves focused by spherical alignment of the piezoceramic elements
e Evaporization of water by discharge of a spark gap. Focusing by a semiellipsoid reflector
f Electromagnetically induced movement of a metal membrane. Focusing by an acoustic lens

arrive at the other focus (F2) after being reflected at the boundary of the semiellipsoid (Fig. 3.**14**). The simultaneous arrival of reflected acoustic energy creates a shock wave at F2 that is located about 15 cm above the rim of the reflector. In order to effect the disintegration of stones, sufficient energy density is provided up to a distance of about 1 cm laterally to F2 and about 5 cm above and below F2. In addition, a direct, unreflected wave will also reach the focus.

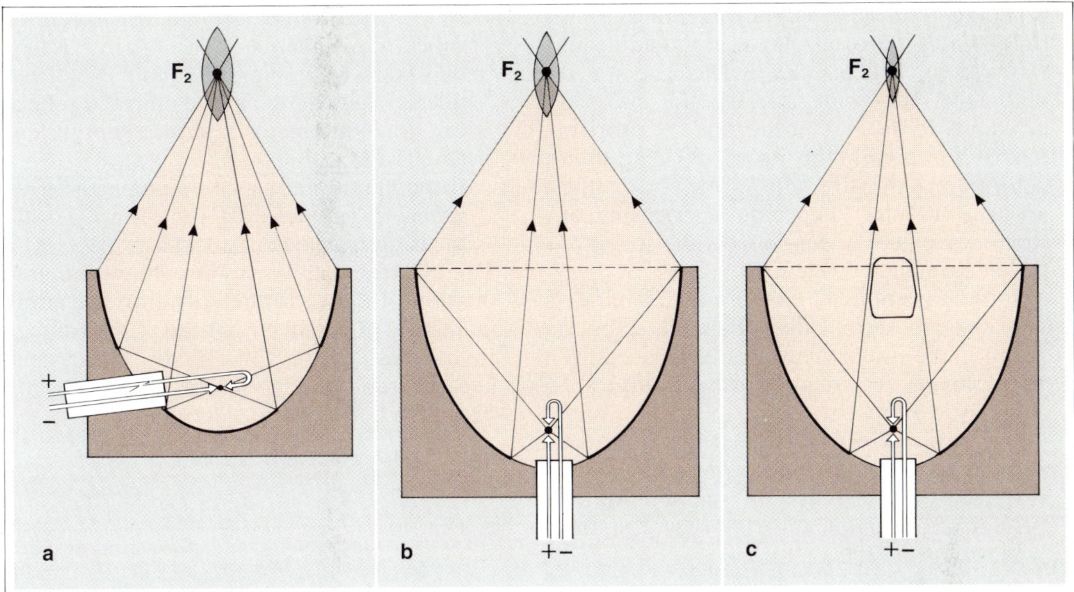

Fig. 3.13   Focusing characteristic of the electrode systems
a   Dornier HM3 (modified)
b   Dornier MFL 5000
c   Dornier MPL 9000 with "in-line" transducer

However, its peak pressure falls inversely with the distance.

One main feature of point sources is the extremely low content of tensile waves due to the asymmetrical pulse shape of the primary shock wave.

2. **Extended sources,** which induce an acoustical plane wave inside the fluid. If the peak amplitude of this wave is high enough, it becomes more inclined during its propagation and results in the formation of a shock front. Extended sources for ESWL are *piezoelectric* and *electromagnetic systems.*

Piezoelectric: When an external electrical field is applied across a crystal made from a piezoelectric substance (i.e., ceramic), it changes the external dimensions of the crystal. Movement of the crystal produces a pressure wave. Such crystals are used as acoustic sources in diagnostic ultrasound probes. Tensile pressures result from the return of the crystals to their original shape, but these can be reduced by suitable electri-

cal and mechanical design (i.e., irregular reflector; Fig. 3.12). Due to the limited power of a single piezoelectric element, 300 to 3000 crystals are necessary for sufficient shock wave pressure. Focusing of shock wave energy is achieved by *spherical alignment of the piezoelectric elements,* with the focus at the center. In both systems used for clinical ESWL, the diameter of the sphere is 50 cm. The large aperture results in a considerable increase of the entrance area and decrease of shock wave pressure on the skin, thus enabling anesthesia-free treatment (Fig. 3.14). Due to the large aperture, the focal zone is considerably smaller than that of the spark gap ellipsoid system of the Dornier HM3.

Electromagnetic: An electric current flowing through a wire generates a magnetic field. Magnetic materials can be attracted or repelled by this field. For shock wave generation, a pulse of current stored in a capacitor is transmitted through a flat copper coil, repelling a flexible copper membrane; it thus creates a pressure wave in the adjacent water (Figs. 3.**11b**, 3.**12**, 3.**15**). The speed of the current rising through the coil, its proximity to the membrane, and the properties of the membrane itself are critical in determining the strength and shape of the acoustic impulse. The type of focusing of shock wave energy depends on the shape of the electromagnetic element.

– In the case of a *flat membrane,* formation of the shock front takes place in a shock tube; the shock waves are focused by employing an acoustic lens with different acoustic properties than those of water (i.e., polystyrol). Nonlinearity will affect focusing behavior, and some energy will be lost by reflection at the lens-water interface and by absorption within the lens (Fig. 3.**12f**).

– In the case of an *electromagnetic cylinder,* shock wave energy is focused by use of two parts of a semiparaboloid metal reflector. As with the metal ellipsoid reflector, this guarantees minimal energy loss (Fig. 3.**15**).

– If the membrane has a shaped array with *spherical geometry,* it represents a self-focusing system (Figs. 3.**11b**).

The electromagnetic system allows the graduation of the peak pressure fran the minimal to the maximal amplitude of the source. In contrast to this, the spark gap system necessitates a minimal generator voltage for discharge between the electrodes.

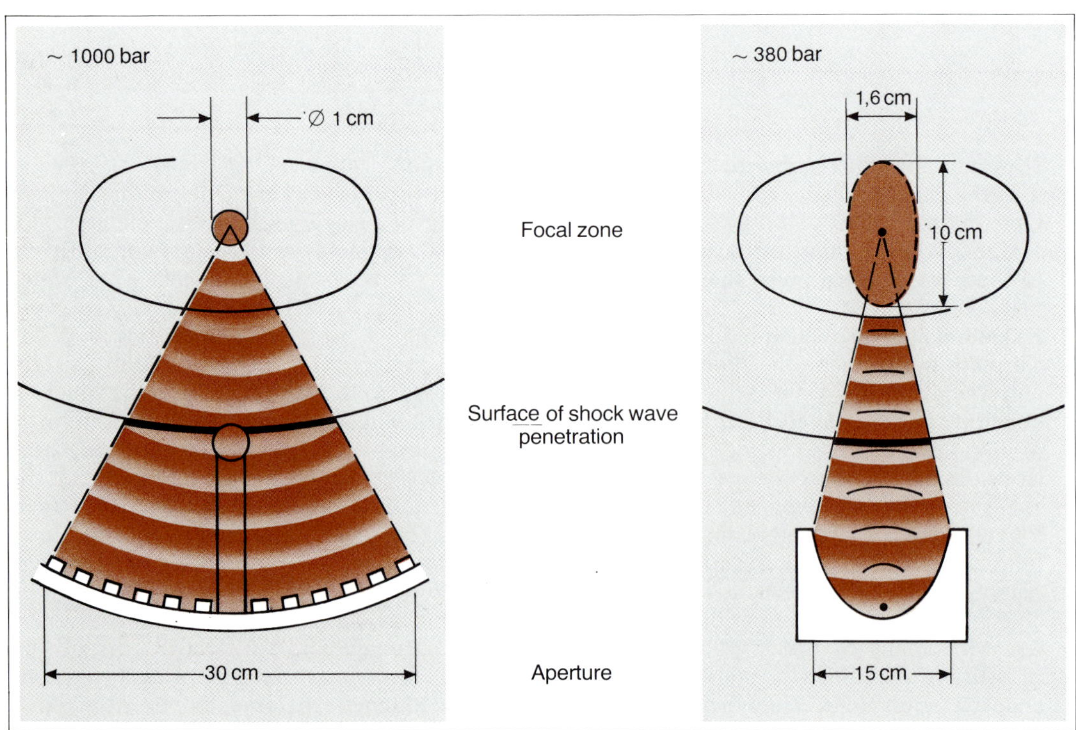

Fig. 3.14 **Comparison of the main technical characteristics of two shock wave generators**

Left: Piezoelectric generator (Piezolith)
Right: underwater electrode (Dornier HM3)

3.6 Shock Wave Focusing

The focusing of shock waves is necessary

- to achieve maximal energy concentration at the stone;
- to ensure minimal damage to surrounding tissue.

Depending on the energy source (Fig. 3.**11b**, 3.**12**), 3.**15** the following principles are applied for shock wave focusing:

- reflection at semiellipsoidal reflector (spark gap, pulsed laser beam, microexplosives)
- Spherical alignment of the energy sources (piezoelectric elements)
- spherical shape of the energy source (electromagnetic membrane)
- lens focusing (electromagnetic diaphragm, piezoelectric system)
- reflection at paraboloid reflector (electromagnetic cylinder)

Physically, all these principles are equivalent. The dimensions of the focal zone depend on the aperture and the geometry of the focusing system.

3.7 Shock Wave Coupling

Optimum shock wave coupling is aimed at keeping the energy loss between energy source and kidney stone as low as possible. Energy-absorbing acoustic interfaces with different impedances should be avoided. The mode of energy coupling is independent of the shock wave generating method. The following possibilities of energy coupling may be employed by use of degasified water (Fig. 3.**16**):

- complete water bath
- partial water bath
- water cushion and gel

On the originally employed complete water bath (bathtub of Dornier HM3), the water bath, as coupling medium, affords the advantage that density and shock wave resistance of water and body tissues (skin, fatty tissue, muscles, renal parenchyma) are very much alike (Table 3.**2**). Therefore, there is minimal energy loss when the shock wave enters the body. However, the system needs considerable space.

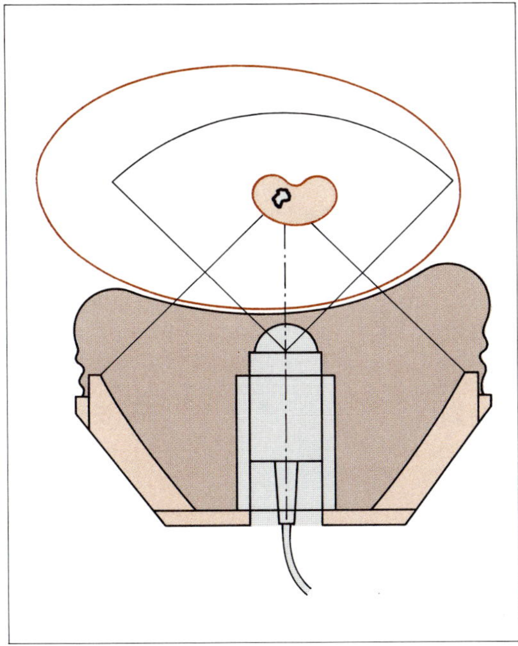

Fig. 3.15 Shock wave generation by an electromagnetic cylinder. Focusing by a paraboloid metal reflector

Table 3.**2** **Physical properties of body tissue** (from Habermann)

Material	Velocity of sound (m/s)	Specific density (g/cm^3)	Impedance (g/cm · s · 10)
Lung	650–1,160	0.4	0.26–0.46
Fatty tissue	1,476	0.928	1.37
Water	1,492	0.998	1.49
Kidney	1,570	1.04	1.63
Muscle	1,630	1.06	1.72
Bone marrow	1,700	0.97	1.65
Bone	4,100	1.8	7.38
Urinary calculi	4,000–6,000	1.9–2.4	5.6–14.4
Iron	5,100	7.9	40.3

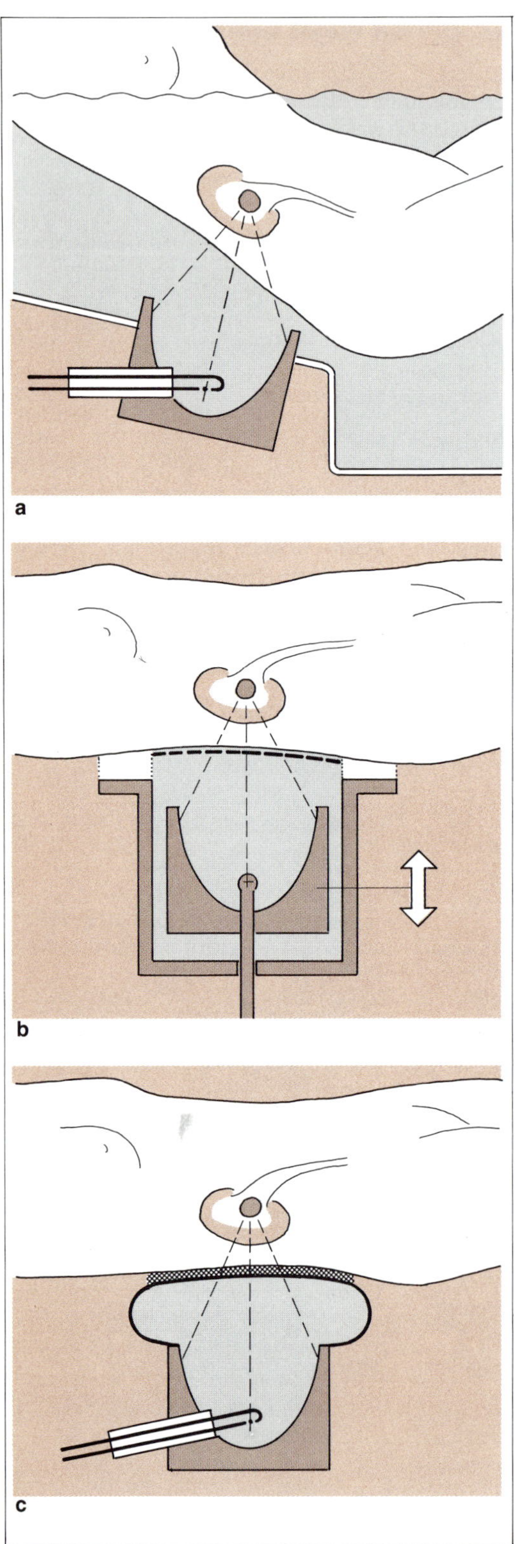

Newly designed lithotriptors use only a partial water bath or, more often, a water cushion together with coupling ultrasound gel for shock wave coupling. The use of a *water cushion* does not signify the absorption of energy. On the contrary, it has lead to a significant space reduction and reduced maintenance of the lithotriptors, allowing the integration of ESWL units into multifunctional urological tables (see Chapter 7). Moreover, the dry coupling together with the reduction of focal site has decreased the risk of the induction of extrasystoles by ESWL. Therefore, the ECG-triggered shock wave application has become dispensible for the majority of patients (except those with cardiac arrhythmia and pacemakers).

3.8 Stone Localization

The localization system of a lithotriptor should meet the following requirements:

- reliable and easy localization of the majority of calculi
- convenient control during therapy
- reliable evaluation of the therapeutic result (i.e., disintegration)
- minimal radiation exposure of the patient

Basically, urinary and biliary calculi can be located by the use of fluoroscopy or ultrasound. Table 3.**3** shows the most important modifications of these imaging systems available at present.

For *clinical use* in combination with the underwater electrode and semiellipsoid (Dornier HM3), X-ray location utilizing **two fixed-image converter systems** whose central beams intersect in focus F2 has proved to be most effective (Fig. 3.**17**). X-ray documentation during treatment can be made by various techniques that make use of an increasing radiation load (normal X-ray, short-term high-current technique, long-term high-current technique).

◀ Fig. 3.**16** **Principles of shock wave coupling**
a Complete water bath ("the tub")
b Partial water bath, mobile ellipsoid
c Water cushion and ultrasound gel

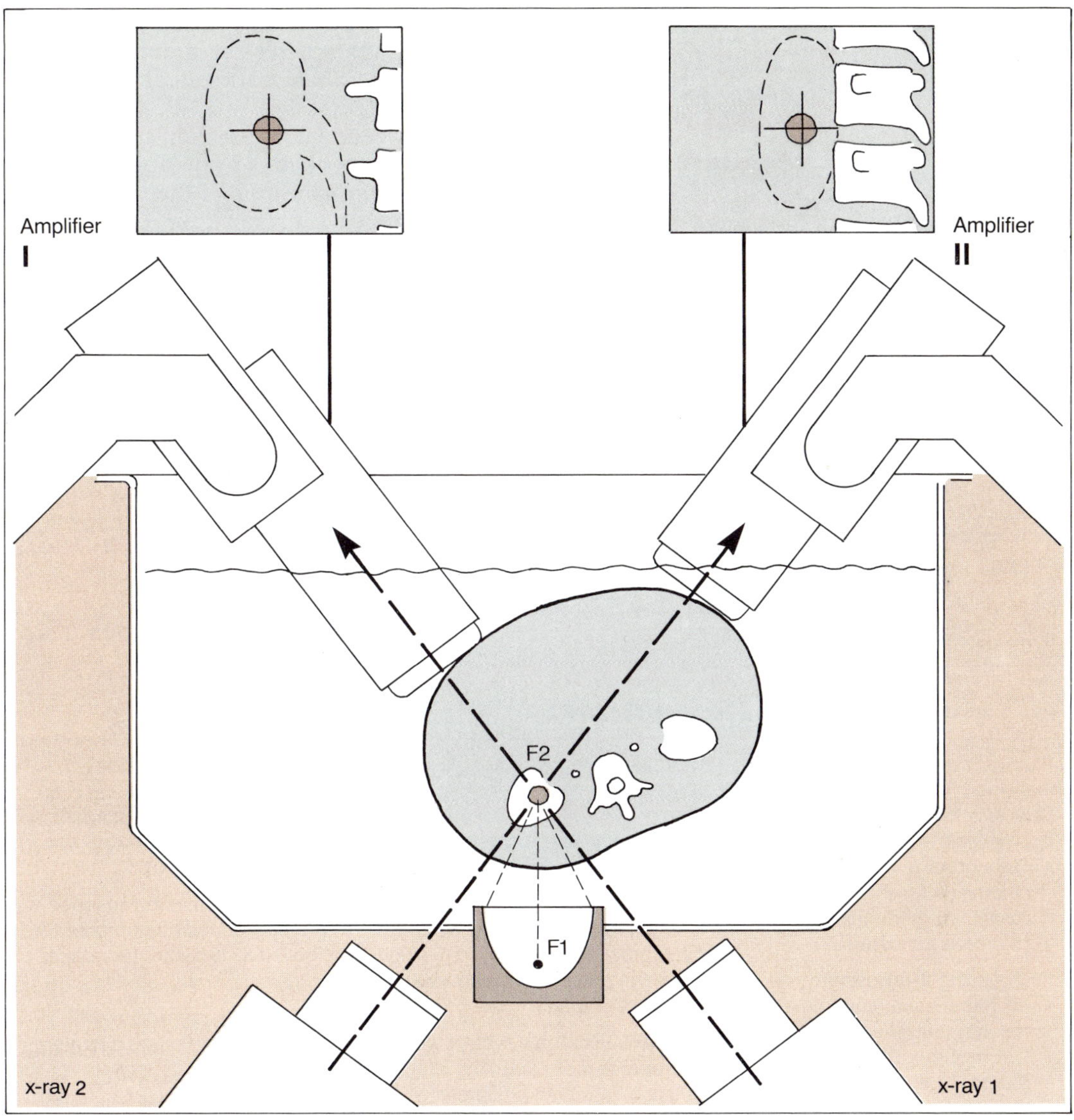

Fig. 3.**17** **Stone localization with the Dornier HM3 using two X-ray converters with intersecting central beams.** The cross-hairs of each monitor correspond to each central beam

The choice of an adequate locating system has become more complicated since the advent of new ESWL machines with modified shock wave generation, focusing, and coupling (Table 3.**3**).

Ultrasonic localization of most of the renal calculi is possible, and the success of the treatment can be assessed sufficiently (Figs. 3.**18**, 3.**19**, 3.**22**). The criteria for stone disintegration on the ultrasound scan are broadening of the stone shadow, increasing inhomogenicity of the stone reflex, and, finally, disappearance of the stone shadow (Fig. 3.**20**). There are several *advantages* of sonographical stone localization.

1. It allows real-time scanning without X-ray exposure. Thus, the stone can be focused by the patients breathing (Fig. 3.**21**).

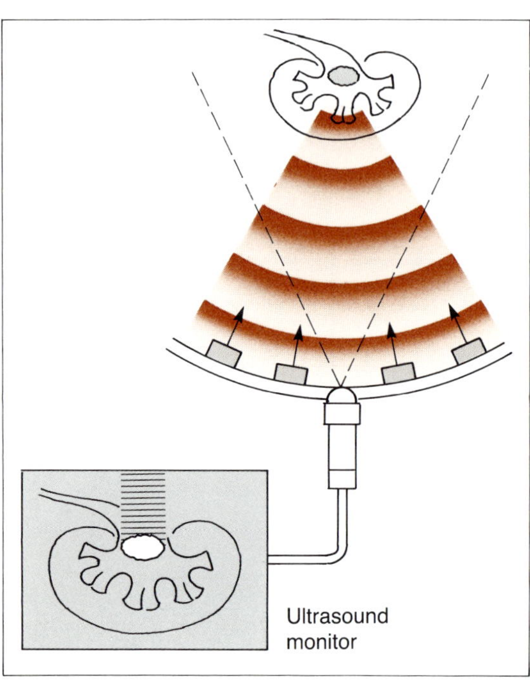

2. Slightly opaque or nonopaque calculi can be localized, thus increasing the range of indications for ESWL, particularly with respect to *gall bladder stones.*
3. In the treatment of smaller calculi, ultrasound provides better resolution than X-ray due to the visualization of the movement of the stone or fragments, or both, during shock wave exposure.
4. It is considerably less expensive than an X-ray system.

◀ **Fig. 3.18   Coaxial Ultrasound localization** (Edap LT01)

Table 3.3   Modifications of stone location for ESWL

Fluoroscopy	Ultrasound	Ultrasound and Fluoroscopy
Dual axis X-ray system with two fluoroscopic units – Orthogonal to the vertebral column (Dornier HM3, HM4) – Axial to the vertebral column (Siemens Lithostar) One rotating X-ray system – Microprocessor-controlled fluoroscopy unit (Dornier MFL 5000) – C-arm (Direx Lithotriptor) – Fluoroscopic ring (Lithoring) Three-dimensional X-ray system (stereofluoroscopy)	One or two coaxial ultrasound probe(s) ("in-line" scanner) (Wolf Piezolith 2300), Edap LT01, Storz Modulith SL10) One lateral ultrasound probe with microprocessor-controlled positioning of the patient (Sonolith 3000, Dornier Compact) Dual axis ultrasonic system with microprocessor-controlled lateral and coaxial scanner (Dornier MPL 9000)	One coaxial ultrasound scanner with an integrated rotating C-arm (Storz Modulith SL20) One coaxial ultrasound scanner with an integrated microprocessor-controlled X-ray table (Diasonics Lithotriptor) One rotating X-ray system with a lateral ultrasound probe (Dornier MFL 5000-u) Dual axis X-ray system with two fluoroscopic units and an independent ESWL head with coaxial ultrasound scanner (Siemens Lithostar Plus) One "in-line" ultrasound probe + one "in-line" X-ray system (Wolf Piezolith 2500) Fluoroscopy + computerized infrared-controlled lateral ultra sound probe (Lithoring, Medstone 1000) Dual axis ultrasonic system with microprocessor-controlled lateral and coaxial scanner combined with a mobile X-ray C-arm (Dornier MPL 9000-x)

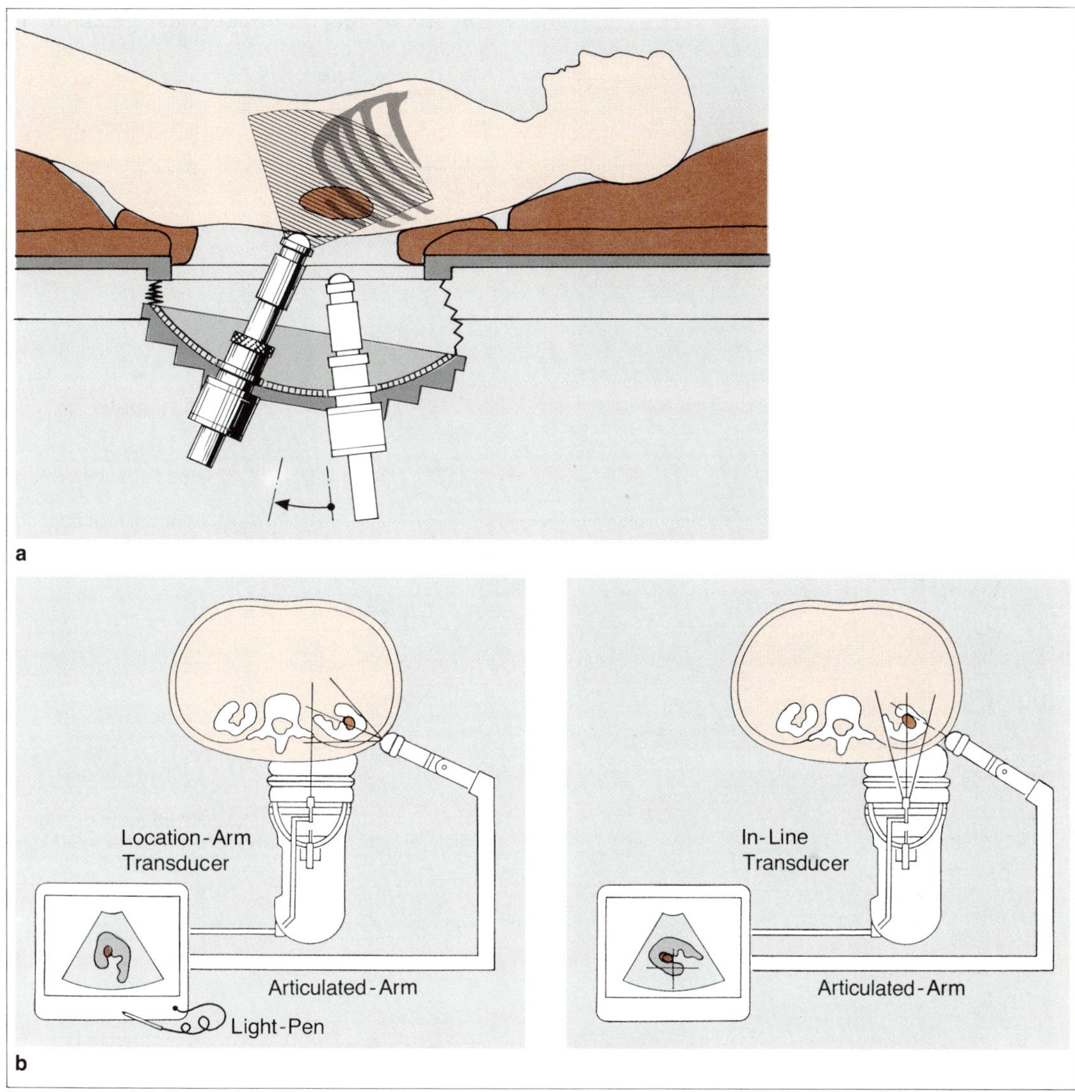

Fig. 3.19 Ultrasound localization in different litho-triptors

a Piezolith 2300: two in-line probes
b MPL 9000: one coaxial and one lateral probe

However, *disadvantages* of ultrasonic stone location have also been determined.

1. Stone localization is difficult and almost impossible in some areas (Fig. 3.**22**). Visualization may be difficult in upper caliceal calculi in cranially located kidneys due to superpositioning of the 12th rib.
The most problematic area for sonographic stone location is the ureter. Only calculi in the upper-third part of a dilated ureter or in the intramural tunnel of the ureter can be located safely. This amounts to about 40%−60% of all ureteral stones (Fig. 3.**22**).

2. Localization of stones may be problematic following the insertion of an indwelling ureteral catheter (Double J-stent) or in the presence of a nephrostomy tube.

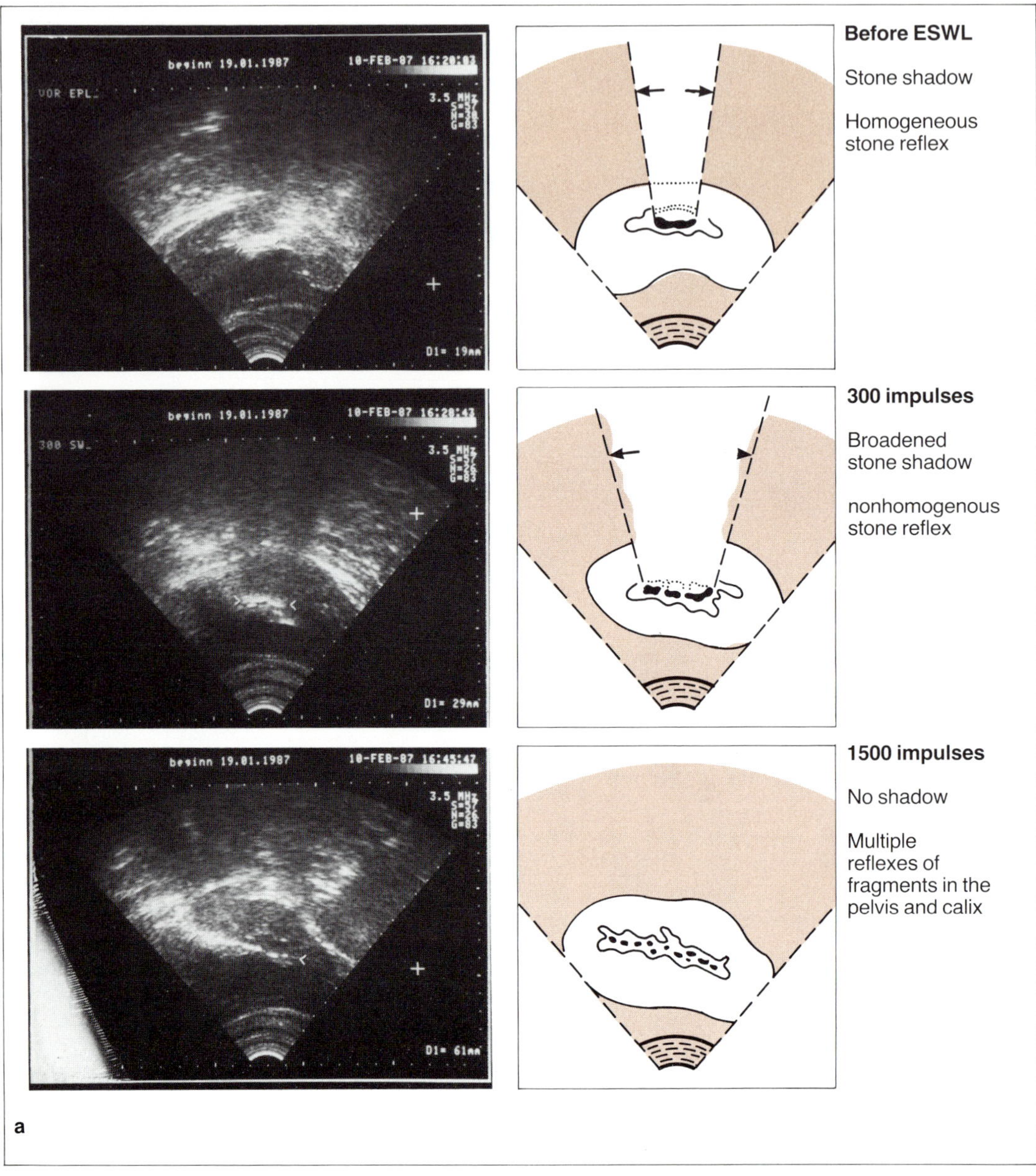

Fig. 3.20   The sonographic criteria for stone disintegration. Ultrasound scan and schematic drawing prior to ESWL, after 300 impulses, and at the end of the treatment (Piezolith 2200)

3. Determination of the size of each individual may not be sufficient due to superpositioned fragments or artifacts.
4. Ultrasound depends mainly on the experience of the operator. This necessitates a prolonged training period.

The final goal is the **integration of fluoroscopy and ultrasound** (Fig. 3.**23**). Apart from the aforementioned criteria, the choice of a localizing system depends on the *design of the lithotriptor*. The problems are

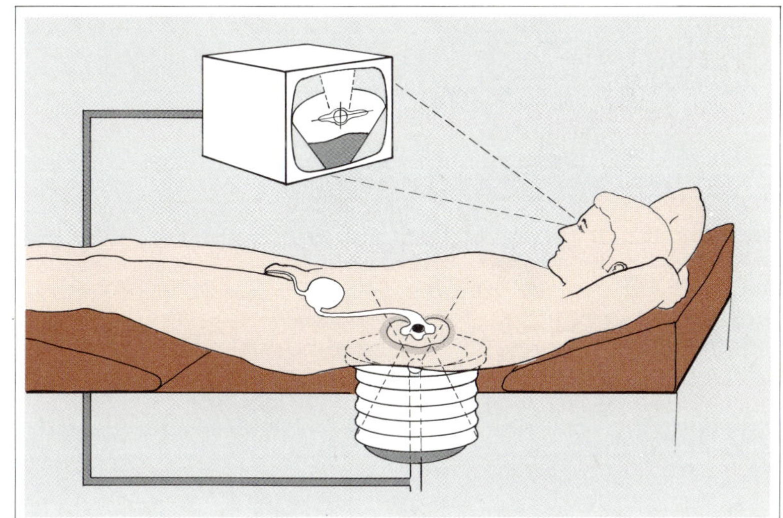

Fig. 3.21 Stone localization by use of coaxial ultrasound providing real-time scanning without fluoroscopy and focusing of the stone by the patient's breathing

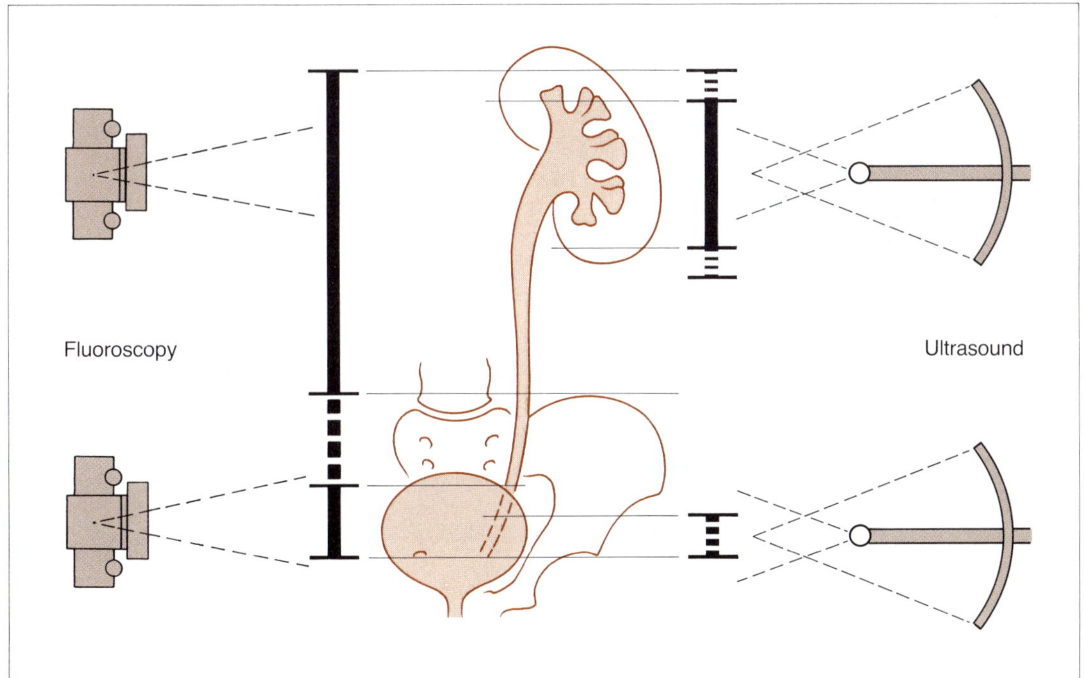

Fig. 3.22 Fluoroscopic versus ultrasonic stone localization. Comparison of areas where stones can be localized

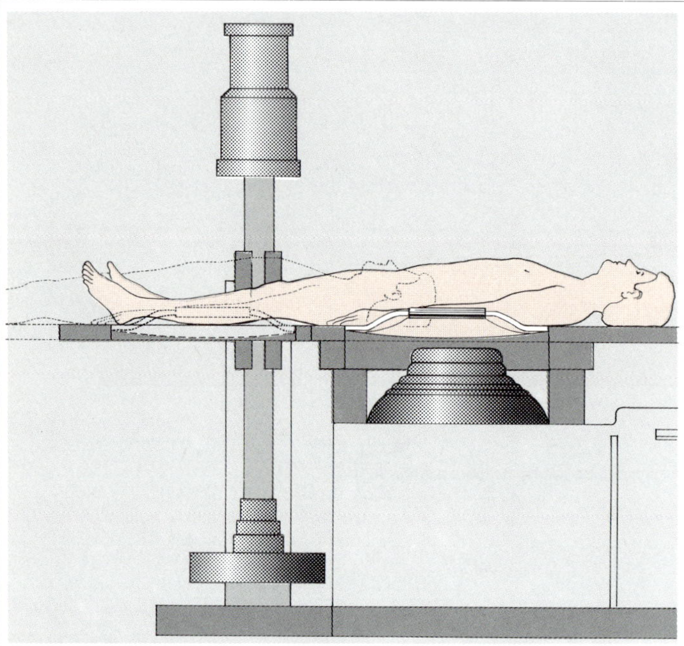

a

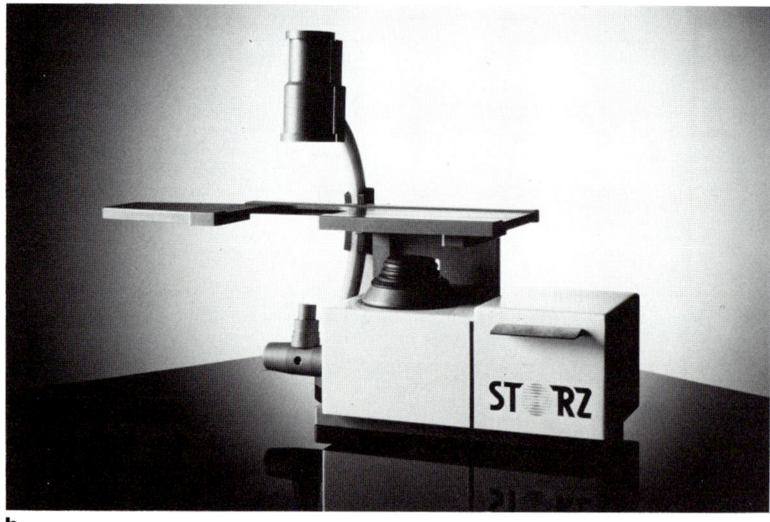

b

Fig. 3.23 Combination of ultrasound and fluoroscopic stone localization

a–c Integrated C-arm with movable table. Fluoroscopic localization using a virtual focus (= isocenter) along y-axis. Subsequently, the patient is moved into the real focus (Storz Modulith SL 20) where coaxial ultrasound is used

d Combination of "in-line" ultrasound and fluoroscopy (Piezolith 2500)

e Combination of x-ray and ultrasound with a mobile fluoroscopic c-arm (Dornier MPL 9000-x)

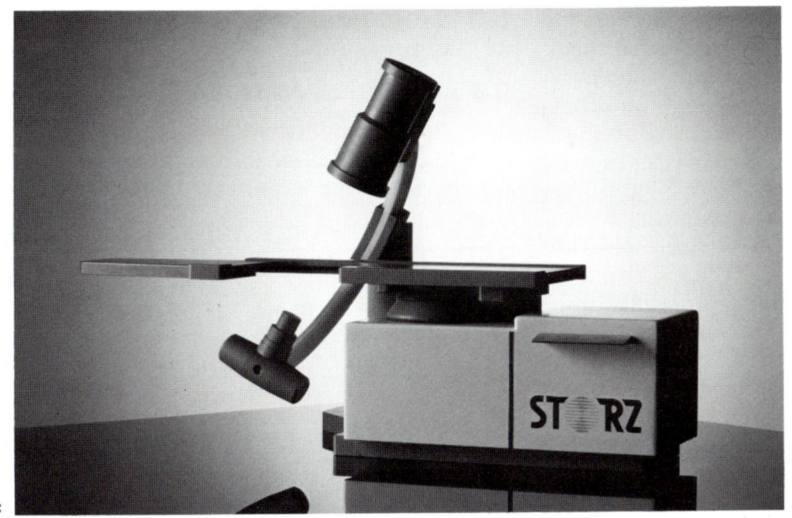

c

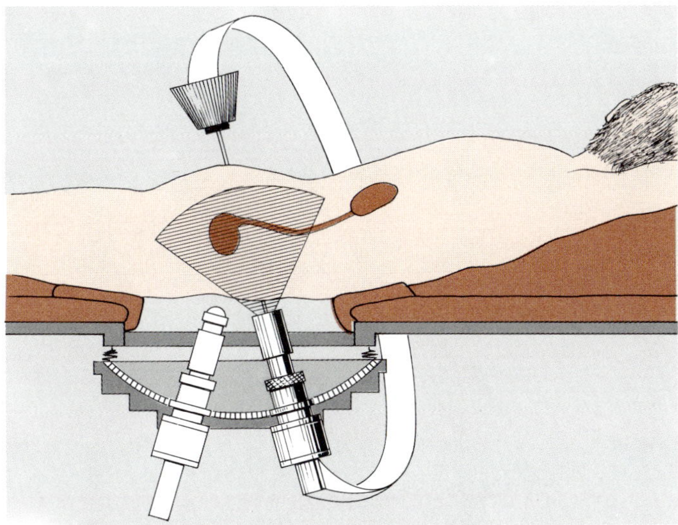

d

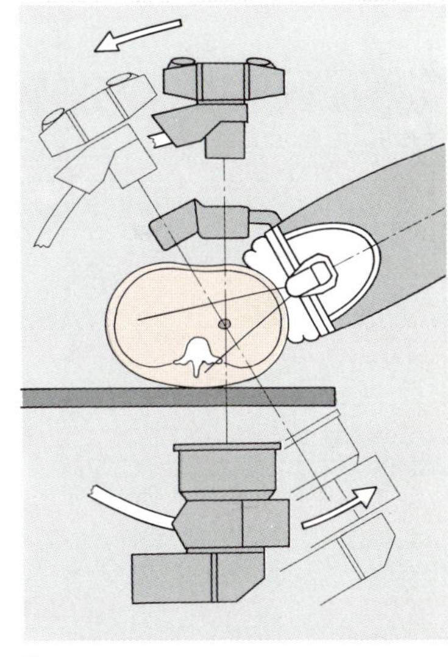

e

- the size of the shock wave source;
- whether the shock wave head is fixed or mobile.

The following factors are important:

1. Energy sources with an aperture of more than 18 cm cannot be integrated in fluoroscopic systems. Therefore, ultrasound must be employed as the primary locating method. The combination with X-ray is only feasible if the patient is positioned into a *"virtual focus (F')"* apart from the shock wave source along the y-axis. After focusing, the patient is moved back over the shock wave source and acoustic coupling is performed (Fig. 3.**23a**).

2. Energy sources of less than 18 cm are necessary in order to integrate them into multifunctional urological tables utilizing one or

two comfortable X-ray units for direct stone localization. On the other hand, such shock wave sources need intravenous analgesia during treatment. The direct real-time combination of ultrasound and fluoroscopic systems in such multifunctional tables has been realized recently (Dornier MFL 5000-u).

3. In the case of shock wave sources with a larger aperture (Fig. 3.**23b**), one solution could be the integration of the X-ray unit in the shock wave generator (= "in-line" fluoroscopy). However, in this case, multifunctional use of the machine cannot be ensured. More over real-time fluoroscopy is not ensured since the x-ray beam is poorly transmitted via the water.

Another possibility represents the oblique coupling of the shockwave source combined with a mobile X-ray C-arm (Fig. 3.**23c**) which allows real-time monitoring with fluoroscopy *and* ultrasound.

However, this solution requires considerable space.

3.9 Biological Effects of Shockwaves

3.9.1 Historical Aspects

The clinical application of shockwaves for contact-free kidney stone disintegration was based on the following experimental results (Table 3.**1**):

– The growth behavior of human lymphocyte cultures remained unaffected.
– The in vitro hemolysis of human blood could not be demonstrated in the peripheral blood under in vivo conditions.
– Shock wave treatment of eviscerated parenchymal organs and muscle tissues of rats (liver, kidney, spleen) did not produce any irreversible lesions.
– A fracture discovered in cadaver bones could not be demonstrated in the case of vital bony tissue.
– Shock wave treatment of eviscerated, air-

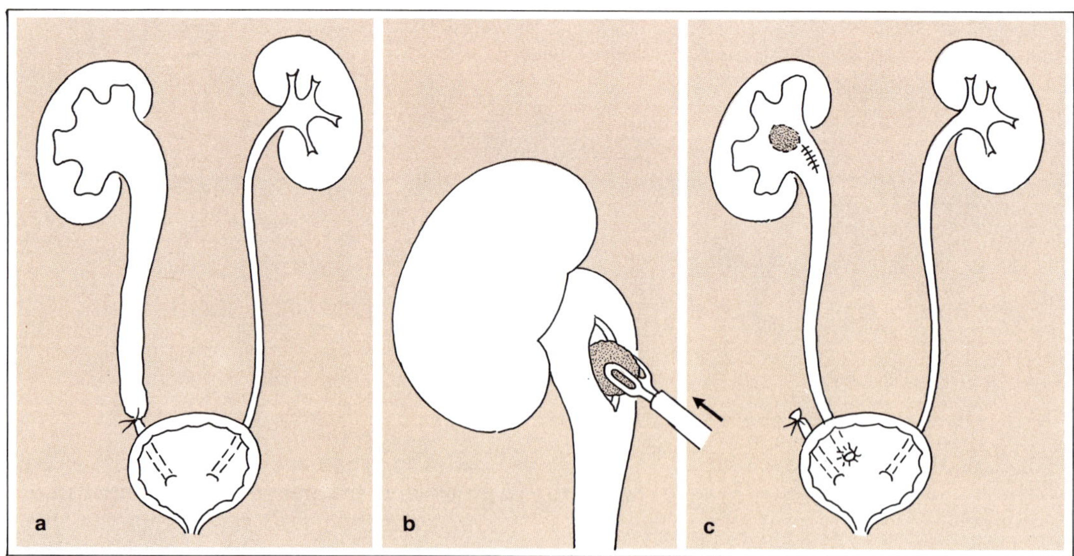

Fig. 3.**24   Canine kidney stone model for experimental studies of ESWL**
a   Prevesical ligation of right ureter inducing dilatation of the upper urinary tract
b   Surgical implantation of human kidney stones in the dilated renal pelvis
c   Reimplantation of the right ureter (Politano-Leadbetter technique)

filled rat intestines lead to petechial hemorrhage. There were no comparable changes with intestines void of air.
- Shock wave application to lung tissue resulted in alveolar ruptures as a result of the different impedance of the alveolar air and the parenchyma.

Using the animal model (dogs) with implanted human kidney stones, disintegration could be achieved by ESWL. Shock wave treatment effected spontaneous passage of stone debris without damage to the experimental animals (Fig. 3.**24**).

As clinical experience progressed very quickly, demonstrating only minimal side effects and a very low complication rate, there was only minor interest in the biological effects of shock waves on experimental models. However, the introduction of second generation lithotriptors and reports on the higher incidence of hypertension subsequent to ESWL has lead to increasing interest and a number of experiments in this field.

Generally, the bioeffects of shock waves are described in the following ways:
- as side effects of clinical ESWL;
- as injury to organs or tissues that have been exposed to shock waves;
- as damage of cells in culture that have been treated with shock waves.

The extent of the lesion depends on the amount of applied shock wave energy, which may be classified physically by the peak positive and negative pressure, focal size, the number of impulses, and the degree of shock wave attenuation by the surrounding tissue or material.

3.9.2 Clinical Side Effects

Today, the side effects of ESWL are equivocally classified as follows:
- pain
- skin petechiae or ecchimosis
- hematuria
- renal injury

Pain. With the Dornier HM3 or a comparable system, general or epidural anesthesia was required because the *pain during treatment* was intolerable. However, modification of the generator and the ellipsoid, as well as the intro-

duction of other energy sources with an increased aperture (i.e., piezoceramic elements), now enables ESWL to be performed without anesthesia (Figs. 3.**15**; 3.**25**).

Principally, two types of pain are experienced during shock wave lithotripsy: (1) a superficial pain at the surface of the skin, and (2) a visceral pain in the kidney. The main factors for the induction of pain are (Fig. 3.**15**).
- the peak pressure of the shock wave in the focus;
- the size of the focal zone;
- the area of shock wave penetration on the skin corresponding to the focusing system.

The most important factor of pain sensation seems to be the distribution of shock wave pressure at the skin. This corresponds to the aperture of the focusing system. The aperture should exceed 20 cm to allow pain-free application.

The size of the focal zone and the peak pressure of the shock wave seems to be responsible for visceral pain. At the start of treatment, the visceral pain is more or less tolerable when working with the new modified lithotriptors. However, after the application of more than one thousand shocks, it may become intolerable; this reflects dose-dependent renal trauma by ESWL.

There are further factors of pain that have not yet been fully investigated (i.e., duration of the shock wave impulse and cavitation at the surface of the skin). The latter may be responsible for local skin *petechiae or ecchimosis* on shock wave entry; this occurs in about 10% − 20% of the patients.

Renal trauma. In contrast to early experimental results, some renal injury resulting from ESWL therapy has been frequently documented using different imaging techniques and laboratory studies (Tables 3.**4**, 3.**5**).

Renal trauma induced by ESWL varies from mild contusion to large perirenal hematoma. Minor renal traumatization reflects in *gross hematuria,* which is apparent in most of the cases. Whereas computed tomography (CT) scans and ultrasound usually fail to detect such lesions, magnetic resonance imaging (MRI) shows minor morphological changes (i.e., loss of corticomedullary demarcation and perirenal fluid; Table 3.**5**).

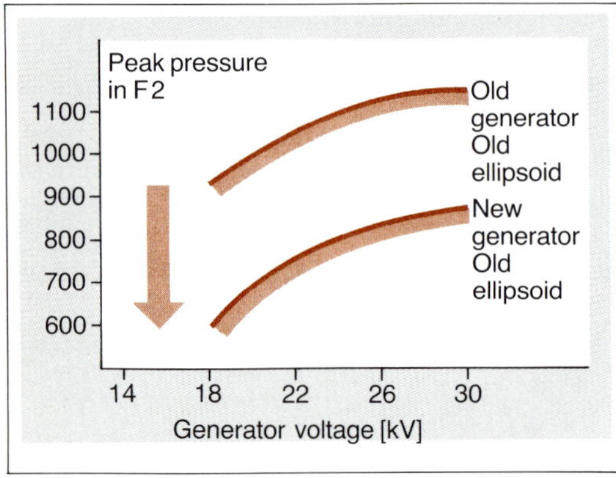

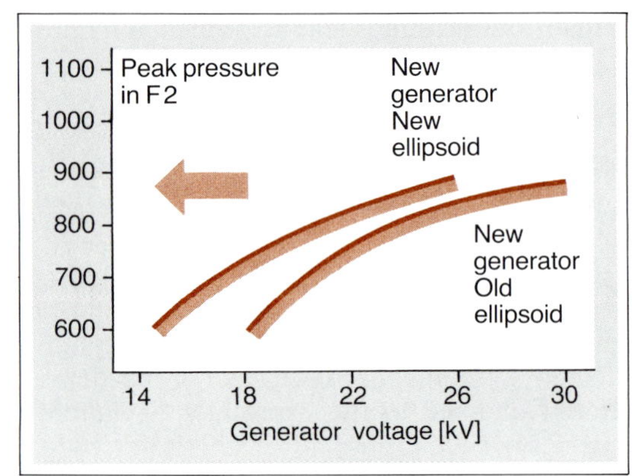

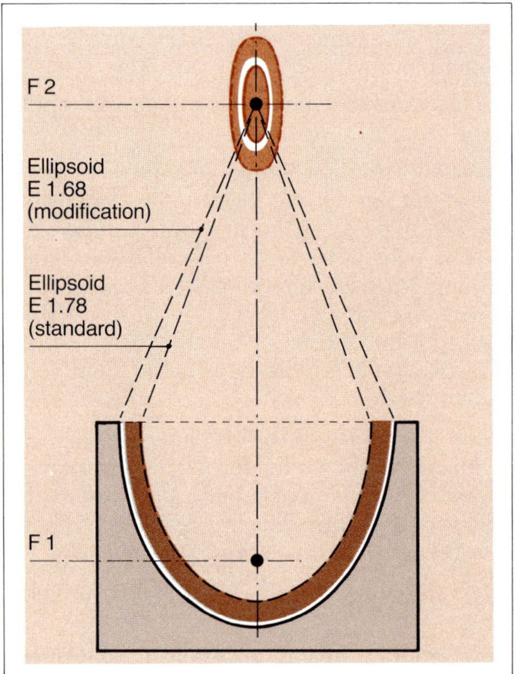

Fig. 3.25 Technical modifications of the standard Dornier HM3 providing low pressure ESWL under intravenous analgesia (= HM3+). All measurements were made with a PCB transducer

a Diagram of peak pressure in F2 using the old generator (80 nF), and the new generator (40 nF) with the old ellipsoid

b Diagram of peak pressure in F2 using the old ellipsoid (15 cm), and the new ellipsoid (17 cm) with the new generator (40 nF)

c Schematic drawing of the two ellipsoids. Increase of the aperture size results in decrease of the size of the focal zone

Due to the low number of cases, no definite correlation could be found to the number of shock waves or generator voltage. However, it seems that patients suffering from hypertension had a greater tendency towards hematomas. The majority of these hematomas were managed conservatively and disappeared within two to three months. A perirenal hematoma, in contrast, occurs in less than 0.5% (Fig. 3.26).

Moreover, temporary increase of cytoplasmic enzymes (i.e., NAG, γGT in blood and urine) or proteins (β-micro-globulin) in urine (Fig. 3.27) demonstrate such injury (Table 3.4).

Table 3.4   Pathophysiological effects of shock waves on the human kidney

Functional Test	Result	Reference	
Renal plasma flow	No or minor difference between treated and untreated kidney	Thomas et al	1988
Renal plasma flow	5% reduced flow in treated kidneys in 33% of cases	Kaude et al	1985
Excreted enzymes and antigens	Alterations of distal tubular epithelium	Schulze et al	1988
Proximal tubular enzymes	Perirenal soft-tissue trauma, possible glomerular dysfunction	Krongrad et al	1988
Lactate dehydrogenase (LDH) N-acetylglucosaminidase (NAG)	Increase in blood and urine, increase in urine	Marcellan et al	1986
Lactate dehydrogenase (LDH) N-acetylglucosaminidase (NAG) Glutamic pyruvic transaminase (GPT)	Transient increase in blood and urine	Kishimoto et al	1986
N-acetylglucosaminidase (NAG) activity	Temporary renal dysfunction	Das et al	1988
Fibrinolytic system	Increase of coagulative fibrinogen	Di Cello et al	1988
Urinary excretion of lysozyme, -glutamyl-transferase	Transient increase; after 6 months the tubular functions had been restored to normal	Jaeger et al	1988
Urinary proteins	Temporary increase of albumin, IgG, beta-2-microglobulin, Tamm-Horsfall protein; alteration of glomerular permeability	Steinmann et al	1988

Table 3.5   Side effects of shock waves (SW) after clinical ESWL

Organ	Result	References	
Kidney	MRI: dose-dependent subcapsular fluid collections and hemorrhages, no serious renal pathologic condition	Baumgartner et al	1987
		Jordan et al	1982
	CT: identical results	Grote et al	1986
		Rubin et al	1987
	MRI: renal contusion, subcapsular hematoma, hemorrhage into renal tissue	Arduan et al	1988
	Hemoglobinuria, decrease in renal function, local contusion, pain, focal fibrosis	Drach et al	1988
Skin	renal contusions	Kaude et al	1985
	Petechial bleeding at areas where SW enter the body	Eisenberger and Rassweiler	1986
		Wilbert	1987
Heart	Incidence of ventricular arrhythmias	Chaussy	1986
		Janssens et al	1988
Blood pressure	Incidence of hypertension (8%)	Steele et al	1988
		Lingeman et al	1987
	No significant incidence of hypertension (3%)	Liedl et al	1989
		Zwergel et al	1989
Intestine	Gastric, duodenal, and colonic erosions	Karawi et al	1987
		Cass et al	1988

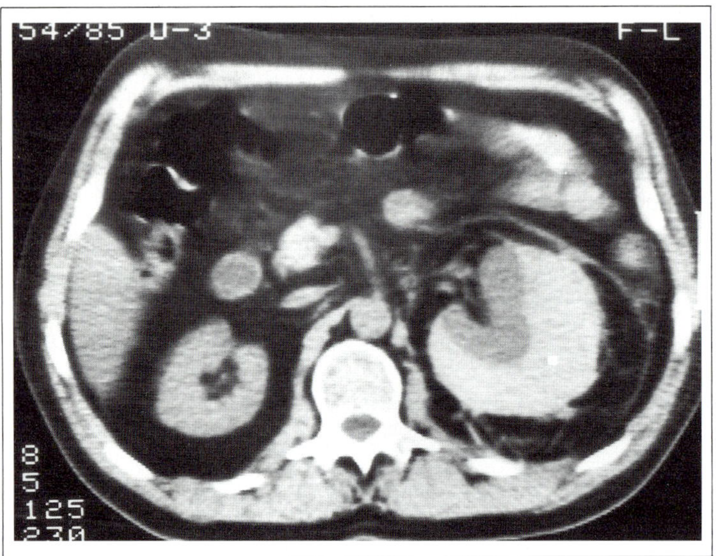

Fig. 3.**26** **Large perirenal hematoma after ESWL showed in CT scan.** Conservative management

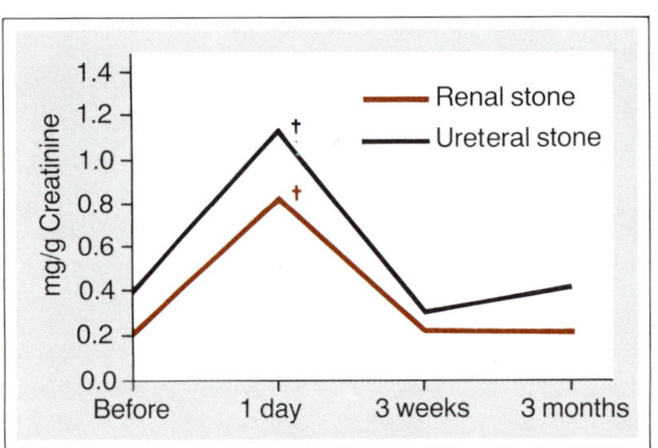

Fig. 3.**27** **Urinary beta-2-microglobulin changes following ESWL of renal and ureteral calculi** (from Yokogama et al., 1988)

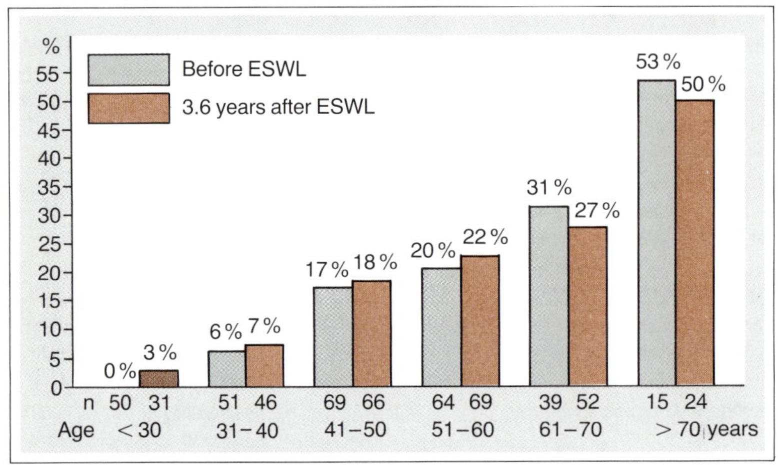

Fig. 3.**28** **Age-dependent prevalence of arterial hypertension prior to and 3.6 years after ESWL.** No significant difference (from Liedl et al., 1989)

Chronic changes subsequent to ESWL could not be demonstrated up to present. The early discovery of a higher incidence of arterial hypertension following ESWL could not be substantiated in further studies (Fig. 3.**28**).

Apart from these observations, *extrarenal injury* has very rarely been observed (i.e., gastric, colonic, or duodenal bleeding due to ESWL-induced erosions or minor pulmonary hemorrhage) (Table 3.**5**).

3.9.3 Experimental Animal Studies

Independent of the animal model, the extent of the renal injury by shock waves strictly depends on the energy applied (Table 3.**6**). Low pressure (or generator voltage) leads to only microscopically detectable lesions (i.e., tubular dilatation, rupture of glomerula), whereas higher peak pressures induce intraparenchymal hematomas (Fig. 3.**29**). The size of the hematoma depends on the focal area and the level of generator voltage. Exceedingly high levels (above 1,000 bar) may even lead to perirenal bleeding. The predominant area of the lesion seems to be the corticomedullary junction, owing to rupture of the arcuated veins. However, on high energy levels interlobular arteries may rupture, too, resulting in a perirenal hematoma. Once a hematoma develops, the increase of impulses does not result in greater injury. On the other hand, staged application of shock waves (interval of two days) is less traumatic than the full dose of shocks in a single session (Table 3.**7**).

The long-term observations show healing of the renal lesions by cicatrization; this results in small interstitial or even segmental fibrosis (Fig. 3.**30**), depending on the shock wave energy applied (Table 3.**7**).

Table 3.**8** summarizes the findings when other tissue was exposed to shock waves. No damage was observed in the ureter, the adrenals, and the ovary; however the liver, the bone, the intestines, and the lungs may be damaged by shock waves (Fig. 3.**29b**). Moreover, alteration of the microcirculation has been found after shock wave application.

3.9.4 Cell Culture Experiments and Tumor Models

There is an increasing number of experiments investigating the effect of shock waves on normal and malignant cells (Table 3.**9**). However, some of these findings seem to be contradictory.

– Preliminary studies showed damage of erythrocytes but no significant hemolysis in vivo. Moreover, no influence on the proliferation of human lymphocytes was detected.

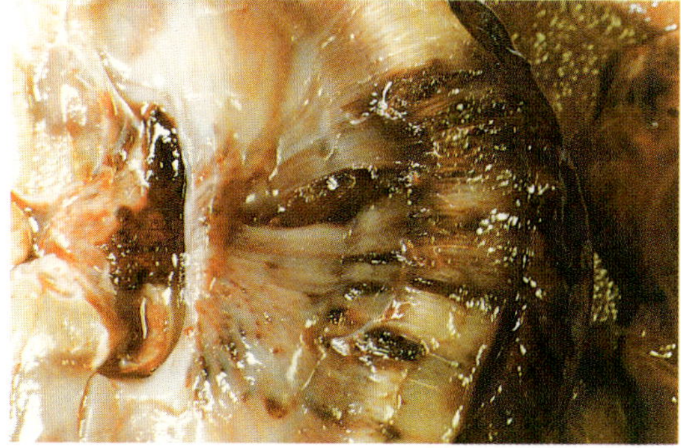

Fig. 3.**29 Acute side-effects in animal studies.**
a Focal intrarenal hematoma (⌀ 1.5 cm) at the corticomedullary junction of a canine kidney after 2,500 shock waves at 15 kV (~ 550 bar) using a laboratory lithotriptor with electromagnetic shock wave generator (Storz Modulith)

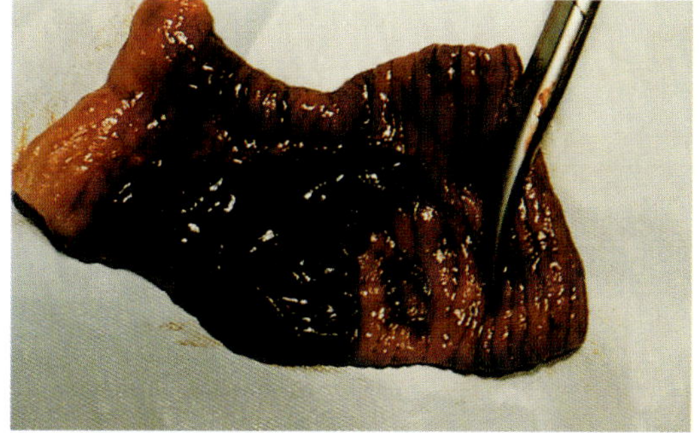

b Colonic erosion observed after 2,500 shock waves exposed to the right canine kidney with 18 kV (900 bar) using a laboratory lithotriptor (Storz Modulith)

Table 3.6   Morphological findings after exposure of canine kidney to different shock wave energy using a new electromagnetic source (Storz Modulith).

a) Acute changes after 1500 SW and 2500 SW

kV	N	Macroscopy	Histology	Grade of lesions
11−13	7	No lesion or parenchymal petechiae	Minimal tubular necrosis	I
14−16	14	Parenchymal hemorrhage	Rupture of venolae and arteriolae	II
17−20	6	Perirenal hematoma	Rupture of Interlobular arteries	III

b) Acute changes at high energy level (20 kV). The impact of shock wave number

SW; number	N	Macroscopy	Grade of lesion
25− 60	3	Petechial bleeding	I
300− 600	4	Parenchymal hemorrhage	II
900−2500	4	Perirenal hematoma	III

c) Long-term findings 10 weeks after 1500 and 2500 SW

kV	N	Macroscopy	Histology
15	3	No residuals detectable	Hemosiderin residues in the medulla, tubular regeneration
16−17	3	Small cord-like scars at the cortex	Hemosiderin residues and wedge-shaped corticomedullar scar formation
20	3	Residues of parenchymal hematoma perirenal fibrosis	Demarkation of the hematoma, wedge-shaped scar formation

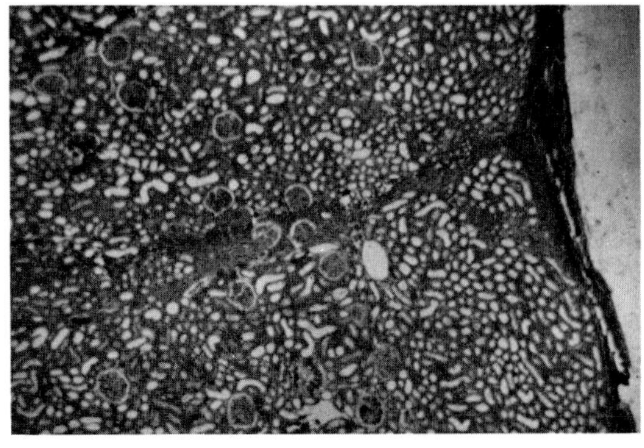

Fig. 3.**30   Long-term changes in the canine kidney.** Segmental fibrosis as a result of healing 10 weeks after a perirenal hematoma due to 2500 shock waves at high-energy level (18 kV) using the Modulith laboratory lithotriptor

Table 3.7   Shock wave-induced renal trauma in experimental studies

Lithotriptor	Animal Model (species)	Energy Setting	No. of Shocks	Short-Term Effect	Long-Term Effect (4–6 weeks)	Author
Dornier HM1	Dog	12–15 kV	500	No damage	No visible damage	Chaussy et al 1977
Dornier HM2	Dog	20 kV	500	Intrarenal hematoma ($\varnothing$ 5 mm)	–	Delius et al 1987
			1,500	Multifocal hematoma ($\varnothing$ 5 mm)		
			3,000	Multifocal hematoma ($\varnothing$ 6–18 mm), venous thrombosis		
			3,000 (burst)	Intrarenal ($\varnothing$ 15 mm) and perirenal hematoma		
Dornier HM3	Dog	18–24 kV	1,600	Intrarenal hematoma ($\varnothing$ 5 mm)	Small fibrosis	Newman et al 1987
			4,500 6,000	Intrarenal hematoma ($\varnothing$ 15 mm) and perirenal hematoma	Interstitia fibrosis	
	Dog	–?–	1,500	Intrarenal bleeding and subcapsular hematoma; glomerular rupture, rupture of peritubular venoles	Interstitial fibrosis	Jäger et al 1989
	Pig	15–30 kV	750–12,000	Dose-dependent damage: intrarenal ($\varnothing$ 10 mm) and perirenal hematoma. No difference between 6,000 and 12,000 shock waves	Segmental fibrosis / Fibrosis of capsule	Muschter et al 1989
	Rat	15 kV	500	Subcapsular and intrarenal bleeding	Interstitial fibrosis	Recker et al 1989
			2,000 5,000	Diffuse hemorrhage and subcapsular bleeding	Segmental fibrosis (severe scarring)	
	Rabbit	14 kV	2,000 + 2,000	Tubular dilatation (2 weeks)	–	Fuchs et al 1989
			4,000	Renal infarction, subcapsular hematoma (2 weeks)	Focal and segmental fibrosis	
	Rabbit	21 kV	500	Intrarenal hematoma ($\varnothing$ 30 mm)	Segmental fibrosis	Morris et al 1989
Wolf Piezolith 2300	Dog	IV	1,000	Subcapsular hematoma (10 mm)	No visible damage	Kopper et al 1986
		IV	2,000 4,000	Subcapsular hematoma Rupture of arcuate veins, lesion of intima of arterials, necroses of papillae		Neisius et al 1989

Table 3.7 Shock wave-induced renal trauma in experimental studies (continued)

Lithotriptor	Animal model (species)	Energy setting	No. of Shocks	Short-Term Effect	Long-Term Effect (4–6 weeks)	Author
	Rabbit	IV	1,000	Subcapsular hematoma (10 mm)	No visible damage	Morris et al 1989
Edap LT01	Dog	100%	6,000 12,000 24,000	Intrarenal hematoma (8–10 mm)	Interstitial fibrosis	Thibault et al 1987
	Rabbit	100%	6,000	No damage	No visible damage	Ryan et al 1989
			24,000	Intrarenal and perirenal bleeding	No visible damage	
Siemens Lithostar	Dog	16–19 kV	500–2,000	Focal intrarenal bleeding	–	Wilbert 1989

Table 3.8 Injury to extrarenal organs if exposed to shock waves in experimental studies

Organ	Animal	Observation	Author	
Liver	Rat	Hepatocellular necrosis	Loening et al	1988
			Mardan et al	1988
	Dog	Dose-dependent hematoma, subcapsular hematoma, and necrosis	Rassweiler et al	1989
			Staritz et al	1989
			Neisius et al	1989
Gallbladder	Dog	Hemorrhage and edema of wall	Neisius et al	1989
Lung	Rat	Petechial bleeding, hemoptysis, pulmonary interstitial cellular infiltration	Eisenberger et al	1976
			Loening et al	1988
	Dog	Hemorrhages, hemorrhages after gallstone destruction	Mardan et al	1988
			Delius et al	1987
Intestine	Rat	Petechial bleeding intestinal hemorrhages	Eisenberger et al	1976
			Loening et al	1988
	Dog	Submucosal hematoma, intestinal hemorrhage	Rassweiler et al	1989
			Jäger et al	1989
Ureter	Rabbit	No damage	Fuchs et al	1989
Adrenals	Dog	No adverse effect on function or morphology	Chinn et al	1988
Ovary and fetus	Rat	No adverse teratogenic effect	McCullough et al	1988
Bone	Rabbit	Aseptic necrosis damage to osteocytes	Graff et al	1987
	Rat	Dose-dependent hemorrhagic lesion	Mardan et al	1988

Table 3.9　Effects of shock waves (SW) on cells in culture

Cells	Results	References	
Full blood	In vitro: dose-dependent hemolysis In vivo: no increase in free plasma Hemoglobin in peripheral blood in dogs	Eisenberger et al	1977
Human lymphocytes	Proliferation unaffected	Eisenberger et al	1977
Human neutrophils	In suspension: cellular disruptions, swelling of mito-chondria, plasma-membrane ruptures; permeability and cytoskeletal changes	Holmes et al	1988
Human melanoma	Reduction in cell viability, decrease in colony formation, selective diminution of cells in G2 and M phases.	Russo et al	1987
	No influence on cell cycle, 10-fold potentiated growth inhibition when treated at 18 °C compared to 37 °C and 42 °C	Berens et al	1988
Human renal carcinoma, normal human embryonic kidney	Dose-dependent reduction of viability, in vitro lysis, total inhibition of multiplication for 5 days after 2,000 SW	Chaussy et al	1989
Human cervix carcinoma	No influence of cell cycle, 10-fold potentiated growth inhibition when treated at 18 °C compared to 37 °C and 42 °C.	Berens et al	1988
	In suspension: dose-dependent damage; immobilized cells: no effect	Bräuner et al	1989
Rat prostatic carcinoma	Reduction in cell viability, decrease in colony formation, selective diminution of cells in G2 and M phases, delay in tumor growth after reimplantation. Mitochondria swollen, distorted cristae, in vivo exposure had no distinct his-topathologic or ultrastructural effect.	Russo et al	1986
	In suspension: growth delay, ultrastructural damages; in vivo: growth delay	Loening et al	1988
	Dose-dependent inhibition of cell viability and colony growth; Cells pretreated with SW became more sensitive to chemotherapy or immunotherapy	Oosterhof et al	1988
	6 day prolonged tumor growth after SW plus cisplatin	McCullough et al	1989
Mouse bladder tumor	Palpable tumors were not affected by 800 or 1,400 SW; 2,000 SW lead to a significant inhibition of growth	Chaussy et al	1989
Mouse leukemia	In suspension: dose-dependent damage, immobilized cells: no effect	Brümmer et al	1989
Mouse mammary tumor	In suspension: dose-dependent damage, immobilized cells: no effect	Bräuner et al	1988

However, later experiments found signifi-cant damage of human neutrophils.
- Several studies using suspensions of differ-ent tumor cells showed dose-dependent cel-lular injury resulting in decrease of viability and colony formation (Fig. 3.**31**).

However, later experiments proved that tu-mor cells, if immobilized in gelatine, were unaffected (Fig. 3.**31**). The same applied to tumor cell spheroids (Figs. 3.**32**, 3.**33**).

The explanation for these different observa-tions may be that the cellular damage in vitro

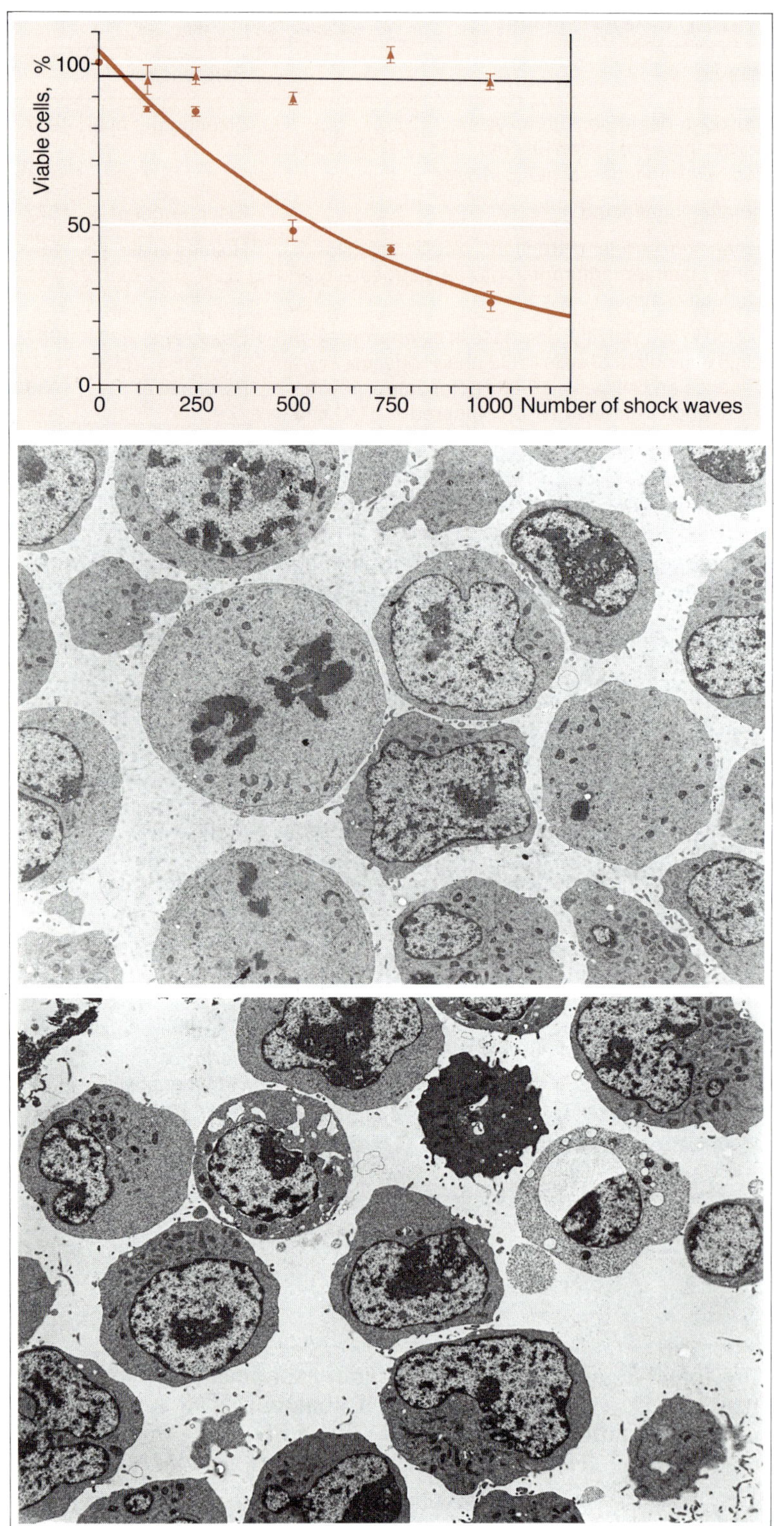

Fig. 3.**31** **Effect of shock waves on viability of L1210 mouse leukemia cells**

a Schematic drawing of viability
   Lower curve: single cell suspension (18 kV, 80 nF, 1 Hz, 21 °C).
   Upper curve: In gelatine immobilized cells (18 kV, 80 nF, 1 Hz, 21 °C).
b Electron-microscopic picture. Control
c Electron-microscopic picture. 500 shock waves (18 kV, 80 nF, 1 Hz, 37 °C). Note fragmented cells, swollen mitochondria, perinuclear cisternae, and vacuolization of cytoplasma.

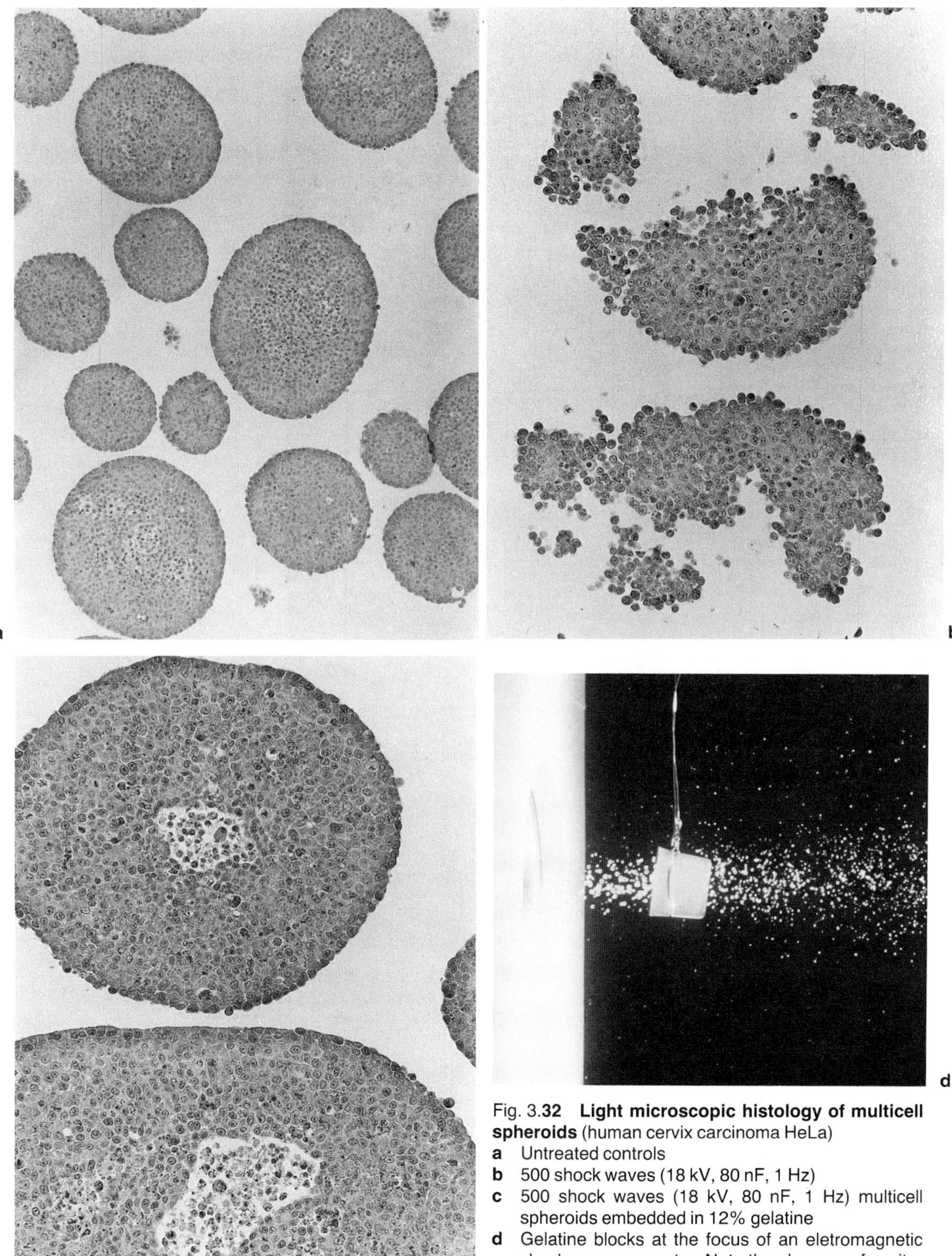

Fig. 3.**32** **Light microscopic histology of multicell spheroids** (human cervix carcinoma HeLa)
a Untreated controls
b 500 shock waves (18 kV, 80 nF, 1 Hz)
c 500 shock waves (18 kV, 80 nF, 1 Hz) multicell spheroids embedded in 12% gelatine
d Gelatine blocks at the focus of an eletromagnetic shock wave generator. Note the absence of cavitation bubbles

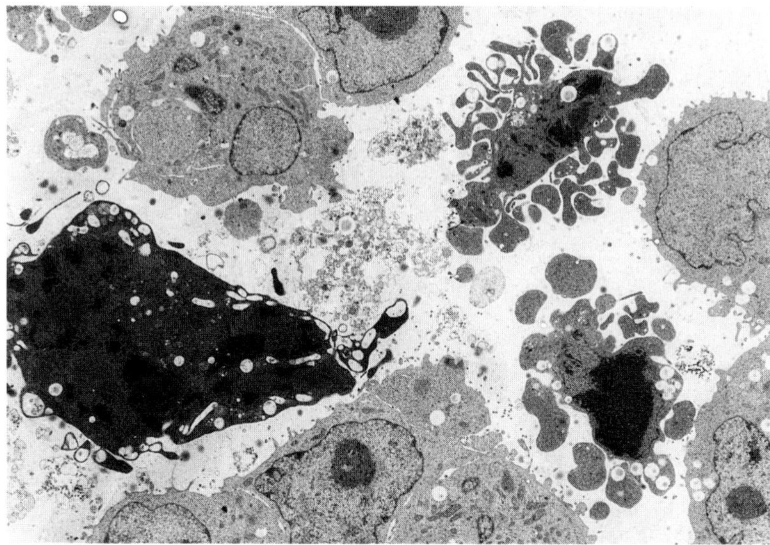

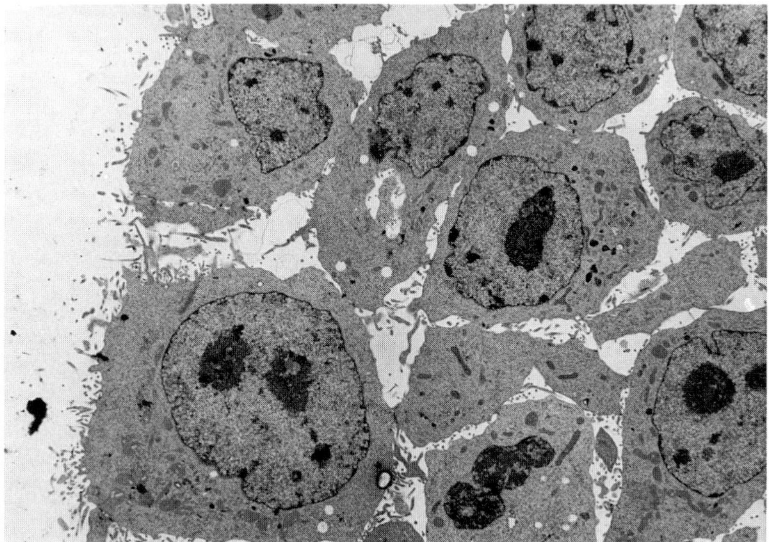

Fig. 3.**33**   **Electron-microscopic histology of multi-cell spheroids** (human cervic carcinoma HeLa)

a   Suspended spheroids after 500 shocks
b   Immobilized spheroids in gelatine after 500 shocks

depends on different mechanisms than the injury of tissue in vivo.

Whereas the peak pressure of the shock wave *in vivo* represents the main factor, *in vitro* (in suspension) secondary effects, due to cavitation and shock wave induced jets, participate in cellular destructions (Fig. 3.**34**). These rapid accelerations of the cells expose them to stress forces and cause collisions.

Immobilization of the cells in gelatine avoids these secondary effects (Fig. 3.**32d**), and thus cellular damage only occurs if very high levels of peak pressure are applied. This observation correlates with the significant attenuation of shock wave efficacy treating impacted ureteral calculi.

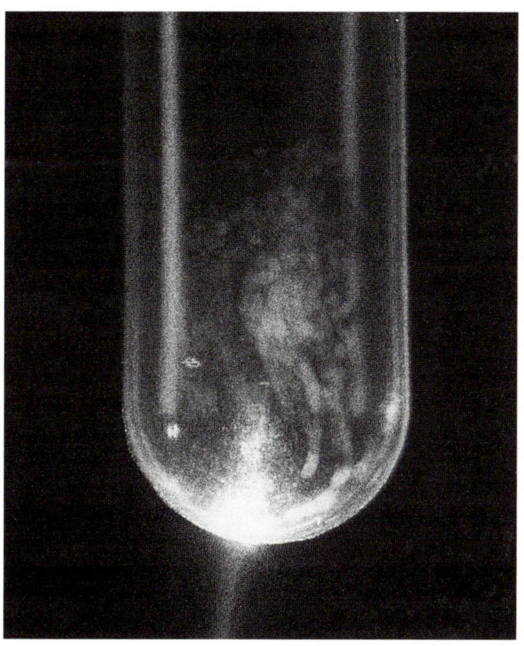

All in vivo experimental tumor models showed some growth delay after shock wave application; however, complete tumor necrosis could not be achieved. Preliminary studies found an increase of chemosensitivity of the tumor when pretreated by shock waves (Fig. 3.**35**). Recently, even a synergistic antineoplastic effect of shockwaves and biological response modifies was observed experimentically (Oosterhof et al. (1990). Nevertheless, all these trials are still a long way from clinical application.

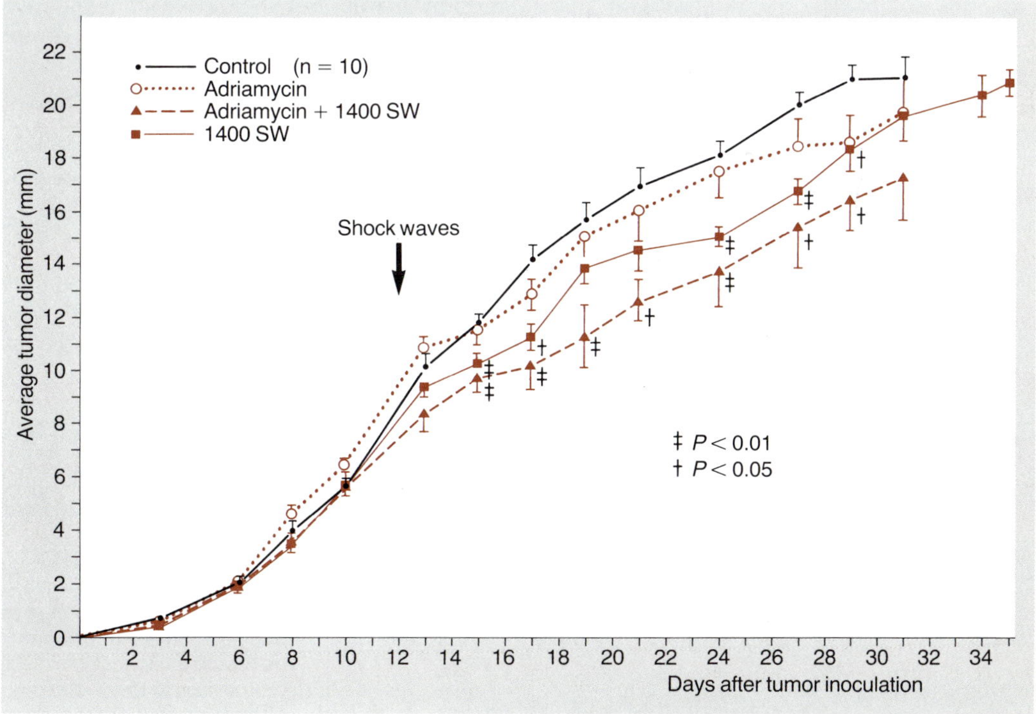

Fig. 3.**34 HeLa multicell spheroids in a polyethylene pipette** (diameter: 1.3 cm) exposed to a single shock wave (18 kV, 80 nF, 37 °C). Stroboscopic illumination

Fig. 3.**35 Synergistic effect of shock waves and chemotherapy in the bladder tumor model (FANFT) of C₃H/HE mice** (from Chaussy and Fuchs, 1989)

3.10 Clinical ESWL

3.10.1 Patient Selection

Absolute Contraindications

- untreated coagulopathy
- gravidity

Relative Contraindications

- untreated UTI
- active tuberculosis
- obstruction of the collecting system distal to the stone (i.e., calciceal diverticulum, infundibular stenosis, UPJ-stenosis, ureteral stenosis)

Technical Problems

- Adipositas permagna (Fig. 3.**36**)
- Children smaller than 100 cm need styrofoam boards to protect their lungs. In some lithotriptors, the stretcher must be modified to fit the patient.

Simulation

All calculi that may be difficult to localize should be simulated the day before treatment to avoid prolonged treatment time and anesthesia. Such calculi are

- *for fluoroscopic stone localization:* stones close to the bones (i.e., ureteral calculi, calculi in horseshoe kidneys or pelvic kidneys, in the case of kyphoscoliosis);
- *for ultrasonic stone localization:* upper and lower ureteral calculi, calculi in dystopic kidneys, residual stones after PCNL.

It should be clarified whether in situ ESWL of the stone is possible or if auxiliary measures prior to shock wave lithotripsy (i.e., ureteral stent, push-back of the stone, use of contrast dye) are required. An additional check should be made to determine whether or not the stone is suitable for ESWL treatment (see Chapter 2).

3.10.2 Indications

1. Radiopaque renal calculi up to a size of 2–3 cm in longitudinal diameter, independent of their position in the collecting system.
2. Radiopaque ureteric stones above *and* below the iliac crest.
3. Residual stones after PCNL or open surgery.

Larger calculi can be treated by ESWL monotherapy as well, but an internal stent should be placed prior to the treatment to avoid complications after ESWL.

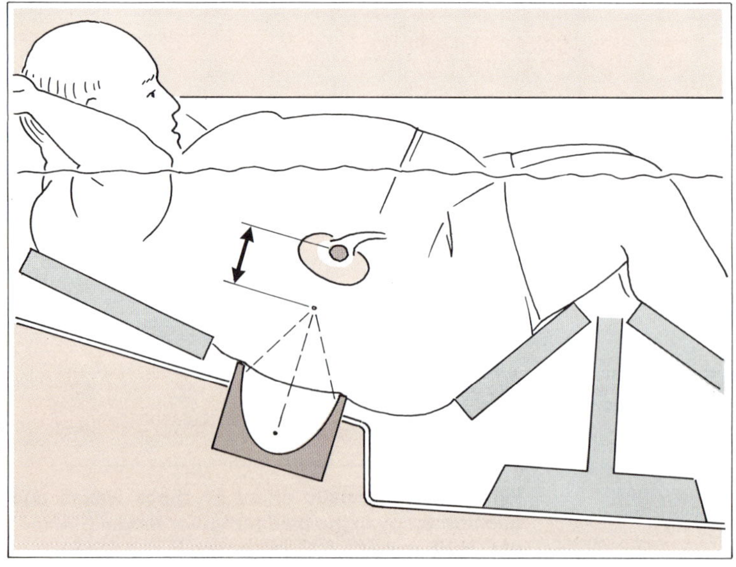

Fig. 3.**36** **In the case of gross obesity, some stones cannot be focused** because the distance from skin to focus exceeds 12 cm. However, most of them can be treated along the "blast path" positioning the stone exactly over F2 on the z-axis (see below)

Radiolucent stones can be located by fluoroscopy only after administration of contrast medium. On the other hand, stone location is simple with ultrasound. However, in the follow-up, the evaluation of treatment success (degree of disintegration) and of complications (i.e., "Steinstrasse") may be problematic. This problem is of minor importance in the case of smaller caliceal and ureteral stones.

Midureteral stones can be located by employing an X-ray system, which necessitates additional administration of contrast dye in some cases. ESWL must be performed in the prone position.

3.10.3 Patient Preparation

As an Outpatient

Intravenous pyelogram (IVP), chest X-ray, ECG, laboratory analysis (blood counts, clotting parameters, electrolytes, serum creatinine).

In order to attain correct determination of the indication, X-ray evaluation should be made by an ESWL-experienced urologist.

As an Inpatient

Urine analysis, urine culture, sonography.

In the evening: laxatives (oral, possibly enema); antibiotics in the case of suspected UTI (urinary analysis!); fasting.

In the morning: 1,500 ml of 0.9% saline solution (renal protection).

Before treatment: unilateral plain X-ray (KUB).

Fasting and administration of laxatives prior to ESWL ensure good imaging during treatment (no overshadowing by intestinal gas). A possible effect of the shock waves on the air-filled intestine is thus prevented (acoustic interface!).

Patient Information

During passage of stone debris, colics may occur in 10%−40% of the cases (dependent on stone size). Additional complications are subcutaneous petechiae (10%) and intrarenal hematoma (less than 0.5%). Auxiliary measures after ESWL (percutaneous nephrostomy, Zeiss loop, URS) are required in 8%−10% of cases. The rate of multiple treatment is between 10% and 40% (depending on stone size and lithotriptor).

3.10.4 Anesthesia

Depending on the technical features of the different lithotriptors (aperture of focusing system, peak pressure, size of focal zone), the following anesthetic procedures are applied:

- epidural anesthesia (catheter)
- general anesthesia
- analgosedation
- intravenous analgesia
- local anesthesia
- no anesthesia

With the standard Dornier HM3 (80 nF generator, 15 cm ellipsoid) *epidural anesthesia* was applied most frequently with the advantage of an indwelling catheter (regional treatment) of colics (multiple treatment).

Table 3.10 **Concept of anesthesia for ESWL**

Criteria	No Anesthesia	IV Analgesia	Epidural/General Anesthesia
Stone size (cm)	< 1.5	> 1.5	Independent
Composition	No cystine No whewellite	No cystine	Independent
Impaction	No	No	Yes
Patient size	Medium−obese	Small−medium	Independent

At some centers, *general anesthesia* was combined with high-frequency jet ventilation (HFJV). This method minimizes the respiratory excursion of the diaphragm, and hence of the kidney and upper ureter, to a minimum, thus resulting in an increased number of impulses hitting their target (by about 30%).

On the modified Dornier HM3+ (40 nF generator, 17 cm ellipsoid), as well as on most second generation machines, the treatment is performed under *intravenous analgesia* or *analgosedation* (Table 3.**10**, Fig. 3.**25**).

Both low-energy shock wave generators and the development of other focusing principles (i.e., spherical alignment of piezoelectric elements) with a larger aperture afford the advantage of ESWL *without any anesthesia*. However, this approach is mainly based on patient cooperation and cannot be applied to all calculi (i.e., impacted ureteral stones). Moreover, the price paid for anesthesia-free treatment is an increase in the retreatment rate (15% vs 40%) and shock wave possession (by about 50%). The solution to this conflict could be the differentiated use of anesthesia depending on stone size, composition, impaction, and size of the patient (see Table 3.**10** and Chapter 7).

3.10.5 Technique and Strategy

The treatment is carried out in three steps: positioning; stone localization; shock wave application. When using the standard Dornier HM3 lithotriptor (or the modified HM3+), the following procedure is recommended.

Positioning

Positioning involves adapting the stretcher to the stone-bearing side and patient size (Fig. 3.**37**). Patients with concrements close to the

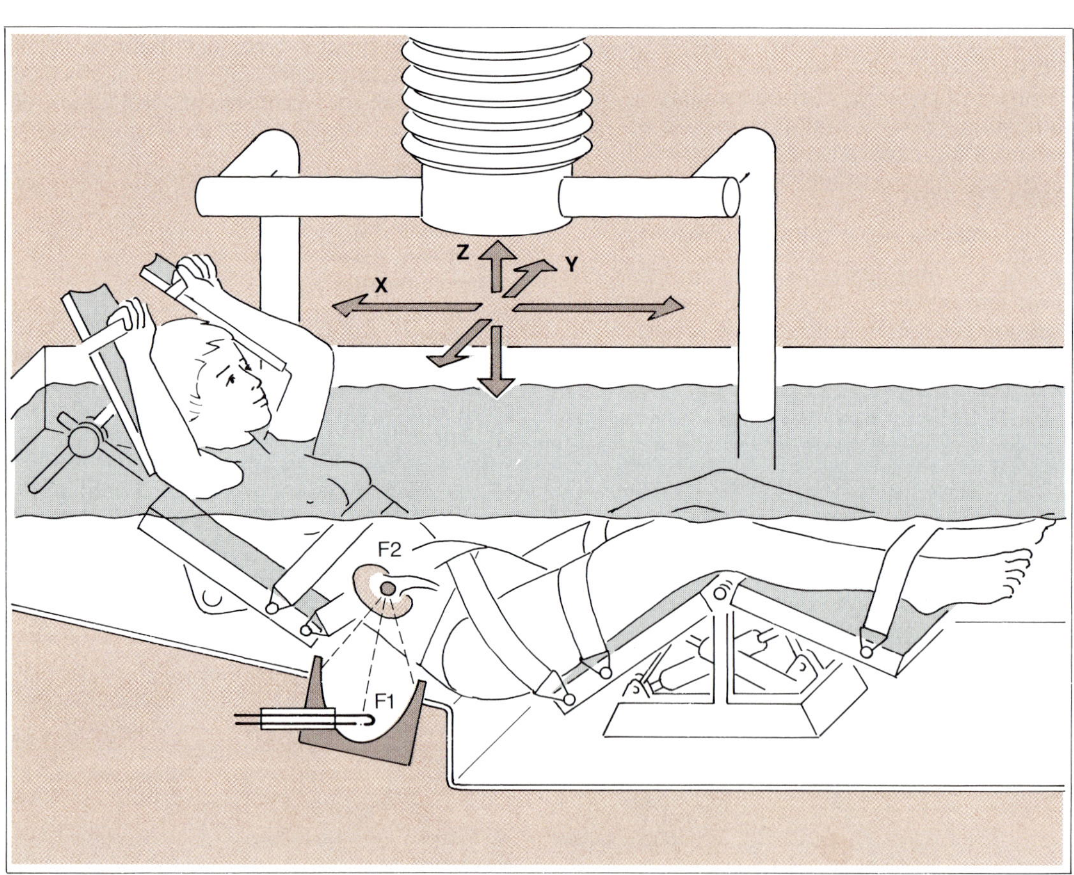

Fig. 3.**37** **Positioning of the patient in the water bath providing best coupling of shock wave energy** (Dornier HM3)

spine should be turned by simultaneously lowering the stone-bearing side (Figs. 3.**38** and 3.**39**). The patient is fixated with straps in order to balance the body's buoyancy in water.

Distal ureteral stones can be treated in two different positions:

Gluteal entrance of shock waves (Fig. 3.**40**) with

– flat position of shoulder and leg segments of the stretcher;
– positioning support by straps crossed at the patient's back;
– turning the patient onto the stone-bearing side.

Perineal entrance of shock waves (Fig. 3.**41** with

– steep position of the shoulder segment and flat position of the leg support;
– sitting position of the patient;
– positioning support by crossed straps.

Stones in the midureter or in pelvic kidneys can be treated in the prone position (Fig. 3.**42**) with

– horizontal position of shoulder and leg segments of the stretcher;
– positioning support by crossed straps;
– low level of water in the tub (just rinsing the abdominal wall of the patient).

On the *multifunctional lithotriptors* with shock wave sources integrated in an X-ray table (i.e., Dornier MFL 5000, Siemens Lithostar, Storz Modulith SL20), there is no further need for a special positioning technique. The X-ray systems have an anteroposterior view and another view after rotation along the vertebral column. This enables easy localization of stones close to the vertebral column.

Nevertheless, *midureteral and most of the distal ureteral calculi* should be treated with the patient in the *prone position* to minimize shock wave attenuation by the bony pelvis.

With those lithotriptors utilizing *coaxial ultrasound* (i.e., Wolf Piezolith 2300, Dornier MPL 9000, Storz Modulith SL10; Edap LT01), a slightly rotated position of the patient to the stone-bearing side is necessary for adequate

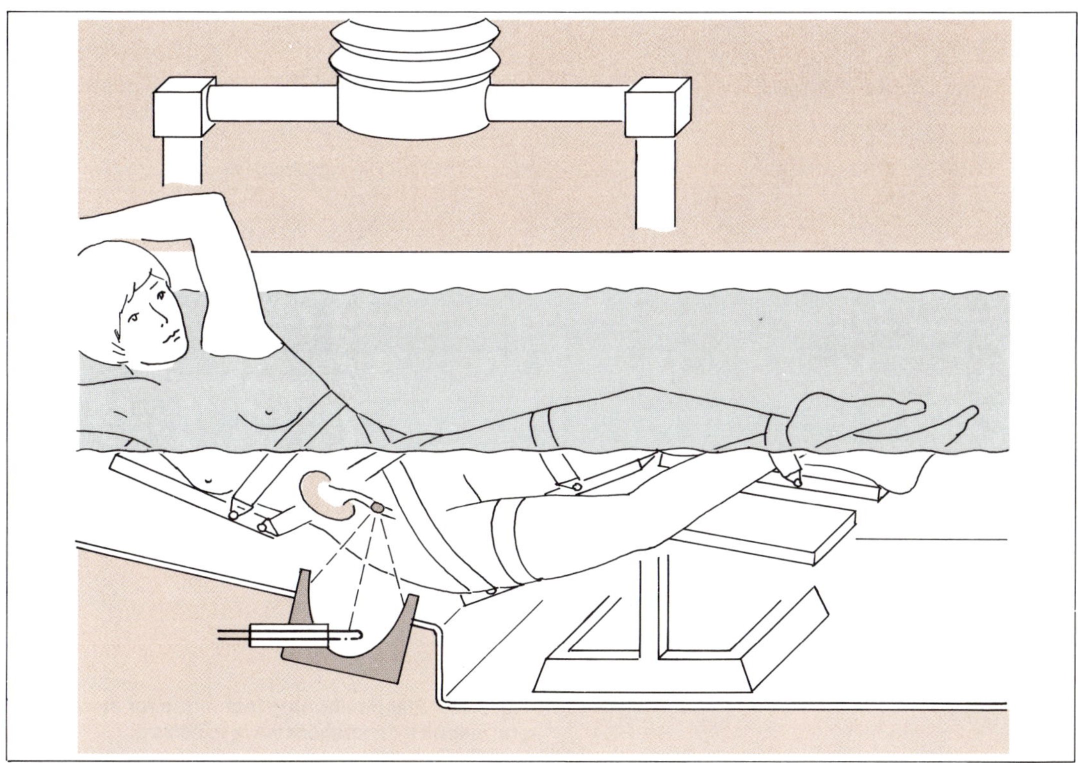

Fig. 3.**38** **Positioning in the case of stones that are close to the spine (i.e., upper ureteral calculi). Rotation to stone-bearing side (crossing of the legs stabilizes the position)**

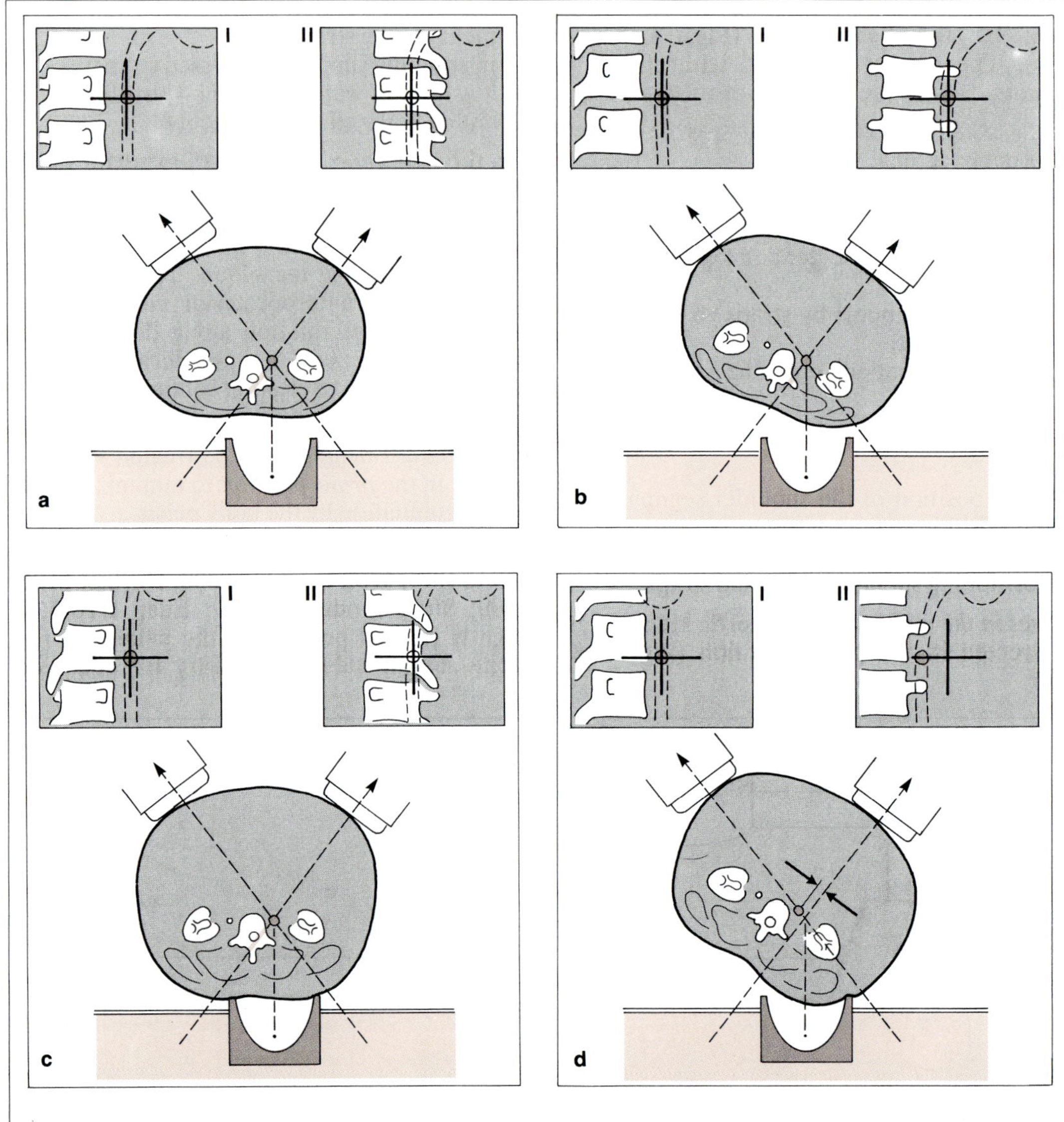

Fig. 3.39 Positioning problems with stones close to the spine

a Horizontal positioning: stones close to the spine are obscured by the vertebral body (monitor II = stone-bearing side)

b Rotation to stone-bearing side: stone can be seen lateral to the vertebral body

c Obese patient, horizontal positioning: stone can be focused but is obscured by the vertebral body on monitor II

d Obese patient, rotated to stone-bearing side: stone cannot be focused any more due to the larger distance between skin and stone (patient lies on the ellipsoid). Treatment has to be performed using the "blast path"

Fig. 3.40 Flat positioning technique for distal ureteral calculi (gluteal shock wave exposure) ▶

Fig. 3.41 Sitting positioning technique for distal ureteral calculi (perirenal shock wave exposure)

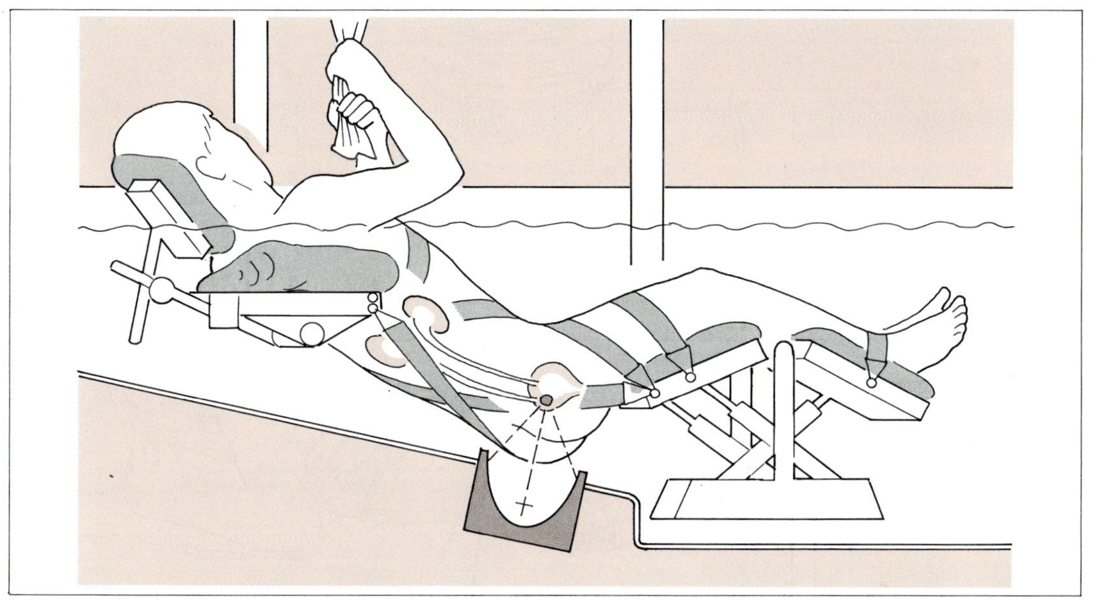

Fig. 3.**40**

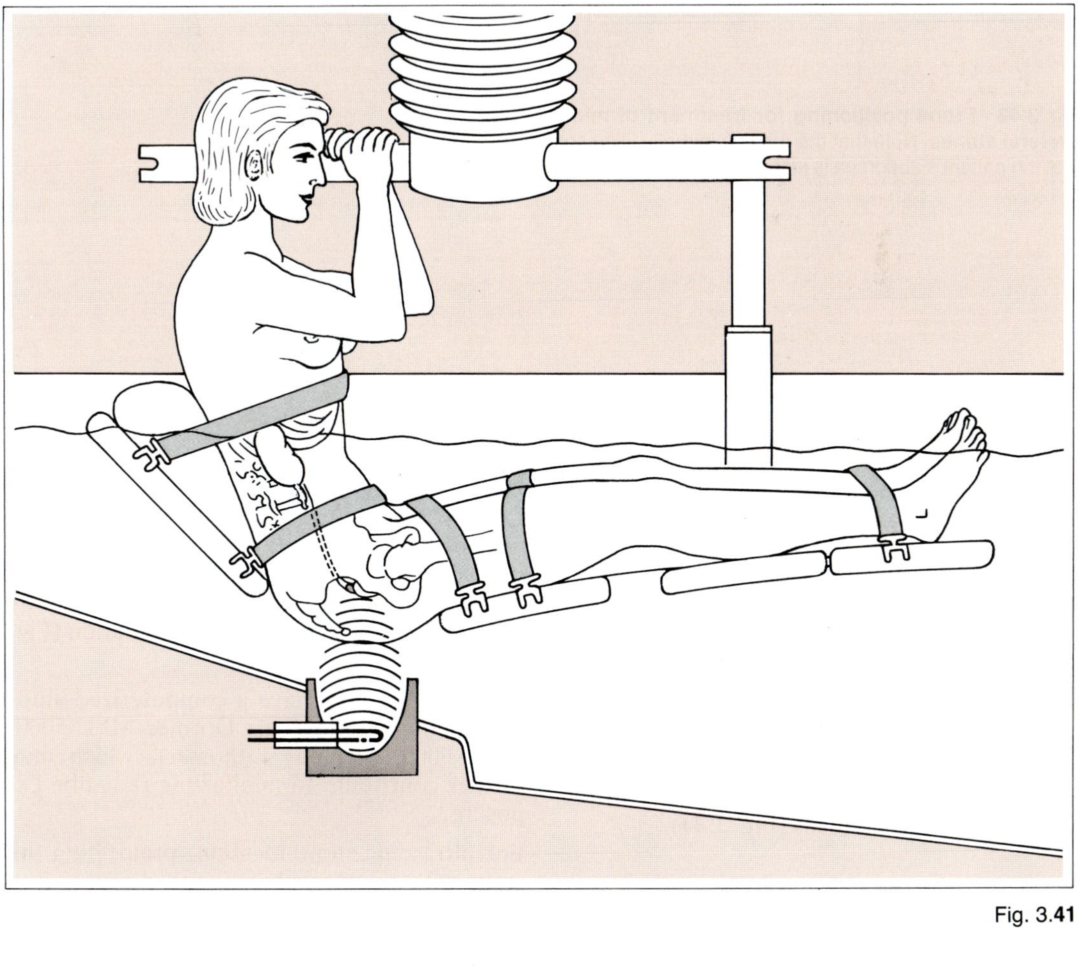

Fig. 3.**41**

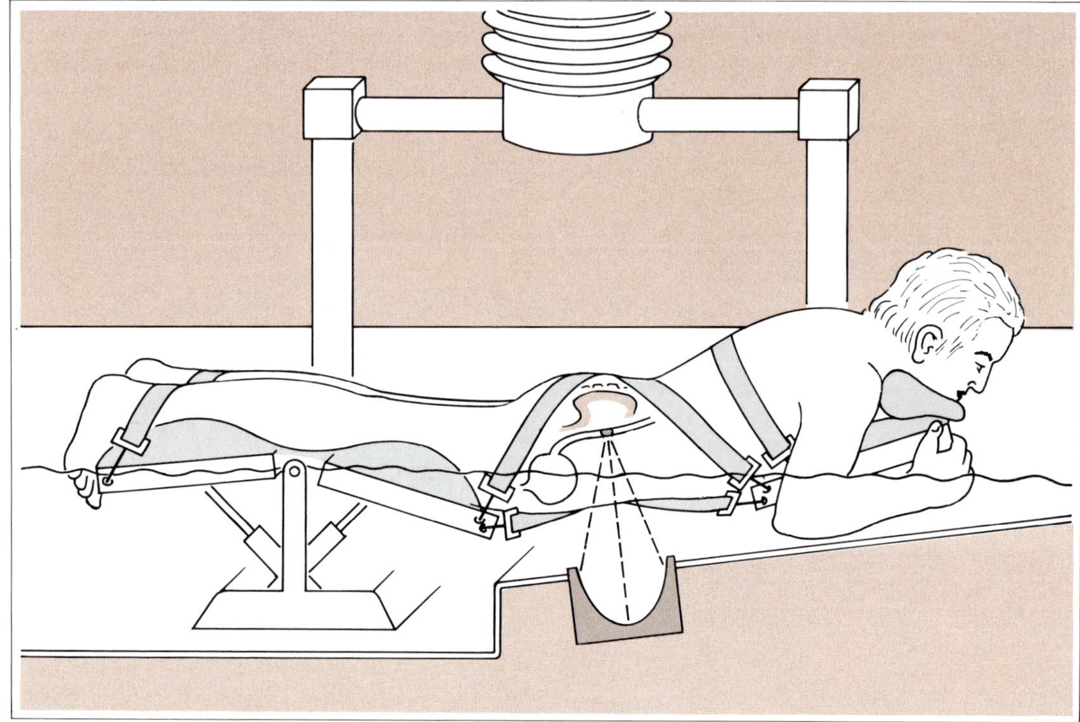

Fig. 3.42 Prone positioning for treatment of mid-ureteral stones. Note that the tub is minimally filled so that the patient's abdomen is just rinsed

location of upper ureteral calculi. Localization and treatment of intramural ureteral stones is also performed in the prone position (Fig. 3.**43**) or with the overhead module of the Siemens Lithostar Plus in supine position.

Stone Localization

With the *X-ray systems* in the fixed position the patient is moved on the hydraulically operated stretcher, which can be moved on three axes, until the stone shows up exactly in the center of the second focus (Fig. 3.**44**).

In order to minimize radiation exposure, positioning should first be made without X-ray control (visual control, coordinates). When the concrements distinctly show up on the monitor, final adjustment can be made by normal fluoroscopy and early collimation (Fig. 3.**45**).

Some lithotriptors have a computerized auto-positioning system (i.e., Dornier MFL 5000, MPL 9000, Siemens Lithostar), which may further contribute to minimizing radiation exposure.

For ultrasonic stone location, prelocating the stone with an external scanner is useful to find

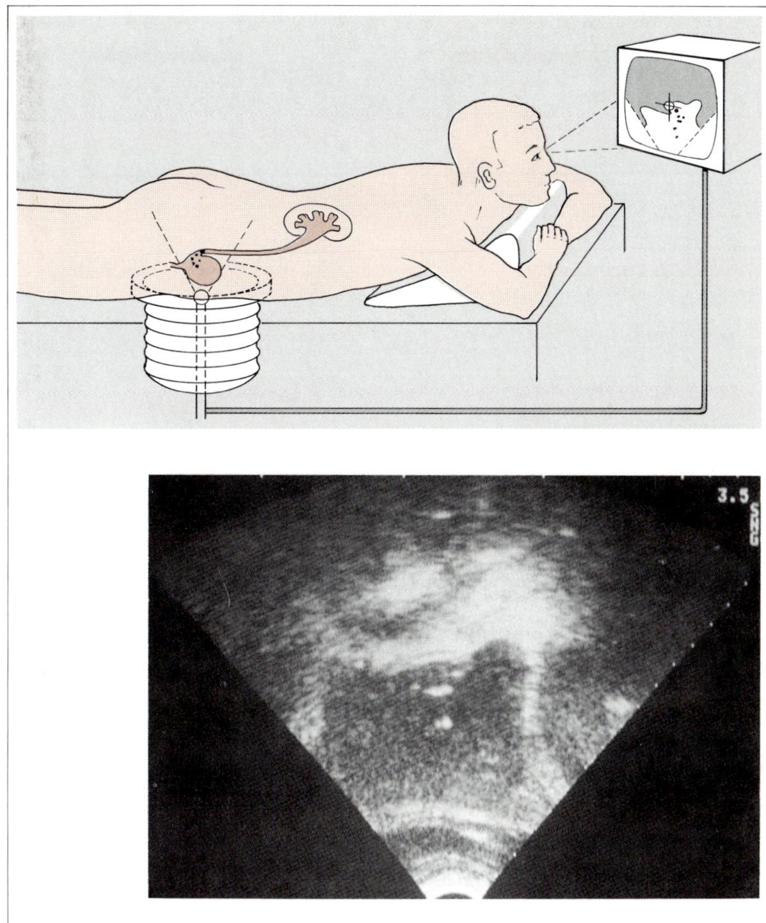

Fig. 3.**43** **Prone positioning technique for ultrasound location and treatment of distal (intramural) ureteral calculi.** The corresponding ultrasound scan shows stone fragments falling out of the orifice (i.e., Dornier MPL 9000, Wolf Piezolith 2300, Storz Modulith SL 10 and 20)

the best acoustic window. For easy orientation on the ultrasound screen, some landmarks (i.e., vertebral processes, liver, spleen) are useful. The exact focusing of the stone can be proven by rotating the ultrasound scanner; the calculus should rotate on the focus. Computerized combination of an external and in-line scanner (Dornier MPL 9000) can be helpful and time-saving (Fig. 3.**46**).

Some lithotriptors (i.e., Dornier HML4, MFL 5000, Siemens Lithostar), provide a *respiratory triggering* (gating) for shock wave application — the impulses are released only in expiration (Fig. 3.**47**) to increase the number of

shock waves hitting the stone. However, this necessitates satisfactory cooperation by the patient. On the other hand, most *ultrasound-guided* lithotriptors (Dornier MPL 9000, Wolf Piezolith 2300, Storz Modulith SL10, Edap LT01) have the advantage of *real-time scanning* during the treatment. This enables autofocusing of the stone by the patient's breathing; this is considerably less expensive. Here again, satisfactory cooperation by the patient is necessary (Fig. 3.**21**).

After 200 shock waves, the course of treatment is checked by fluoroscopy, employing the high-current technique ("quick pic") if neces-

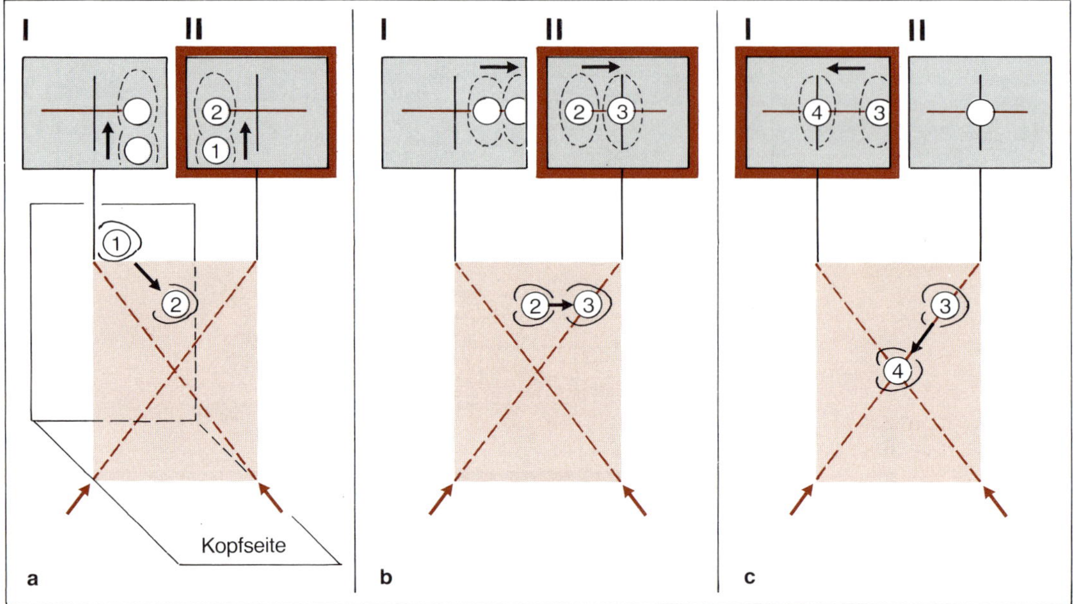

Fig. 3.44 Fluoroscopic stone localization with Dornier HM3 and HM4

a Lowering the patient on z-axis into the tub. The patient is then moved along the x-axis until the stone has reached the horizontal axis of the cross-hair (= intersection of the X-ray beams)

b Moving the stone into the cross-hair along the horizontal axis of the patient (y-axis)

c Focusing of the stone using the "diagonal" button. The patient is moved along the central beam of the contralateral X-ray tube

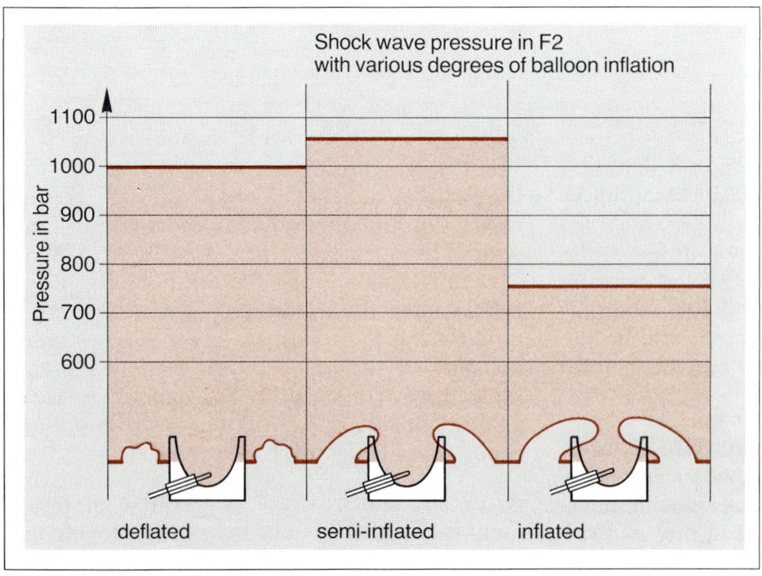

Fig. 3.45 Optimal fluoroscopic checking during ESWL with semi-inflated balloons provides maximal shock wave pressure and sufficient imaging in most of the cases. Thus, time-consuming inflation and deflation of the balloons can be avoided (Dornier HM3)

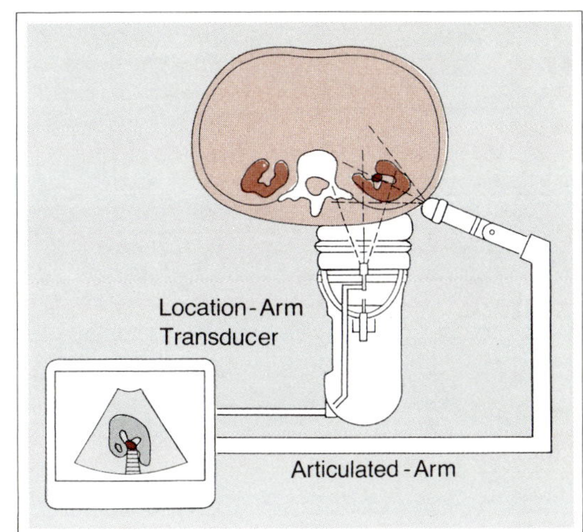

Fig. 3.46 In-line and external ultrasound probe for stone localization and automatic positioning as used in the Dornier MPL 9000

sary. This clearly shows the degree of stone disintegration (Fig. 3.**48**). The screening of stone position is performed by fluoroscopy with semi-inflated balloons (Fig. 3.**45**). In the case of ultrasonic monitoring, shock wave release should be interrupted after 200−300 impulses to allow for the disappearance of shock wave-induced air bubbles that may disturb the exact evaluation of stone fragmentation due to artifacts.

Shock Wave Application

The energy required for stone disintegration is controlled by changing the voltage of the generator. The level of generator voltage depends on the shock wave source. If a wide range of shock wave energy is provided (i.e., Dornier HM3, MPL 9000, Storz Modulith), it is recommendable to start on a low voltage to avoid early scattering of larger fragments, particularly in the case of brittle calcium oxalate dihydrate stones. Calculi that are resistant to shock waves (i.e., cystine, calcium oxalate monohydrate, cholesterol), or impacted stones (ureter, calyx), should be treated on the upper level to crack the stone. Once the stone is broken, further treatment can continue on a lower level (Table 3.**11**).

Shock wave application can be performed by

– ECG triggering (Single or twin pulse);
– constant frequency (1 Hz, 2 Hz);
– respiratory triggering (Fig. 3.**47**).

ECG triggering was necessary on the Dornier HM3 to avoid shock wave-induced arrhythmia. On the new lithotriptors with a partial water bath or only a water cushion and smaller focal zone, the shock waves can be applied on a constant frequency in most of the cases or else the twin-pulse technique can be used (Fig. 3.**49**). Only patients with pacemakers or cardiac arrhythmia should primarily be treated with ECG triggering. However, ECG monitoring during ESWL is still mandatory.

The minimum number of shock waves applied depends on the energy source. For most lithotriptors, the upper limit is between 2,500 and 3,000, whereas on the piezoelectric machines (i.e., Wolf Piezolith 2300, Edap LT01), up to 4,000 and 6,000 shockwaves, respectively, are applied in one session. The average duration of treatment is 40 to 50 minutes.

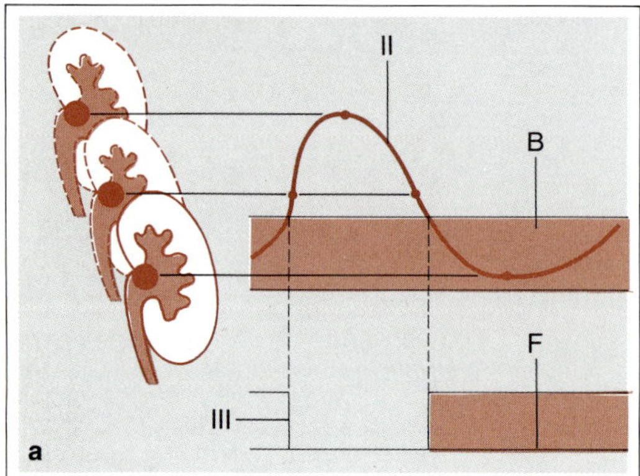

Fig. 3.**47** **Schematic drawing of respiratory triggering in accordance with the inspiration and expiration of the patient** monitored by use of a respiratory belt around the thorax. After two courses of inspiration and expiration (= gating), the shock waves are only released during expiration (Lithostar, MFL 500)
a Movement of kidney during respiration
b Respiratory triggering. ECG, respiration and gating of shock were release
c ECG plus respiratory triggering of shock wave release

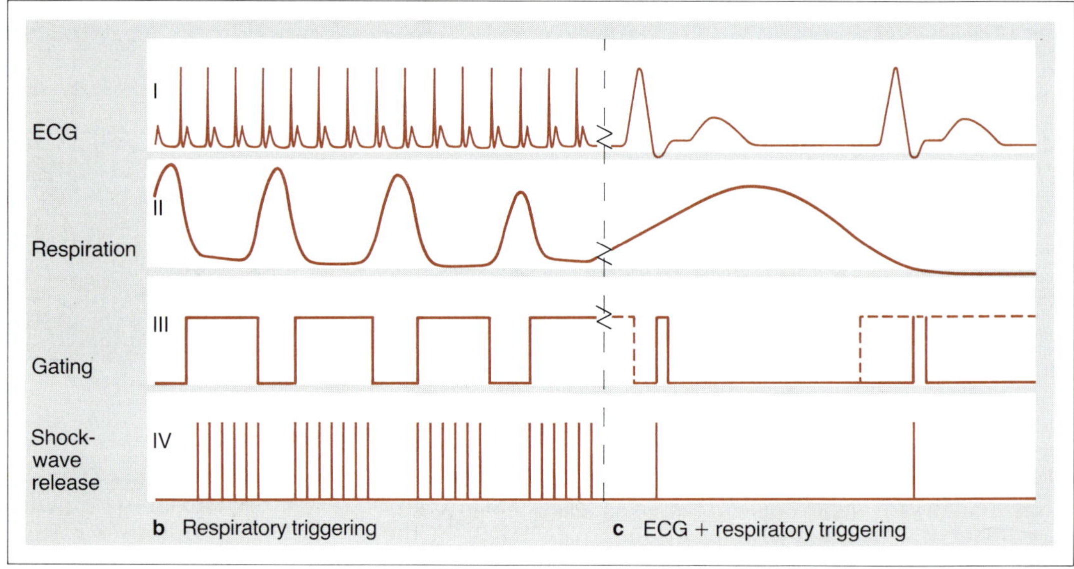

Fig. 3.**48** **ESWL treatment and follow-up of a right ▶ infundibular calculus**
a   KUB prior to ESWL
b–g Fluoroscopic imaging ("quick pic") during ESWL (high-current technique) showing increasing disintegration of the stone. The treatment starts with the upper part of the stone (optimal interface stone-urine, see Table 3.**10**)
h–k Follow-up after ESWL
h   1st day after ESWL: Complete disintegration of the stone
i   2nd day: Stone fragments in kidney and ureter ("Steinstrasse")
j   6th day: Prevesical remnants
k   10th day: Patient is stone-free

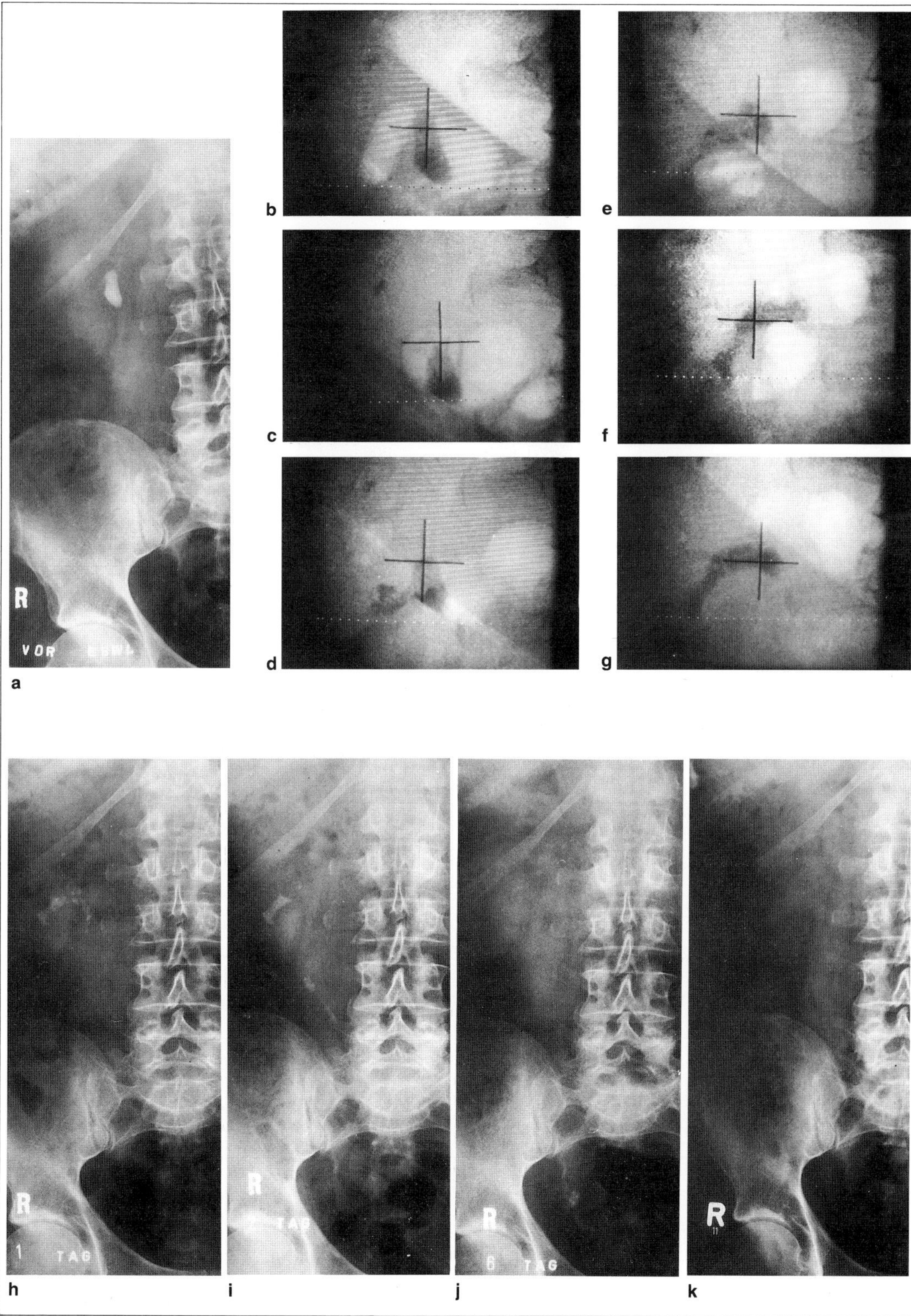

Table 3.11 Therapeutic recommendations for ESWL therapy

ESWL in one session	
"Crystalline" renal pelvis stone (calcium oxalate dihydrate)	– Start with low energy
Impacted calyx stone or ureter stone (calcium oxalate monohydrate)	– Start with high energy
Multiple kidney stones	– Start with smallest concrement – Start treatment at caudal end and continue in cranial direction
Borderline stone or partial staghorn calculus	– Start with stone part in the renal pelvis
Big, obstruent ureteral stone	– Focus on cranial stone rim
Ureter stone that is difficult to localize	– Apply contrast medium by intravenous route
ESWL in several sessions	
Residual fragments of a complete staghorn calculus after PCNL	– Start with stone fragments in the upper calyx groups
ESWL monotherapy of staghorn calculus	– Start with stone fragments in renal pelvis and upper calyx groups
Maximum shock wave hit quota per treatment (Dornier HM3)	
Solitary renal pelvis and calyx stones	2,000–2,500
Multiple stones, staghorn calculi	2,500–3,000
Ureter stone	3,000

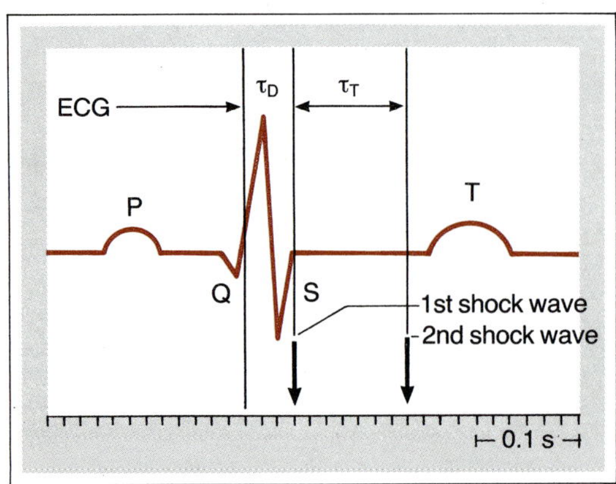

Fig. 3.49 Twin-pulse technique of shock wave application (Dornier HM3+, MFL 5000). Due to the short interval between both impulses, this time-sparing technique can also be used on patients with pacemakers

3.10.6 Complications

Complications during treatment very rarely occur (<1%). Side effects described were cardiac arrhythmia, loss of hearing, hypotonic syncopes, and nausea in the case of peridural anesthesia.

No ESWL-related deaths occurred in the authors' patient population, which comprised more than 10,000 treatments. In a total of 80,000 treatments reported worldwide, only three resulted in fatal outcome (pulmonary embolism, myocardial infarction).

Severe complications during the follow-up phase are also very rare. The incidence rate of clinically relevant intrarenal or perirenal hematomas (Fig. 3.**26**) is below 0.5% and has decreased still further following the introduction of low-pressure lithotripsy.

Petechial skin hematomas were observed in 10% of the patients treated with the Dornier HM3. They seem to occur more frequently with electromagnetic lithotriptors and in case of dry coupling.

The incidence rate of colics and fever after ESWL, as well as the number of auxiliary measures, depends on the size of the stone (Table 3.**12**).

Follow-up as an inpatient

- early mobilization of the patient
- ultrasonic controls on the first, third, and if necessary on the fifth day
- plain X-ray on the first day, followed by additional controls if required

If the first follow-up X-ray check shows complete disintegration of the stone, additional X-ray controls are dispensable. The degree of urinary obstruction and the position of the stone fragments in both kidney and ureter can be sufficiently assessed by ultrasound checks (Fig. 3.**50**).

- colic prophylaxis (i.e., by papaverine hydrochloride or Urol).

If necessary, differentiated *spasmoanalgesic therapy* should be administered, for example

- Diclofenac, intramuscular
- Metimazol, suppository or intravenous
- Intravenous morphine and parasympathicolytics (i.e., hydromorphine-HCl + atropine sulfate)

Table 3.12a   Morbidity after ESWL

Stone size <2 cm		Stone size >2 cm
24%	Colic	34%
5%	Fever	36%
6%	Auxiliary measures	28%
0%	Mortality	0%
4 days	Hospitalization (after treatment)	10 days

Table 3.12b   Auxiliary measures after ESWL

Stone size <2 cm		Stone size >2 cm
5%	Intervention at ureter (Stent, Zeiss loop, URS)	22%
1%	Percutaneous nephrostomy	4%
–	Open surgery	2%

Auxiliary Measures

Retrograde mobilization of ureteral calculi before ESWL is indicated in the following cases:

- emergency situations (continuous colic, urinary obstruction)
- positioning problems
- unsuccessful in situ ESWL

Percutaneous nephrostomy *before ESWL treatment* is indicated in the following:

- infected hydronephrosis (fever, leukocytosis), if placement of a Double-J stent impossible.

An internal ureteral stent (Double-J) *before ESWL* is indicated in the following cases:

- major stone burden (>2.5 cm longitudinal diameter)
- after retrograde mobilization of an ureteral stone
- inflammatory obstruction of the UPJ (stone bed) with hydronephrosis (Fig. 3.**51**)

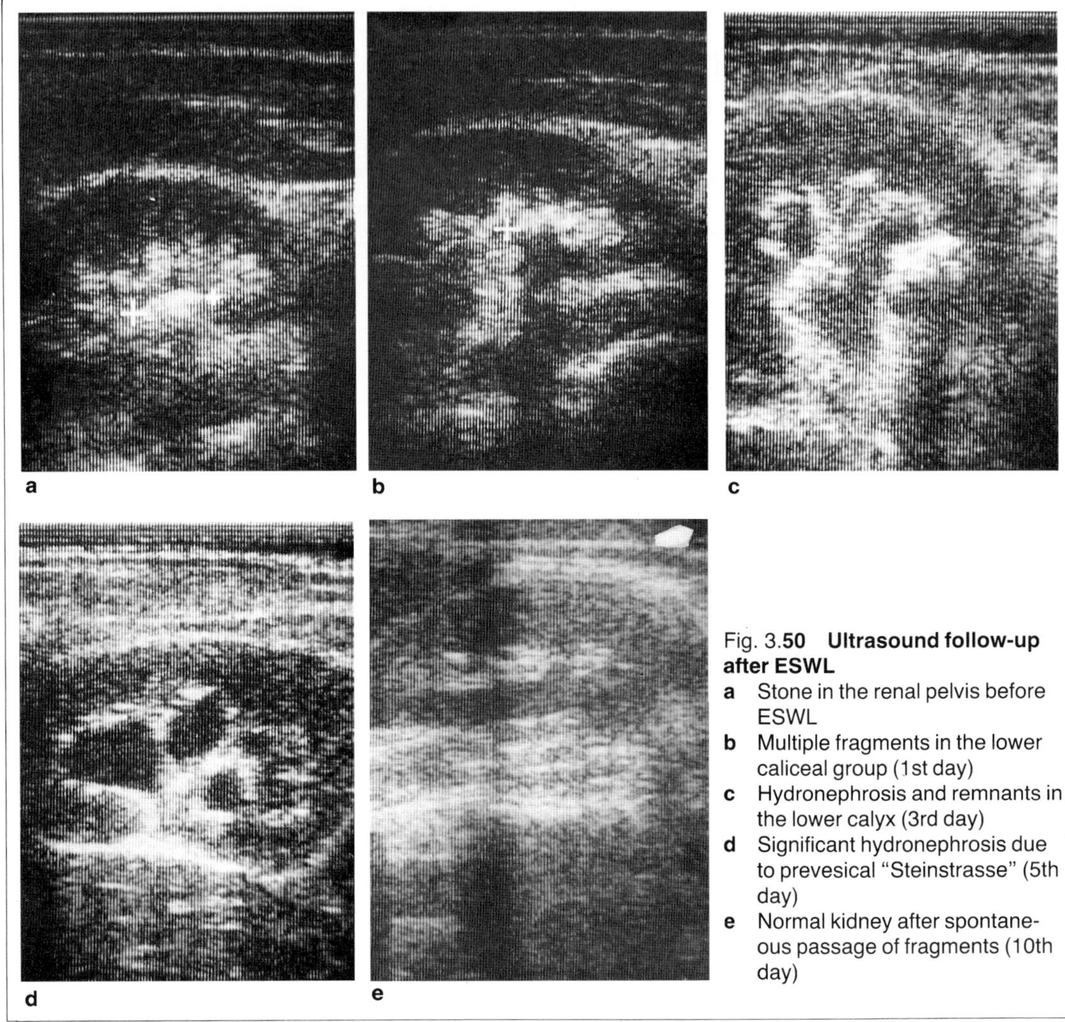

Fig. 3.50   Ultrasound follow-up after ESWL

a   Stone in the renal pelvis before ESWL

b   Multiple fragments in the lower caliceal group (1st day)

c   Hydronephrosis and remnants in the lower calyx (3rd day)

d   Significant hydronephrosis due to prevesical "Steinstrasse" (5th day)

e   Normal kidney after spontaneous passage of fragments (10th day)

Indications for an intervention *after ESWL* treatment are obstructive stone fragments ("Steinstrasse") with

– infected hydronephrosis;
– continuous colic;
– sustained urinary obstruction (for more than 6 weeks).

One alternative for all cases is *percutaneous nephrostomy* (Fig. 3.**52**). In the case of infected hydronephrosis, it ensures safe drainage of the urinary tract system. Additionally, pressure relief normalizes ureteric peristalsis by simultaneously facilitating the spontaneous passage of the stone fragments. It has been found that normal peristalsis is more important than

the hydrostatic pressure exerted on the concrements in the ureter (Wepp et al., 1987).

A *Double-J* stent represents the other alternative. Together with a specially designed co-axial ureteral catheter dilator set, the "Steinstrasse" can be passed and the ureteral stent positioned (Fig. 3.**51**). The Double-J catheter dilates the ureter so that some fragments pass via the stent, and the rest pass spontaneously after removal of the stent (2–3 weeks later). Another possibility is flushing the fragments back up into the kidney using the ureteral dilator, followed by insertion of a Double-J stent. Moreover, due to the dilatation of the orifice, a Double-J stent makes ureteroscopy easier if it becomes necessary.

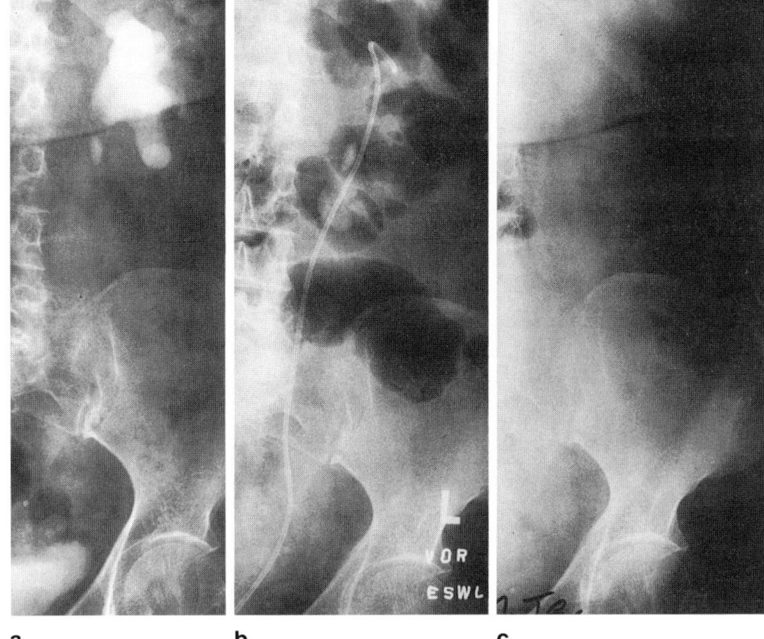

Fig. 3.**51**   **Insertion of a Double-J stent as an auxiliary measure prior to ESWL**

a   Large left upper ureteral stone with hydronephrosis, fever, and leukocytosis

b   The stone cannot be pushed back into the renal pelvis but is bypassed with a Double-J stent providing drainage of the obstructed kidney

c   After successful in situ ESWL, the Double-J stent was withdrawn on the 2nd day

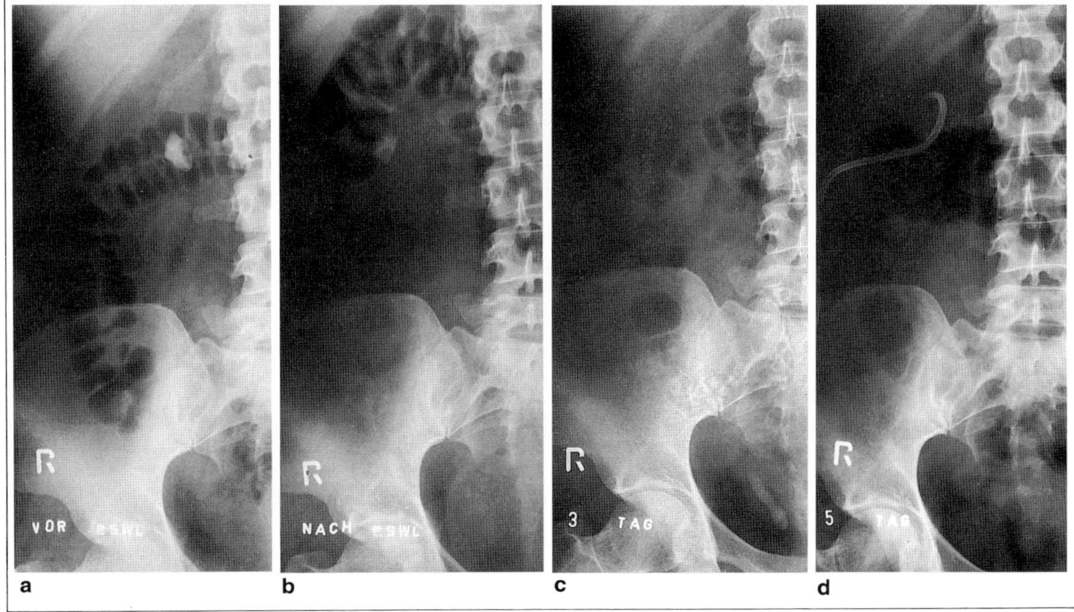

Fig. 3.**52**   **Percutaneous nephrostomy as an auxiliary measure after ESWL**

a   A large stone in the renal pelvis prior to ESWL

b   Stone fragments in the kidney immediately after treatment

c   Persistent prevesical "Steinstrasse" with colics (3rd day)

d   Percutaneous nephrostomy, relief of pain and spontaneous passage of fragments (5th day)

From the technical point of view, retrograde rigid ureteroscopy for the management of "Steinstrassen" is difficult, as it is very time-consuming and does not effect complete elimination of the stone fragments. Postoperative swelling of the ureteral mucosa impairs the passage of stone residues. Such interventions should, therefore, be reserved for "resistant Steinstrassen" (4−6 weeks). The introduction of laser lithotripsy may improve the results of ureteroscopy in the management of "Steinstrassen".

Retrograde manipulations by Zeiss loop or ureteral catheter are ineffective. Ureteral meatotomy is indicated in the case of a narrow orifice. Open surgery is required only in very rare cases.

The rate of auxiliary measures required after ESWL is clearly correlated to the stone volume (see Table 3.**12**).

Follow-up as an outpatient

A total of 70% to 80% of the cases are discharged with stone fragments in the kidney and ureter. The patients are followed in accordance with the conservative management of spontaneous passable ureteral calculi.

- Symptom-free patients should undergo weekly sonography checks or laboratory controls.
- In the case of pain and colics, checks should be made in 2−3 day intervals.

The indication for auxiliary measures corresponds to inpatient follow-up.

If sonography does not reveal any striking findings, such as stone fragments or urinary obstructions, a final IVP can be made by the urologist if required. The follow-up results obtained so far have not shown any signs of renal dysfunction after ESWL. Blood pressure controls should be performed to exclude ESWL-induced hypertension.

Results

To date, more than 2,000,000 treatments have been carried out world wide. A total of 63%−87% of the patients are stone-free within 3 to 6 months after treatment; 10%−25% of the cases exhibit stone fragments that are likely to pass spontaneously and, therefore, do not require treatment; 5% of the patients treated require further treatment (Table 3.**13**).

Table 3.13a Distribution of indications in 1,811 stone patients

− Solitary stone (renal pelvis, calyces)	51%
− Multiple stone	20%
− Borderline stone (> 2.5 cm)	4%
− Partial staghorn calculus	4%
− Complete staghorn calculus	5%
− Ureter stone	16%

Table 3.13b Therapeutic result 3 months after ESWL (n = 1,811). The range of variation is dependent on the stone size

− Stone-free	75%	(63%−87%)
− Stone residues:		
Not requiring treatment	20%	(10%−25%)
Requiring treatment	5%	(2%−12%)
− Multiple sessions	13%	(6%−36%)
− Auxiliary measures	13%	(4%−38%)

The therapeutic result is dependent on the stone size, localization, and the anatomy of the collecting system. Once the stone is fragmented correctly, the results seem to be independent of the type of lithotriptor used.

Long-term results after 2 years or more show a stone-free rate in 67%−78%, with a recurrence rate of 6%−11% (Table 3.**14a**). In these series, the stone-free rate for lower caliceal calculi drops down to 57% and 58%, respectively (Table 3.**14b**). This correlates with the authors' observation after ESWL monotherapy for staghorn stones (Fig. 3.**53**). After a follow-up of 36 months, 60% were stone-free, 33% still had remnants, and only 7% showed recurrent stone formation.

In conclusion, a 90%−100% stone-free rate is not to be expected after ESWL. Factors that reduce the likelihood of achieving a stone-free status are

1. stone burden (>2 cm, multiple calculi)
2. reduced clearance of fragments
   - lower calix location
   - reduced contractability of the collecting system (i.e., hydronephrosis, pyelonephritis)

Table 3.14 Long-term results after ESWL

a) Overall statistics

Stone-free	Residual stone	Recurrent stone	Follow-up (year)	Author	
78%	15%	7%	3.6	Liedl et al	1989
67%	20%	11%	2	Lingemann et al	1989
76%	18%	6%	1.6	Graff et al	1988

b) Stone localization (follow-up 1.6 and 2 years)

	% Stone-free	
Location	Lingemann et al 1988	Graff et al 1988
Pelvis	84%	83%
Upper calix	73%	77%
Middle calix	67%	76%
Lower calix	57%	58%

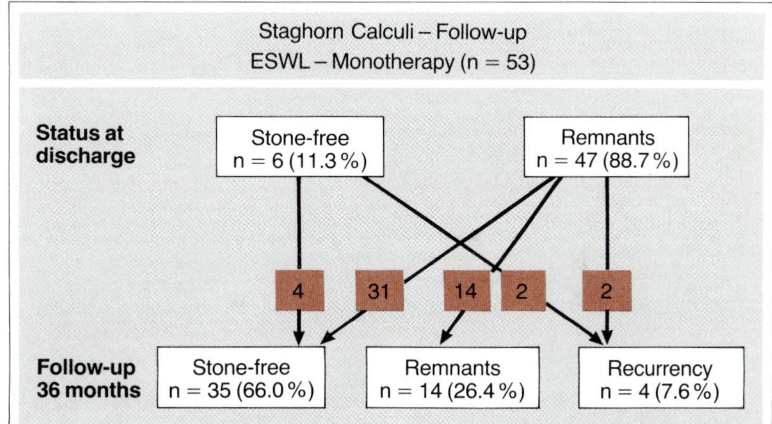

Fig. 3.53 Long-term results after ESWL monotherapy for staghorn calculi

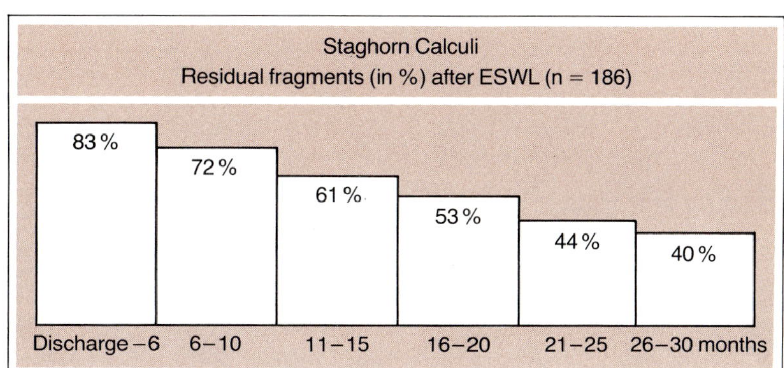

Fig. 3.54 Residual fragments after ESWL monotherapy for staghorn calculi

- caliceal diverticulum
- horseshoe kidney
- medullary sponge kidney
3. Stone composition
  - cystine
  - strucrite

Even though long-term results have shown a much higher rate of remnants than reported at the beginning, the authors believe that their concept of minimal invasiveness and morbidity with ESWL and endourology has been confirmed in the long run. This is mainly due to

- the lack of invasiveness of ESWL;
- the reproducibility of the method;
- the small and mostly asymptomatic remnants;
- the significant reduction of UTI after treatment;
- the still-continuing tendency to pass residual fragments (Fig. 3.**54**).

4 Percutaneous Nephrolithotomy (PCNL)

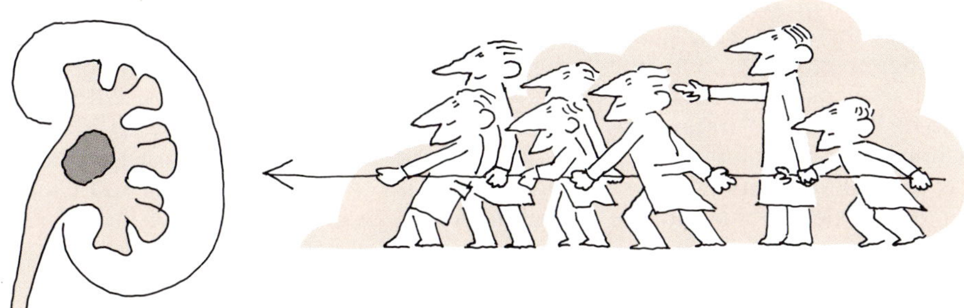

Definition

Endoscopic removal of stones from the kidney following percutaneous puncture of the collecting system and dilatation of the puncture channel.

4.1 Patient Selection

- Absolute contraindications: untreated clotting disorder
- Relative contraindications: untreated UTI, untreated tuberculosis, pregnancy, high-risk patients
- Higher degree of technical difficulties: kidney anomalies (horseshoe kidney, malrotated kidney, dystopic kidney), skeletal anomalies (kyphoscoliosis), narrow RCS

4.2 Indications

Stones can, in general, be removed from all parts of the RCS by a percutaneous approach. However, the actual range of indications for PCNL can only be defined under consideration of the indications of ESWL. As a noninvasive and low-complication method, ESWL currently covers about 90% of the "stone spectrum" (see Chapters 2 and 3). The following indications still apply to PCNL:

- stones in caliceal diverticular
- stones in conjunction with a stenosis at the UPJ, requiring surgical correction
- partial or complete staghorn calculi; solitary or multiple stones, if fragment passage after ESWL is likely to be problematic (large stone burden; dilated or dysplastic RCS)

4.3 Patient Preparation

The following tests are performed prior to PCNL: IVP, thoracic X-ray, ECG, laboratory data (clotting factors!), urine analysis, urine culture, and sonography.

Intravenous infusion of 1000 ml NaCl in the evening and 1000 ml NaCl in the morning prior to surgery provides "renal protection" by better hydration of the kidney.

A 24-hour antibiotic prophylaxis is begun in the case of normal urine analysis or negative urine culture. Established UTIs should be treated for at least 48 hours before surgery with appropriate medication.

If there is any suspicion of an obstructive pyelonephritis, the following two-step approach should be pursued to minimize the risk of septicemia:

1. Percutaneous nephrostomy and intravenous antibiotic therapy.
2. Dilatation of the channel, and stone removal. The second session should not be scheduled until the clinical symptoms (e.g., fever) have ceased and the urine gained from the percutaneous nephrostomy shows no evidence of a UTI.

4.4 Patient Information

The patient must be informed about the following possible risks associated with the planned intervention: hemorrhagic complications, infection and septicemia, damage to adjacent organs or the kidney itself, emergency surgery (including nephrectomy!), and the possibility of several sessions also encompassing other methods of treatment (ureteroscopy, ESWL). It is important to point out that this intervention is a "real" operation, whose complications and difficulties should not be underestimated.

4.5 Anesthesia

Epidural anesthesia by catheter has the following advantages:

- low pulmonary and cardiac strain
- possibility of multiple treatments without repeated puncture of the epidural space, thus reducing the stress to the patient

General anesthesia constitutes an equivalent alternative, if

- the condition of the patient does not produce any cardiac or pulmonary risks;
- only one treatment session is to be expected;
- there are contraindications for peridural anesthesia.

If percutaneous surgery is expected to take more than two hours, general anesthesia should be preferred; for patients under epidural anesthesia, the prone position often becomes inconvenient after 1½−2 hours.

The intervention can also be performed under local anesthesia, thereby requiring good patient compliance and mostly additonal sedoanalgesia (e.g., Thalamonal). Even if local anesthesia is applied carefully, surgery can often not be performed completely pain-free, especially if the manipulations take too much time (>1 hour).

The technique of local anesthesia is as follows: to cover a large area of infiltration, 1% Scandicaine is diluted with NaCl to yield a 0.5% solution. A total of 40−50 ml is injected for anesthesia. It is essential to infiltrate the entire operative tract up to the kidney surface.

4.6 Surgical Anatomy

The topographic position of the kidney in the retroperitoneum can be seen in Figure 4.**1**. The "window" for a retroperitoneal, straight tract to the RCS is cranially delimited by the 12th rib, laterally by the ascending or descending colon, caudally by the iliac crest, and medially by the paravertebral muscles. Although an intercostal approach is possible, it is associated with additional risks, such as pneumothorax or hydrothorax (see "Risks and Complications"). A dystopic position of the kidney (pelvic kidney) may complicate a percutaneous access or may even make surgery impossible.

The periphery of the kidney is supplied with arterial blood by five radiary segmental arteries, which divide into the interlobar arteries (Fig. 4.**2**). Since the papillary region is poorly vascularized, this area is best suited for direct puncture.

The RCS divides into ventral and dorsal calyces (Fig. 4.**3**). Since the axes of the dorsal calyces are in the direction of the aforementioned "window" (60° in dorsal direction to the lateral body axis), they are best suited for puncture. It is difficult to approach the renal pelvis via a ventral calyx because of the angle between puncture channel and caliceal axis.

Only a "peripheral" puncture (i.e., puncture at or immediately behind the calyceal apex) ensures a "waterproof" occlusion between instruments and kidney. Due to the risk of vascular damage and extravasation, direct puncture of the renal pelvis must be avoided (Fig. 4.**4**).

4.7 Technique and Strategy

The entire intervention encompasses the following steps: preparation of the patient; puncture; dilatation; nephroscopy; and stone manipulation.

It has generally been accepted to carry out these steps in one session. However, in special cases (such as infected hydronephrosis) treatment in two sessions is indicated.

4.7.1 Preoperative Adjuvant Measures

The patient is positioned in the lithotomy position on an urological X-ray table (alternative:

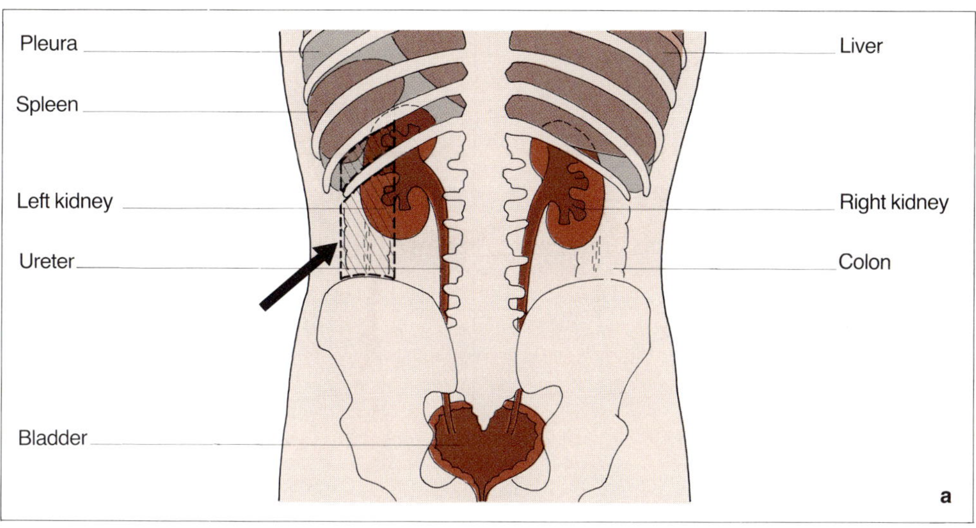

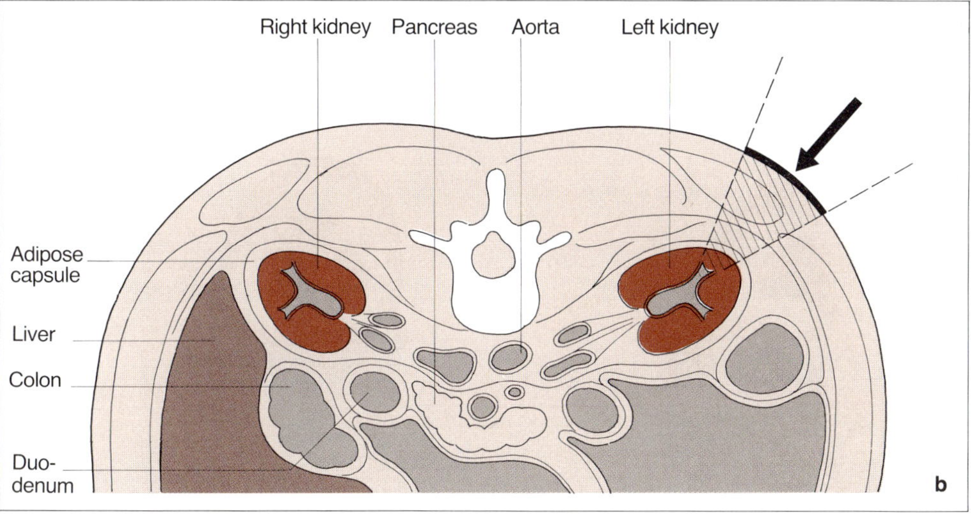

Fig. 4.1

a Position of kidney in relation to adjacent organs (dorsal view). The "window" for a straight percutaneous tract to Kidney is outlined on the left side

b Schematic cross-section at the level of the renal hilus. The angle range for the percutaneous tract is outlined on the left side

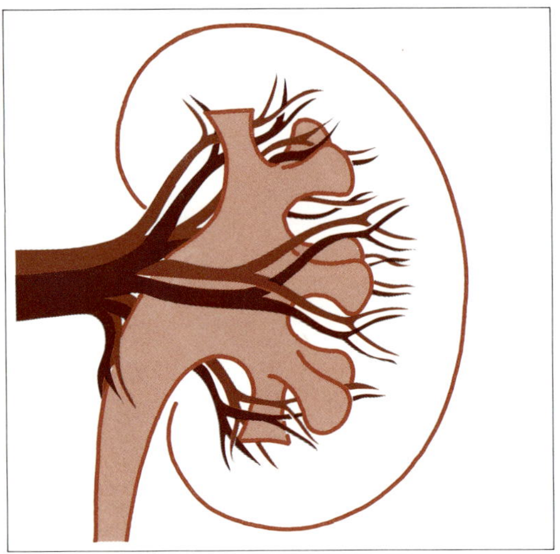

Fig. 4.**2** **Schematic representation of renal vascularization**

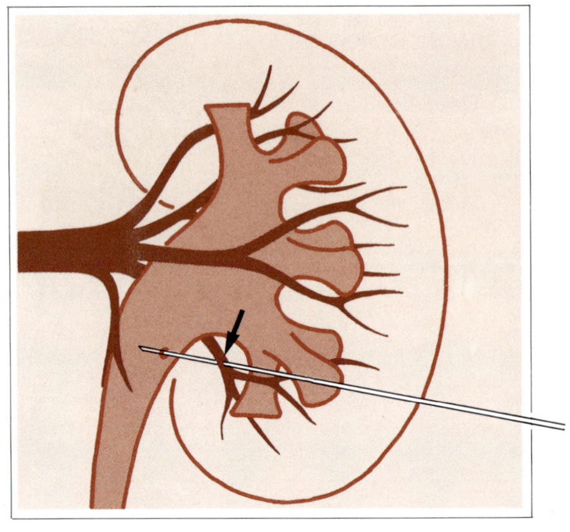

Fig. 4.**4** **Puncture the calyx only!** Puncture of renal pelvis involves risk of extravasation and vascular damage

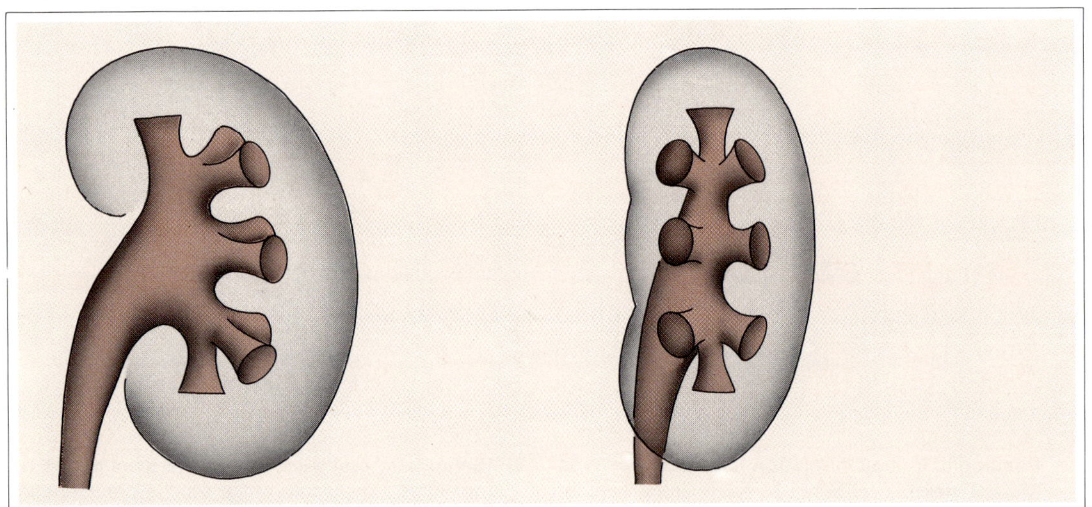

Fig. 4.**3** **Schematic three-dimensional representation of RCS with anterior and posterior row of calyces**

conventional operation table plus C-arm). Following cystoscopy, a balloon-tipped ureteral catheter (5−7 Fr; Fig. 4.**5a**) is introduced into the orifice of the ureter. Stone position and the course of the ureter are documented by plain X-ray and retrograde pyelogram. Subsequently, the ureteral catheter is advanced to the renal pelvis. The balloon is blocked by about 2 ml, and the RCS is filled with contrast medium (Fig. 4.**5b**). A balloon catheter (12 Fr) is inserted into the bladder to ensure drainage during surgery (Fig. 4.**5c**).

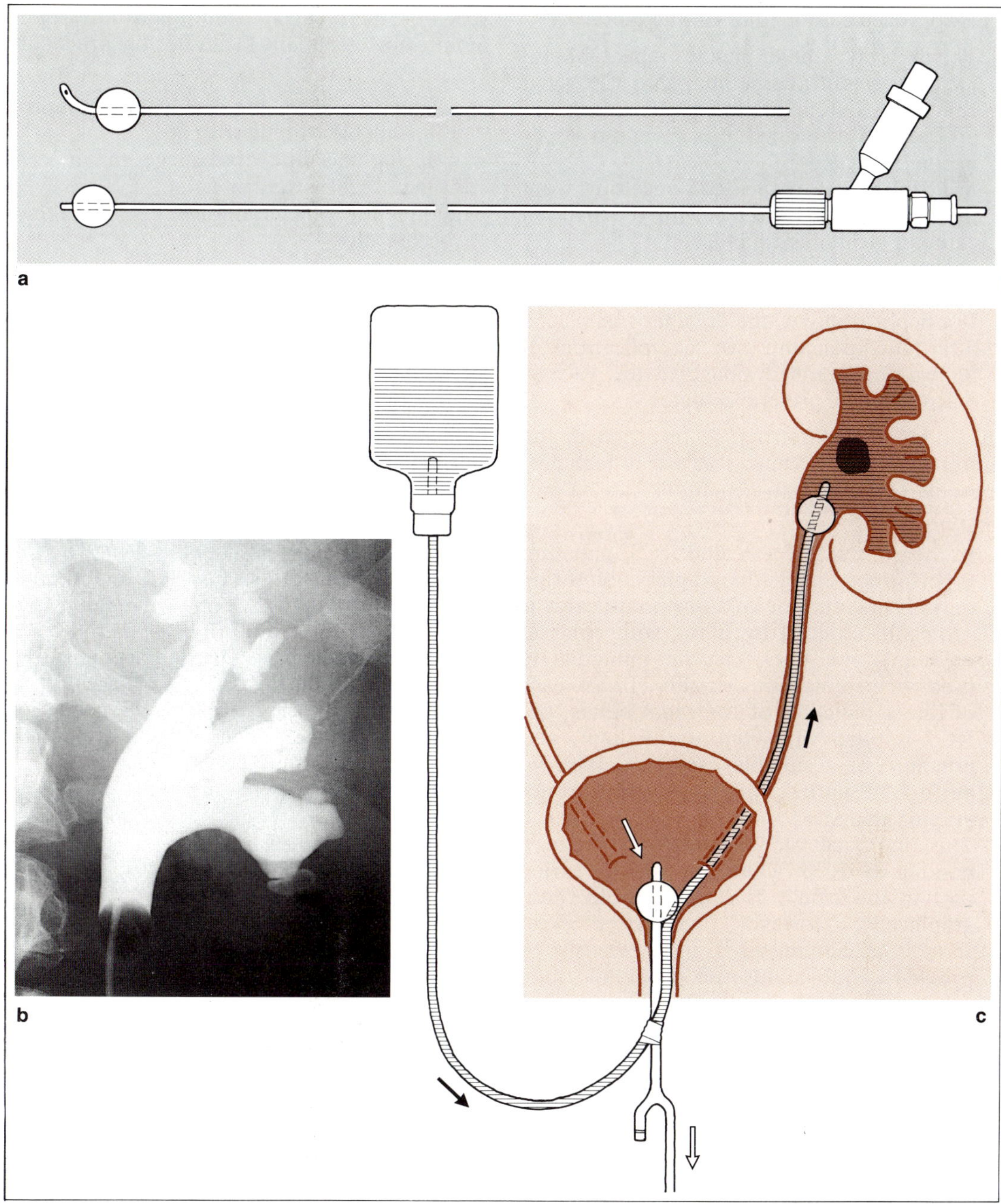

Fig. 4.**5**

a   Balloon ureteral catheter (5 Fr) with single terminal perforation, angled or straight tip and removable connecting port

Advantages: selective filling of contrast medium distal to the balloon. The short tip enables placement of balloon straight under the stone. After placing the catheter, the cystoscope can be removed without difficulty. In the case of difficult retrograde manipulation (kinking in the ureter), balloon catheter with angled tip (top) should be used

b   Slightly dilated RCS filled with contrast medium. The balloon catheter provides complete obstruction of ureter

c   Schematic representation of situation before puncture. Ureteral and bladder catheters in situ. Contrast medium infusion through ureteral catheter

This approach has the following advantages:

- The ureteral catheter enables repeatable injection of contrast medium into the renal collecting system at any time during the procedure (in contrast to intravenous application of the dye).
- Mild dilatation of the RCS resulting from the blocking of the UPJ with the balloon catheter facilitates puncture.
- Dislocation of stone fragments into the ureter during stone manipulation is prevented.
- If a nephrostomy catheter cannot be placed after failed puncture (see "complications"), at least minimum drainage of the RCS is ensured by the ureteral catheter.

In the event that retrograde insertion of the ureteral catheter is impossible due to technical reasons, two alternative methods can be employed:

1. In the presence of a dilated RCS, puncture is performed under sonographic monitoring only. If puncture of an appropriate calyx is successful (control by filling with contrast medium), the track can be immediately used for percutaneous surgery. In the case of direct puncture of the renal pelvis, the RCS is filled with contrast medium, and puncture of a suitable calyx can then be performed under fluoroscopic and sonographic guidance.
2. This approach can also be pursued in a nondilated RCS when the stone-bearing part of the kidney is clearly visible sonographically. However, contrast medium should be administered intravenously to provide additional fluoroscopic monitoring.

4.7.2 Patient Positioning

After retrograde manipulation, the patient is positioned for the percutaneous intervention in a prone position. Lumbar lordosis is compensated by means of a foam wedge or cushion (Fig. 4.**6a**).

After surgical skin disinfection the patient is sterilely covered, preferably using a waterproof disposable set with integrated foil and water bag (Fig. 4.**6b**).

4.7.3 Puncture

High resolution fluoroscopy is the most important prerequisite for a successful puncture of a specific renal calyx. Additional ultrasound monitoring essentially facilitates the procedure by

- providing a three-dimensional orientation, not available with fluoroscopy;
- reducing the risk of damage to adjacent organs such as the intestine, spleen, liver, and pleura, which cannot be visualized fluoroscopically;
- reducing the radiation exposure as a result of quicker puncture.

The sonographically controlled puncture is facilitated by using a biopsy transducer (e.g., linear scanner with central puncture aid, sector scanner with lateral puncture aid). The scanners are either gas-sterilized or coated with a sterile film (Fig. 4.**7a**).

4.7.3.1 Practical hints. The lower pole of the kidney is imaged by ultrasound scanning (Fig. 4.**7b**). While being telescoped, fine and hollow needles (Fig. 4.**7c**) are inserted under sonographic control until they reach the kidney surface. Brief X-ray monitoring shows the direction of the needle axis. The fine needle is then introduced into the desired calyx (Figs. 4.**7d,e**; movement of the calyx wall on the needle tip hitting the surface!). The draining of contrast medium confirms the correct position of the needle tip.

Exceptions:

- Narrow, undilated urinary tract system. In this case, the needle tip may touch the calyx wall. Careful of injection of a small amount diluted contrast medium (beware of extravasation!) confirms the correct position of the needle tip.
- Stone-bearing calyx. In this case, direct contact with the stone can be felt with the needle tip.

After introducing the hollow needle over the fine needle into the calyx, and after repeated position control, a guide wire (Fig. 4.**8a**) is advanced into the renal pelvis or upper calyx (Fig. 4.**8b,c**).

In the event of an unsuccessful puncture, the fine needle is completely withdrawn from the kidney. After slight correction of the entire needle set, puncture is repeated.

4.7.3.2 Alternative puncture techniques. If fluoroscopy is the only monitoring method at

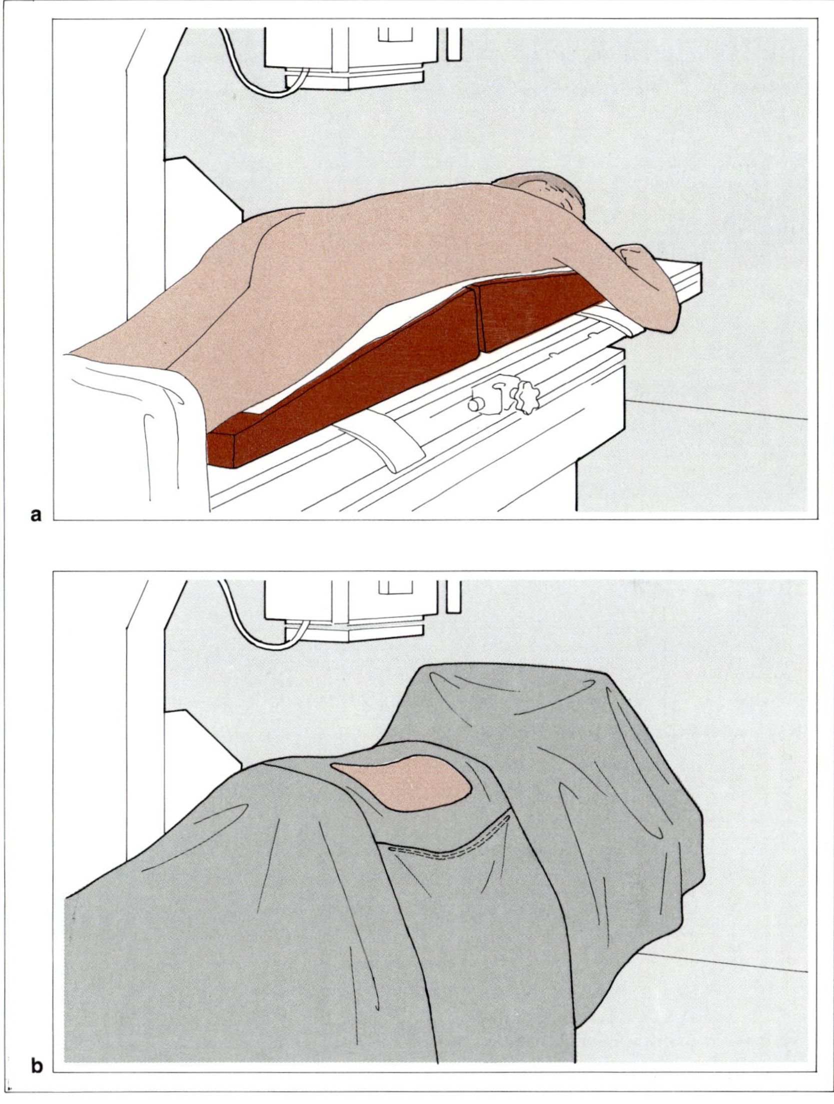

Fig. 4.**6**

a Positioning of patient in prone position on a radiolucent foam wedge for compensation of lumbar lordosis

b Patient covered with disposable set with integrated foil in the puncture field and bag for irrigation liquid

hand, the entire needle set is first advanced to the kidney surface (movement of the kidney is seen on the monitor when the needle tip touches the surface) and is then scanned by the pointless cannula. At the point of maximum convexity, the fine needle is advanced to the desired calyx. Failed puncture is corrected as described above. The disadvantage of this technique is that an interposition of adjacent organs in the puncture channel cannot be safely excluded.

An alternative approach is to place the patient in a 30° oblique position (Fig. 4.**9**) so that the dorsal calyces are perpendicular to the horizontal plane. The needle is then introduced

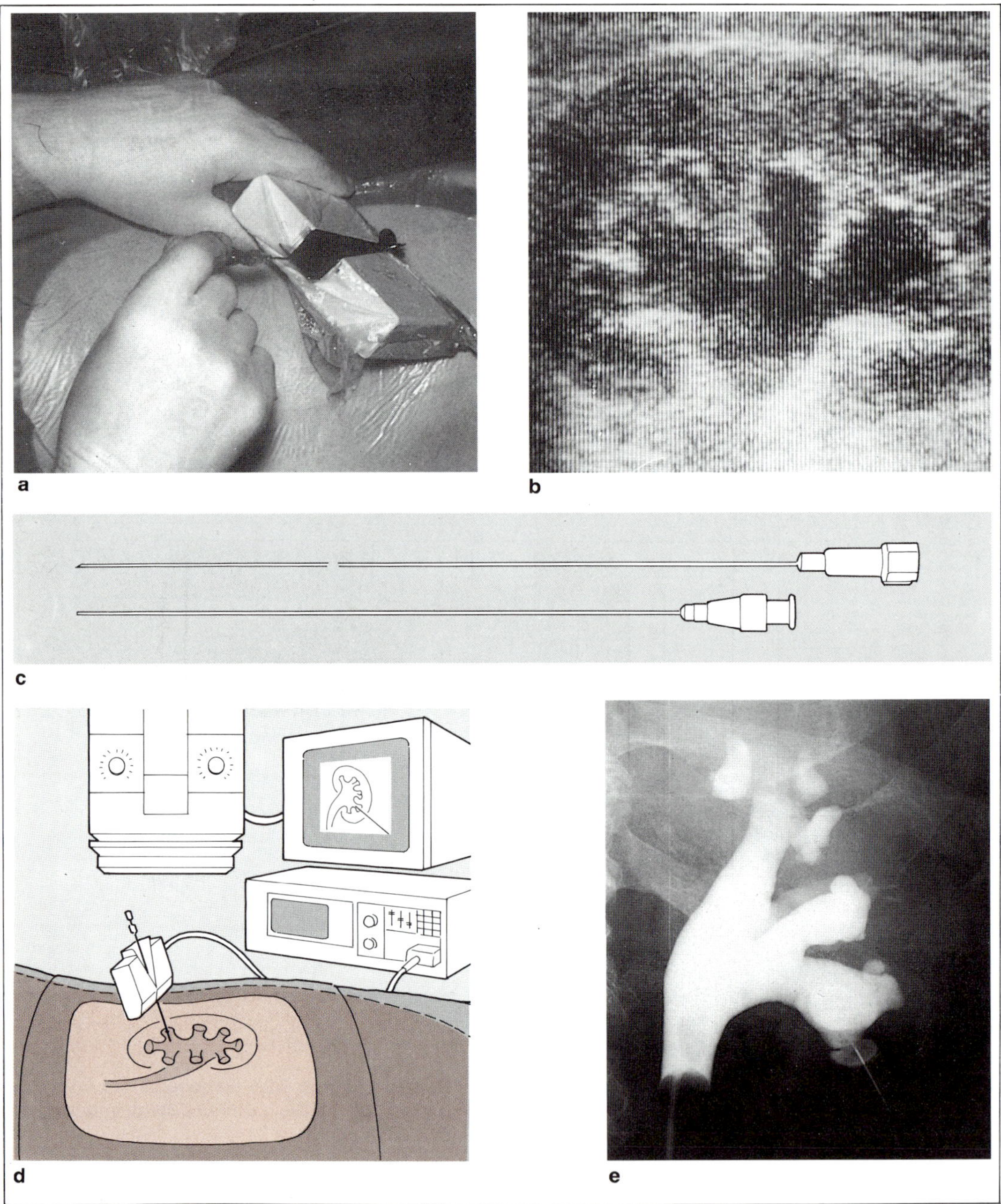

Fig. 4.7
a **Linear scanner coated with sterile foil and equipped with puncture aid**
b **Sonographic longitudinal-section of kidney with dilated RCS**
c **Puncture needles:** Fine needle (0.7 mm) for primary puncture (minor traumatization!); cannula (1.3 mm) for coaxial advancing over the fine needle. A guide wire can be forwarded into the renal system through the cannula
d **Schematic representation of a puncture under combined sonographic and fluoroscopic monitoring**
e **Primary puncture of lower calyx group using fine needle**

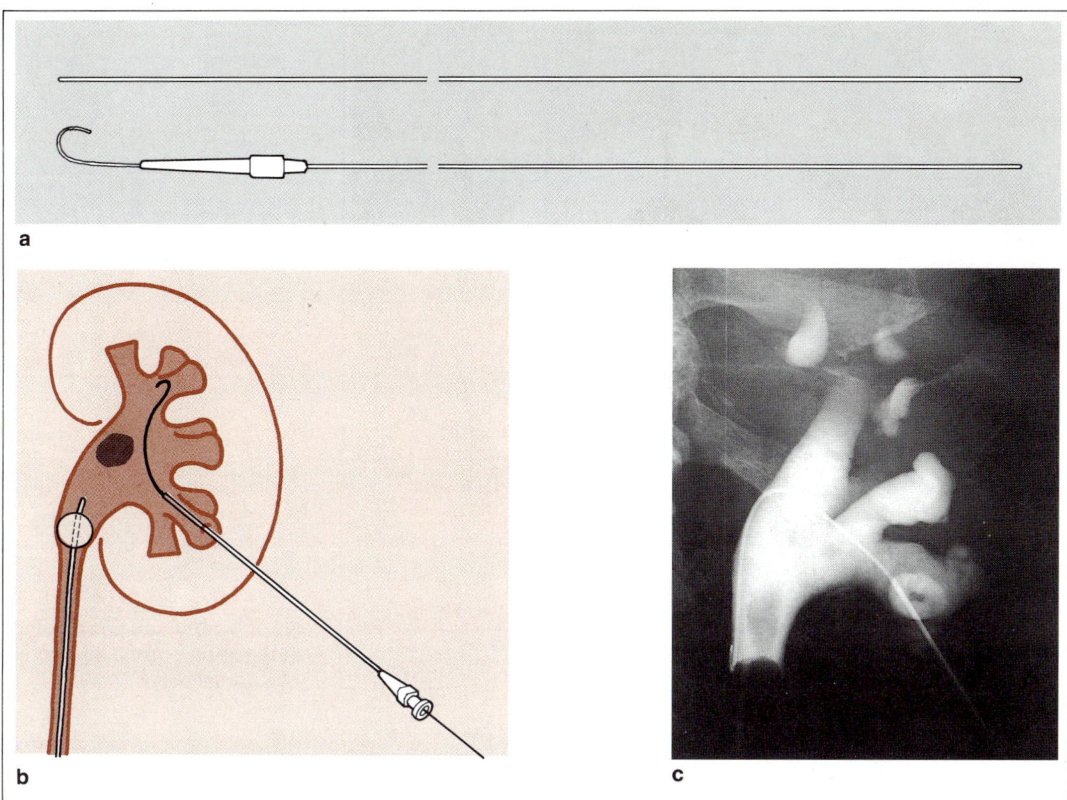

Fig. 4.**8**

a **Guide wires:** soft Seldinger wire (top), Advantages: minor traumatization of urinary tract system; no risk of perforation. Disadvantage: risk of kinking during primary dilatation procedure. Lunderquist wire (bottom) with floppy tip and rigid sheath. Advantage: safe guiding during dilatation. Disadvantage: higher risk of perforation

b **Schematic representation of introduction of guide wire through the cannula**

c **Cannula and guide wire in situ**

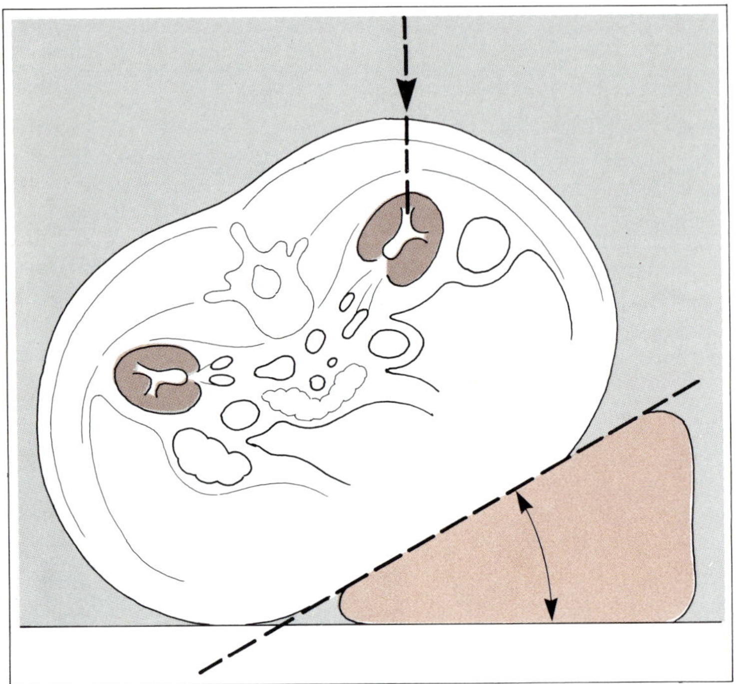

Fig. 4.9 **Oblique positioning of patient for vertical puncture of a dorsal calyx**

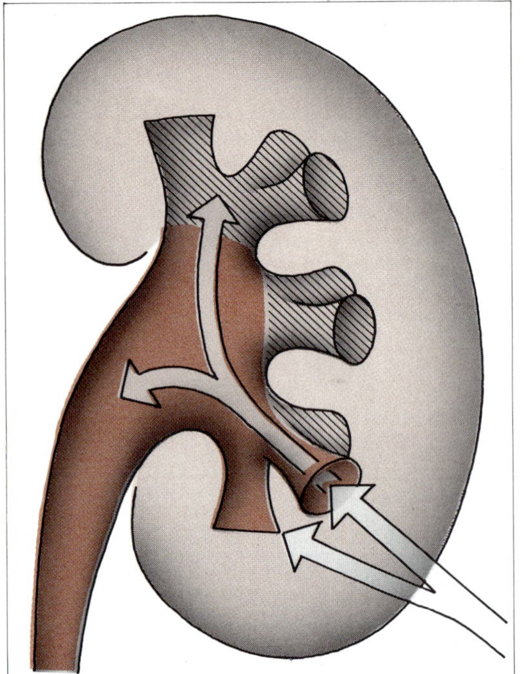

Fig. 4.10 **The major part of the RCS can be reached via the posterior dorsal calyx.** Insertion of rigid nephroscope into the upper calyx is occasionally possible, depending on individual anatomic situation

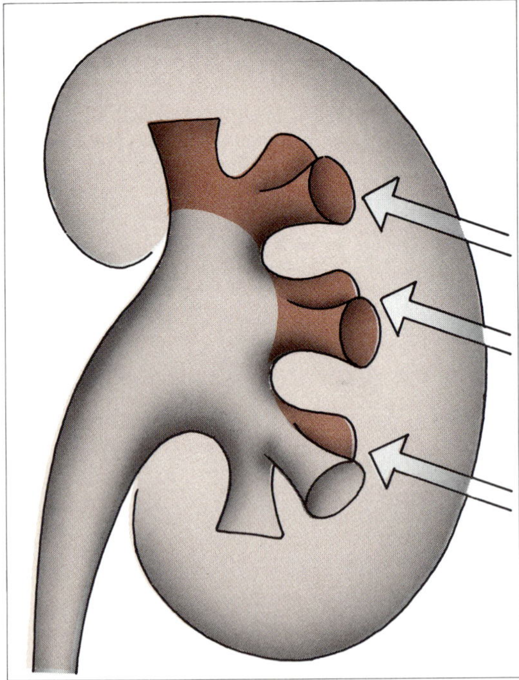

Fig. 4.11 **Direct puncture of calyx stones or calyceal branches of staghorn stones**

coaxially with the X-ray beam. Subsequently, either the patient or the X-ray tube is moved in order to safely assess the exact depth of the needle point. The disadvantage is that the hands of the operator are repeatedly exposed to fluoroscopy during puncture if no "needle-holder" is used.

4.7.3.3 Selection of the puncture channel. The site of the percutaneous tract is essential for the success of the intervention, and should therefore be carefully adapted to stone position and anatomy of the RCS.

In about 80% the cases, puncture of the lower dorsal calyx is appropriate (lower caliceal stones, proximal ureteral stones, renal pelvic stones, upper caliceal stones in selected cases only; Fig. 4.**10**). Exceptions are solitary stones in a middle or upper calyx, which must be approached by direct puncture of the stone-bearing calyx (Fig. 4.**11**). Direct puncture is also applied in the case of ventral calyces, as access to the stone from the adjacent dorsal calyx is difficult. Successful stone removal from the upper calyx through a tract from the lower calyx is occasionally possible, depending on the individual anatomy of the RCS.

4.7.4 Dilatation

Dilatation of the percutaneous tract is performed in 2 steps:

1. Primary dilatation by a conical metal bougie up to 9 Fr (Fig. 4.**12a**), followed by insertion of a safcty wirc through the metal cannula (Figs. 4.**12b,c**). In the case of dislocation of the nephroscope, the RCS can be safely re-entered with the aid of this safety guide wire.
2. Definitive dilatation of the tract by the telescope bougie set (Fig. 4.**13a**), which can be used in all cases, even in the presence of pronounced cicatrization of the perirenal tissue (as a result of previous surgeries!).

4.7.4.1 Practical hints. Skin and fascia are incised with a scalpel. When starting dilatation, care should be taken to introduce the bougies in coaxial direction with the guide wire (check fluoroscopically!) to avoid kinking of the wire (Fig. 4.**12d**). This risk is reduced by the application of a Lunderquist wire (see Fig. 4.**8a**) with its rigid sheath.

The individual dilators of the bougie set are progressively telescoped by slight turning movements (Fig. 4.**13b**). The resistance at the fascia or kidney surface should be carefully overcome without any undue force. Fixation of the central rod of the bougie set with one hand prevents perforation on the oppsite renal pelvic wall during dilatation. For the last step, the sheath of the nephroscope or an Amplatz sheath is advanced over the telescope bougie set (Fig. 4.**13c**). The use of an Amplatz sheath (26 or 28 Fr, depending on the size of the nephroscope) has the following advantages:

– Big stone fragments resulting from the lithotripsy of hard stones can be quickly extracted, thus considerably speeding up the entire intervention.
– In addition to the permanent suction system of the double sheath nephroscope, the Amplatz sheath provides drainage of the RCS during surgery, thus preventing a hazardous rise of pressure within the kidney. However, the introduction of an Amplatz sheath may be difficult in the case of a narrow RCS or in the case of branched calculi leaving minimal space in the calyx for instrument manipulation.

4.7.4.2 Alternative dilatation methods

– *Semirigid fascia dilators*
  Advantage: Low risk of perforation.
  Disadvantage: Each dilator has to be withdrawn before the next one can be inserted. This results in repeated bleeding from the percutaneous tract.
– *Balloon dilators*
  Advantage: Minimal traumatizing effect; no risk of perforation.
  Disadvantages: Expensive system since it can only be re-used to a limited extent; unsuitable in the case of perirenal cicatrization.

4.7.5 Radiation Protection

During puncture and dilatation, both patient and urologist are exposed to radiation by intermittent fluoroscopy. The extent of the actual radiation exposure depends on various factors, as follows:

– technical standards of the X-ray system
– weight of the patient
– experience and skill of the operator

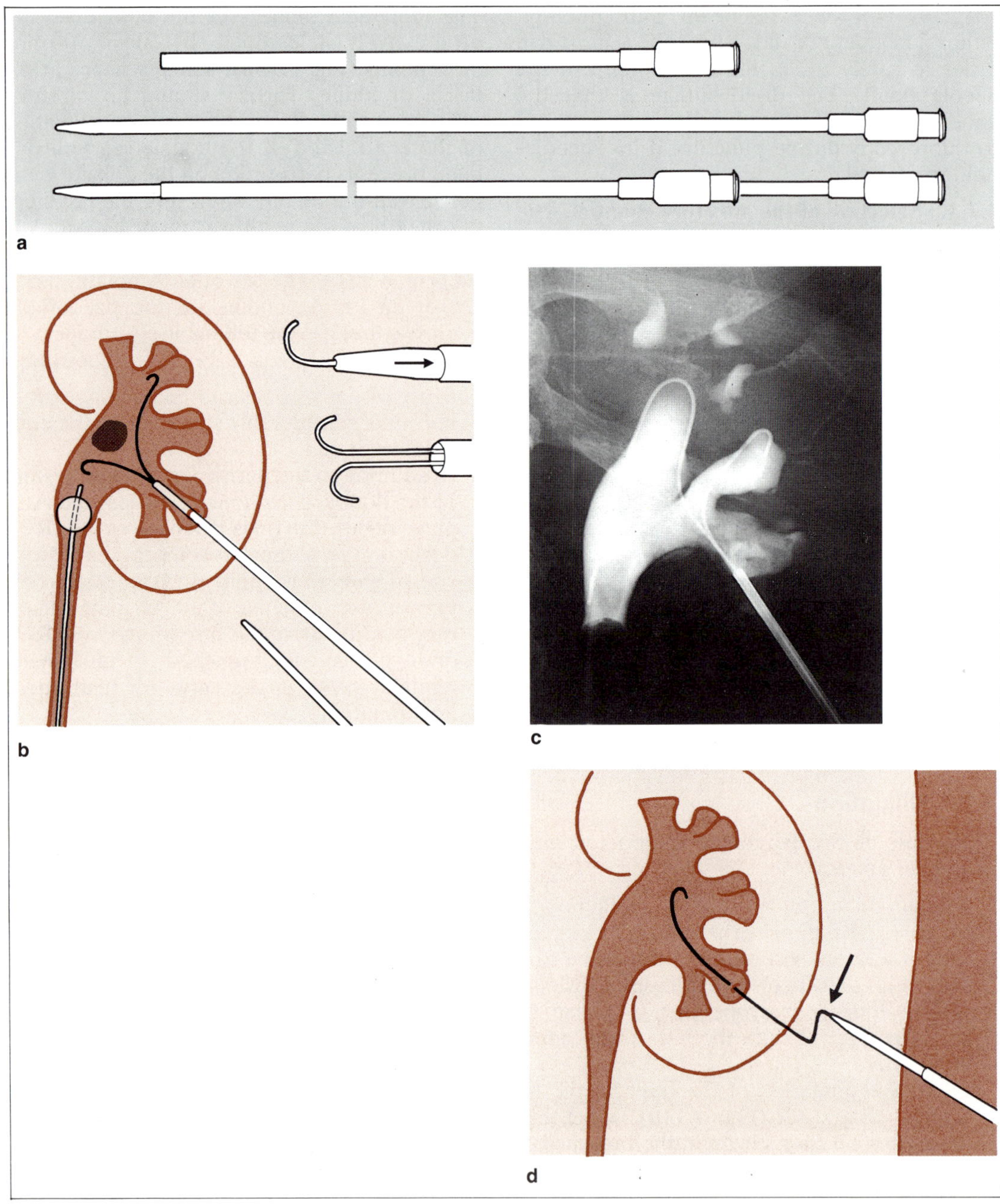

Fig. 4.**12**

a **Set for primary dilatation.** Middle: Metal bougie (9 Fr) with conical tip. Top: Metal cannula that is passed over the bougie (bottom) to enable insertion of two guide wires

b **After primary dilatation, a second wire is inserted through the cannula**

c **Metal cannula with two guide wires in situ**

d **Attention: Angulation of guide wire in course of primary dilatation.** In such an event, remove bougie, reinsert cannula, and exchange guide wire

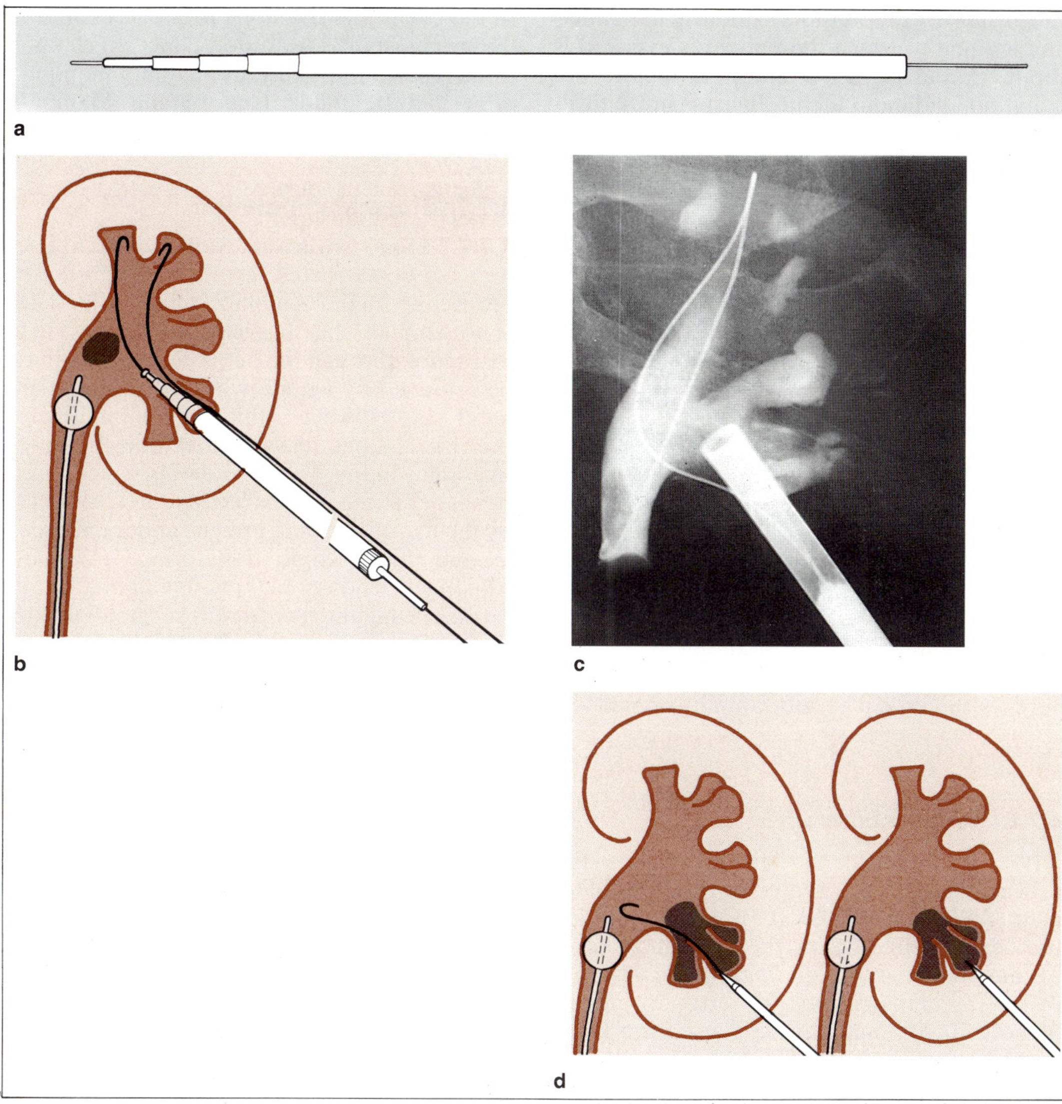

Fig. 4.**13**

a **Metal bougie set for dilatation of operative channel**

b **Step-wise dilatation with telescope bougies set.** Note safety wire beside bougie set

c **Nephroscope sheath in situ after removal of bougie set**

d **Peculiarities of puncture and dilatation in the case of staghorn calculi.** If the caliceal branch cannot be passed with the wire, stone is first fixed with needle tip and then with rigid tip of guide wire. The tract is then dilated by the wire up to stone position (Warning: danger of dislocation of the wire and consecutive "via falsa" of the dilators)

According to the authors' studies, the radiation loading to which the patient is exposed is about 15 rad. Due to many variables, the radiation loading to the urologist is more difficult to assess. The loading to the hands, which are most exposed, should be determined with the aid of a ring dosimeter.

An array of protective measures is available, the regular application of which is highly recommended.

– Use of filters for the X-ray tube
– Fade-in of monitor image, if possible
– Lead aprons for patient (genital region!) and urologist
– Withdrawal of the hands from the direct X-ray beam during fluoroscopy
– Lead glasses and thyroid protection for the urologist (scattered radiation in the case of an over-the-table X-ray arrangement)

As a general rule, it may be said that fluoroscopy time should be as long as required but as short as possible. In the case of uncomplicated percutaneous surgery, a time period of three minutes should not be substantially exceeded.

4.7.6 Nephroscopy

After introducing the nephroscope (Fig. 4.**14a**), the RCS is irrigated to rinse out blood clots. As irrigation fluid, 0.9% NaCl should be used exclusively. During the procedure, variable amounts of irrigation fluid will be absorbed by the vascular system or the retroperitoneum, or both. If sodium chloride is used, no hypotonic hyperhydration (TUR-syndrome) but rather isotonic hyperhydration occurs, the latter being far less harmful. As an additional prophylactic measure, repeated administration of diuretics during the operation is useful to minimize serious side-effects of hyperhydration (edema of the lungs!).

Subsequent endoscopic scanning of the RCS comprises identification of the renal pelvis, including ureteral pelvic junction (balloon ureteral catheter!), identification of the calyces, and, above all, identification of the stone (Figs. 4.**14b,c**). Naturally, the maneuverability of the rigid instrument within the RCS is limited. The application of too much "tilting force" creates the risk of parenchymal damage with subsequent considerable bleeding.

In the event that the stone is not accessible via the tract installed (unsuited puncture channel, stone dislocation), various auxiliary manipulations can be made (see "Stone Manipulation").

4.7.7 Stone Manipulation

4.7.7.1 Stone extraction. Stones of up to 8–10 mm can be extracted directly through the nephroscope or the Amplatz sheath (Fig. 4.**15**). If no Amplatz sheath is used, stones too big for extraction through the nephroscope sheath can be removed by withdrawing the entire instrument set. However, this procedure involves the risk of stone dislocation within the operative tract. In this event, a new approach should be made, fixing and extracting the concrement by the use of grasping forceps under endoscopic and fluoroscopic monitoring. (Warning: prolonged endoscopic manipulations in the retroperitoneum may lead to substantial extravasation of irrigation fluid.) Alternatively, the stone may be extracted with a conventional stone forceps solely under fluoroscopic control.

4.7.7.2 Stone disintegration. Currently three methods for stone disintegration are available:

1. Mechanical lithotripsy (stone punch);
2. Electrohydraulic lithotripsy (EHL);
3. Ultrasound lithotripsy (USL).

However, laser lithotripsy is now increasingly beeing used in a clinical setting; it may become an equivalent or even superior alternative in the near future (see Chapter 8).

Mechanical disintegration of renal pelvic stones with the stone punch is difficult for two reasons: (1) Due to the narrow viewing angle, the operative area cannot be clearly viewed. (2) The space for manipulation in the renal pelvis is limited, compared with that of the urinary bladder. Since USL and EHL can easily be used, mechanical lithotripsy is rarely a valid alternative and therefore seldom used in conjunction with percutaneous surgery (Fig. 4.**16**).

Disintegration with EHL provides the advantage of enabling the use of a flexible probe (3 or 5 Fr). Its disintegration power and speed is slightly higher when compared with USL. It is therefore particularly suited for the treatment of hard stones (calcium oxalate monohydrate,

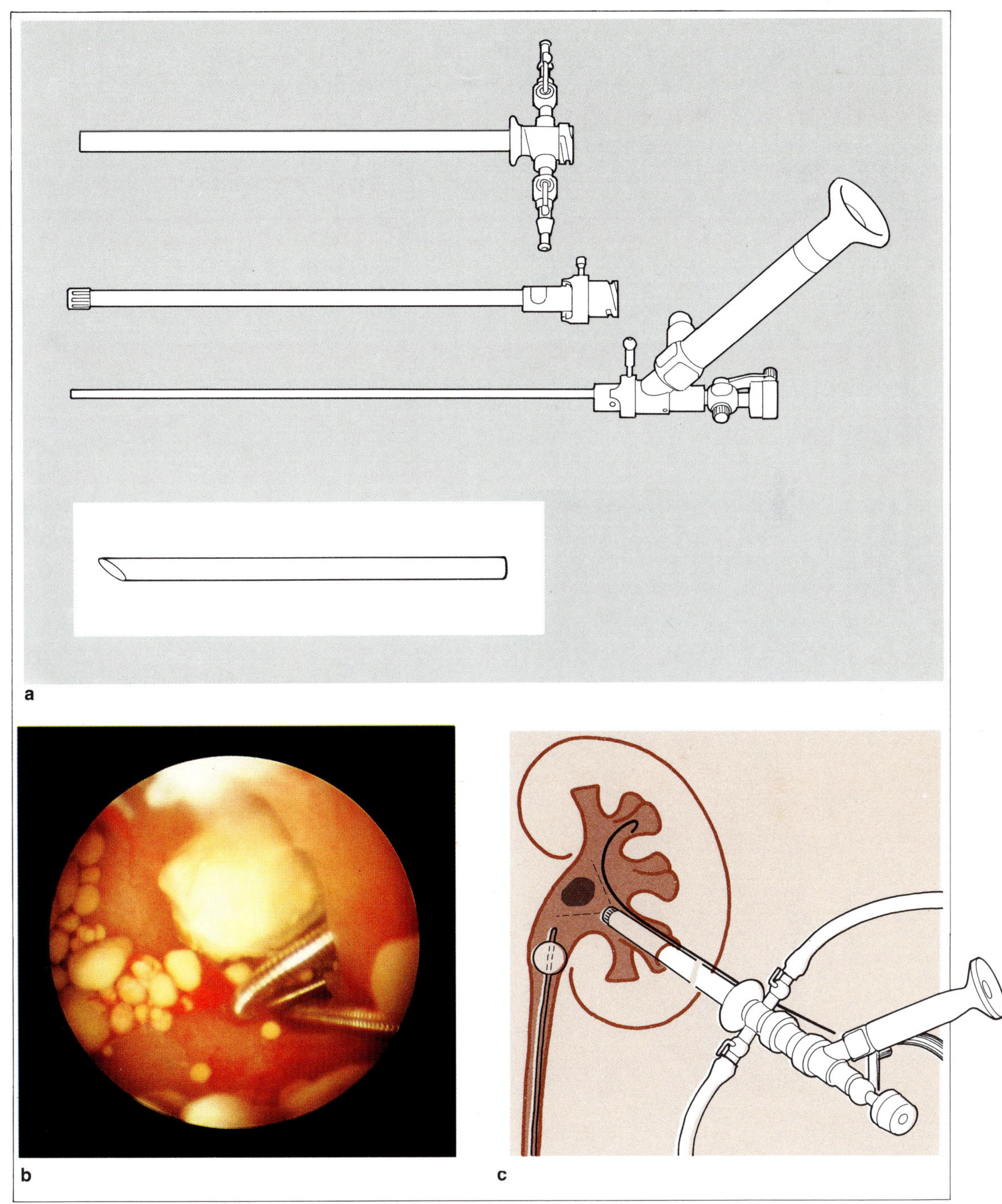

Fig. 4.**14**

a   **Nephroscope (26 Fr) with double shaft for low-pressure irrigation, oblique optic, and straight working channel** (courtesy Storz). Amplatz sheath for easily repeatable introduction of the nephroscope for stone extraction (bottom)

b   **Nephroscopy: Stones and safety wire in the RCS**

c   **Schematic representation of nephroscopy;** low-pressure irrigation through continual rinsing and suction of the irrigation liquid

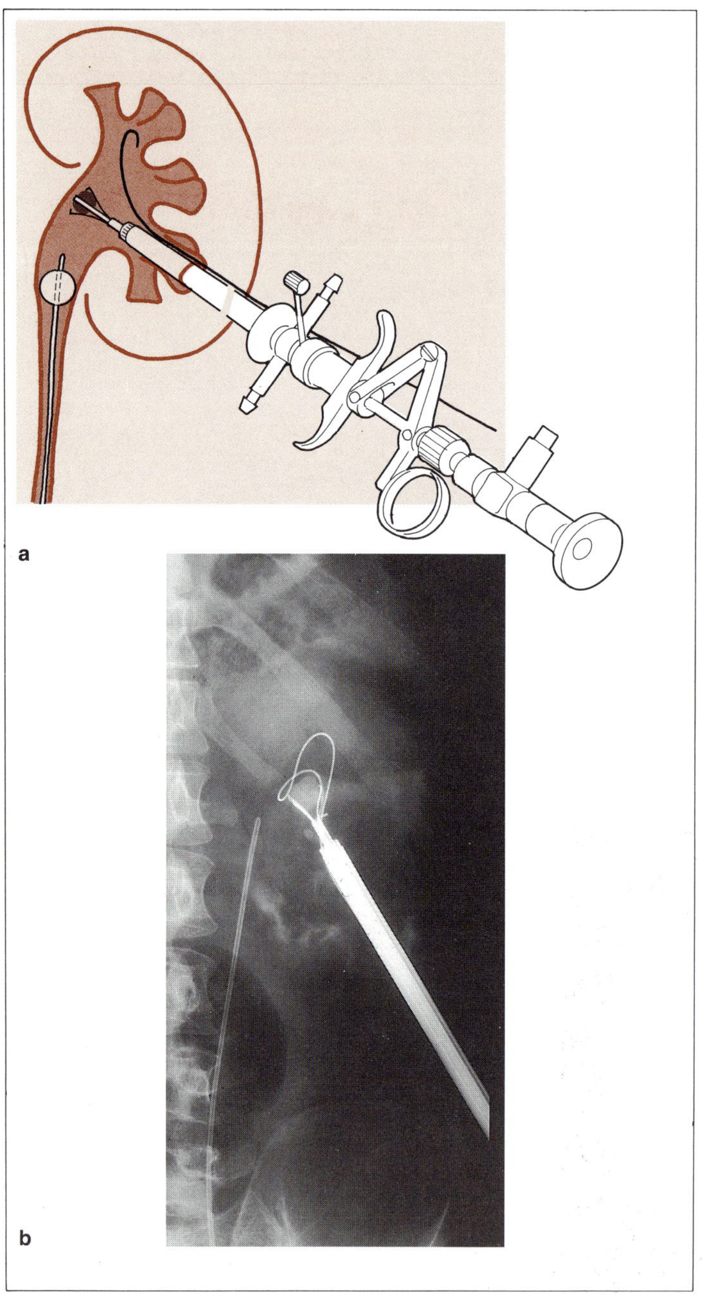

Fig. 4.**15**

a   Extraction of small concrements by means of forceps

b   Pelvic stone engaged in three-branch grasping forceps. The concrement is removed through the tract by withdrawing complete instrument set

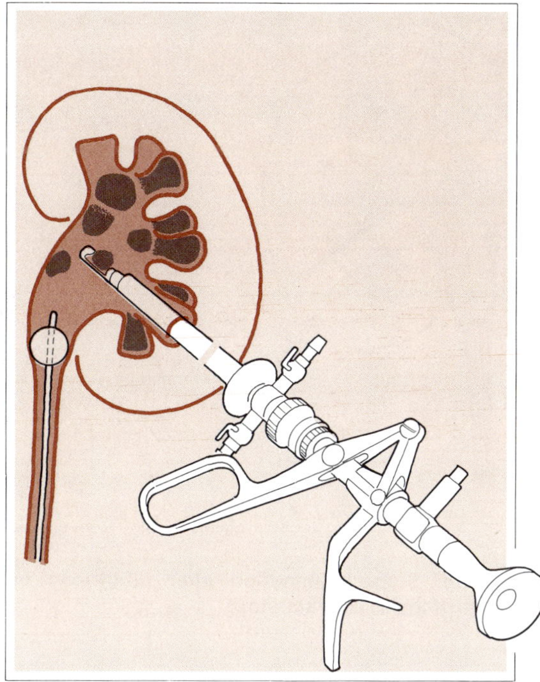

Fig. 4.**16** **Stone punch for mechanical disintegration of renal concrements**

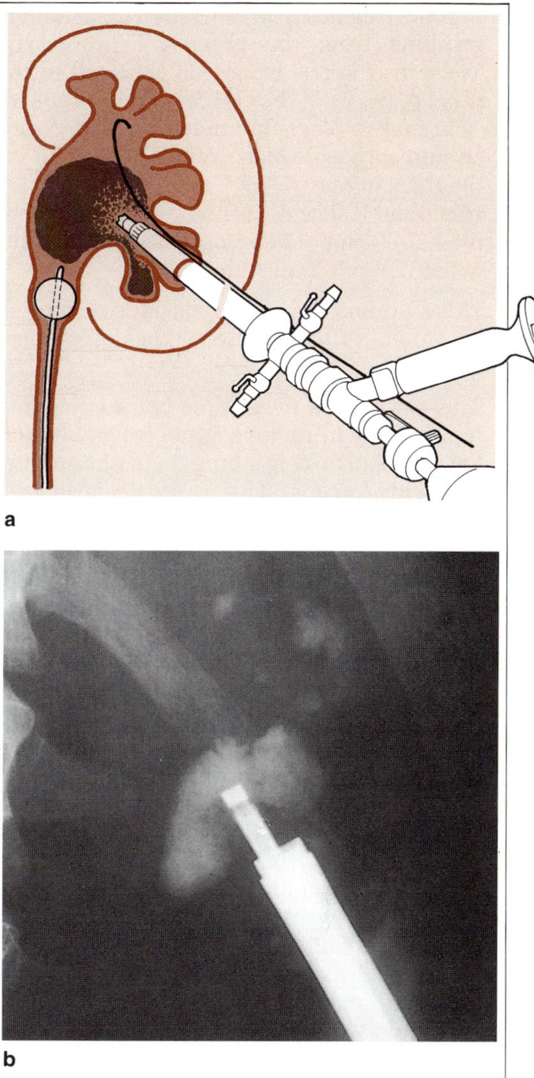

Fig. 4.**17**
a **Disintegration of large renal pelvis stone by ultrasound probe**
b **Ultrasound probe and nephroscope in situ.** Note dislocated stone fragments in the upper calices

cystine). Another advantage of EHL is that it can be used in conjunction the flexible nephroscope when the 3 Fr probe is utilized.

Disadvantages of EHL are that dislocation of stone fragments is difficult to control and that a discharge of the probe close to the urothelium may lead to perforation. Moreover, discharge close to the instrument tip may damage the lens.

The advantages of USL (Fig. 4.**17**) are that stone debris can immediately be removed by sucking out the fragments through the central channel of the probe and that there is no risk of immediate perforation when the probe is used close to the urothelium. However, the disintegration of hard stones with this method may take more time than with EHL.

The authors routinely use USL since, in their opinion, it represents the optimal compromise between safety and efficacy of all methods currently available. Other methods for stone disintegration are applied by the authors in exceptional cases only.

4.7.7.3 Retrieval of residual stone fragments.
Following USL or EHL, multiple stone fragments may be left in the RCS. Two types of residual concretions can, in general, be differentiated:

1. Mobile fragments of various sizes, mainly resulting from the precedent lithotripsy. These fragments are mostly situated in the renal pelvis or in the calyces where lithotripsy has taken place, but may also be dislocated into calyces, which are not accessible via the track in use.
2. Immobile caliceal stones, which, due to their size, cannot be removed from the calyx without previous disintegration.

Various options must be considered for the management of the different types of residual stones.

- The safest but most time-consuming and tedious way to remove stone fragments following lithotripsy is taking them out one-by-one with forceps. This is particularly true when the stone has been broken up into multiple tiny fragments. Thus, when hard stones are to be dealt with, it is wiser to produce larger fragments that are just small enough to pass through the Amplatz or nephroscope sheath. This greatly speeds up the entire procedure. Very tiny fragments or fragments of soft, brittle stones (e.g., struvite stones) are better continuously disintegrated and sucked out through the hollow ultrasonic probe, which can be used like a vacuum cleaner in this setting.
- Another way to remove these type of fragments is by carefully using the Ellik Evacuator (Fig. 4.**18**). However, this approach should be avoided when infected stones are to be dealth with, as there is a risk of septicemia caused by the "high pressure" irrigation.
- Dislocated mobile fragments can sometimes be mobilized by targeted irrigation using a ureteral or an angiographic catheter. However, it is difficult to place the irrigation catheter in the appropriate calyx.

Techniques suitable for the removal of immobile residual stones, which are not accessible with the rigid nephroscope through the percutaneous tract in use, should naturally also be considered for mobile fragments when the aforementioned techniques are unsuccessful.

- The easiest and safest way to deal with residual concrements in unaccessible calyces is to use an extracorporeal lithotriptor three to six days after the percutaneous procedure (Figs. 4.**19b,c**). However, the residual

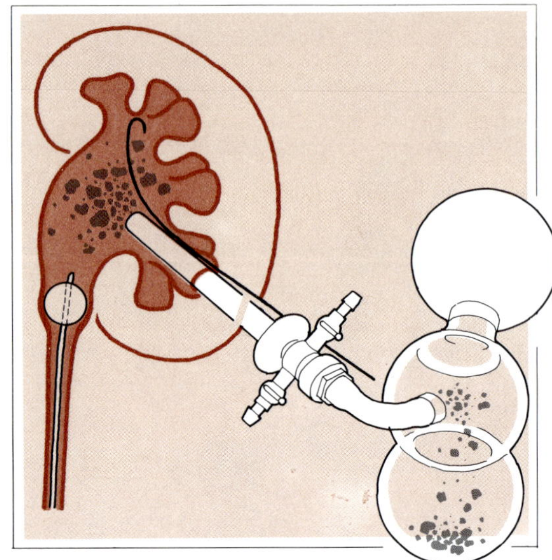

Fig. 4.**18 Stone elimination after lithotripsy by means of the Ellik evacuator**

stone mass should be kept as small as possible in order to yield good results with this approach. In general, a stone-free rate of 55%−90% (Lingeman, 1987; Eisenberger, 1987) can be expected with the combination of PCNL and ESWL.
- Installation of additional percutaneous tracks is another option. This approach is particularly attractive if complete stone removal can expectedly be achieved in one treatment session (Figs. 4.**19d,e**). On the other hand, additional operative tracks involve the risk of additional complications, particularly if an upper calyx has to be punctured via the intercostal route. To minimize the risk of pleural damage and resultant hydropneumothorax, these punctures should be made exclusively under combined ultrasound and X-ray monitoring.
- Another option is flexible nephroscopy. Technical advances have brought about a general increased use of flexible scopes in urology. The flexible nephroscopes (Fig. 4.**20a**) come with a caliber of 16−18 Fr and a single working and irrigation channel of about 3−5 Fr. The modern fiberoptic systems provide a good view. Since the tip of the nephroscope can be deflected actively in two directions up to an angle of 180° (Fig.

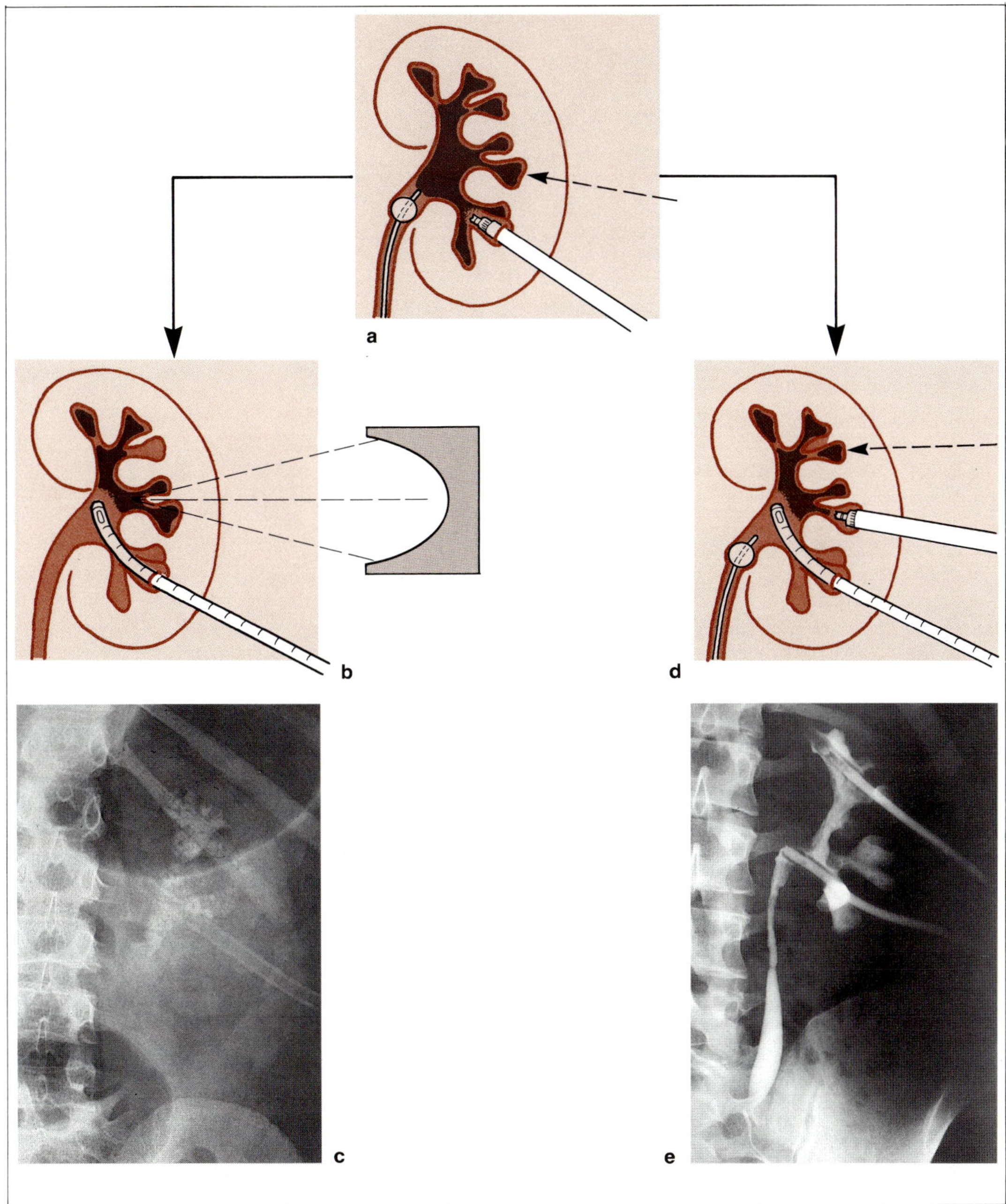

Fig. 4.19 Treatment of staghorn calculi

a First session: PCNL for stone debulking

b Combination of PCNL and ESWL. Residual concrements are disintegrated by ESWL

c X-ray check of staghorn calculus after percutaneous pretreatment and ESWL. Stone fragments dispersed in the urinary tract system. Nephrostomy catheter in situ

d Installation of additional tracts for complete percutaneous elimination of a staghorn calculus

e X-ray after percutaneous operation of a staghorn calculus via two channels; two nephrostomy catheters in situ

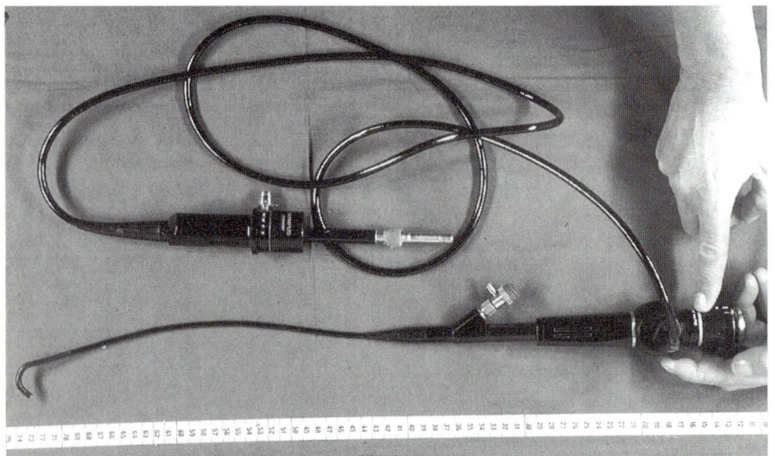

Fig. 4.**20**
a Flexible nephroscope
(16 Fr., courtesy
Olympus)

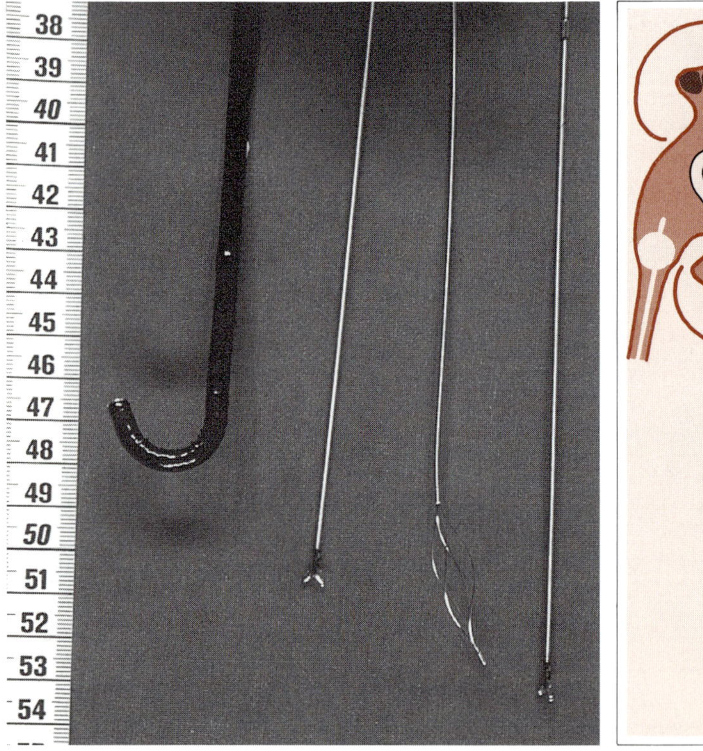

b The steerable tip allows deflection up to 180°.
Auxiliary tools for stone removal

**c Insertion of flexible nephroscope through outer
sheath of rigid instrument**

4.**20b**), these instruments have an excellent maneuverability. Thus, access to all parts of the RCS is normally feasible via one percutaneous channel.

Unfortunately, stone manipulation is still rather limited with the flexible nephroscopes, due to the narrow working-channel. For example, if the 3 Fr electrohydraulic probe is used, irrigation and, as a consequence, vision are considerably compromised. Furthermore, only very tiny stone-grasping instruments are available (Fig. 4.**20b**), which are generally unsuitable for removal of the larger stone fragments.

For the future, the 200 μm laser fiber holds promise in combination with flexible nephroscopes. If clinical experience continues to indicate the laser being an efficient and safe tool for lithotripsy (Dretler 1986, 1988; Watson, 1987), this could have a major impact on flexible nephroscopy. Thus, the desired combination of flexible nephroscopy with efficient lithotripsy under good vision may become a clinical reality in the near future (Fig. 4.**20c**).

— Irrigation for percutaneous litholysis is also an option. Certain stones (uric acid, struvite, cystine; see Chapter 1) can be resolved by percutaneous irrigation. However, depending on the stone size, this procedure is rather time-consuming (3−4 weeks); it should only be employed when all other methods of stone elimination have been attempted.

When the urinary tract is continously irrigated using appropriate substances (bicarbonate, renacidin, N-acetyl cysteine), a two-way nephrostomy catheter or two nephrostomies should be employed to ensure permanent, steady drainage of the RCS. Particularly with renacidin, a pressure rise should be avoided to prevent the risk of renal damage.

4.7.8 Auxiliary Percutaneous Operations

Percutaneous "pyeloplasty" has recently been more widely used for both congenital and secondary stenoses of the UPJ (see Chapter 2).

Access to the RCS is gained through a middle or lower calyx (Fig. 4.**21a**). The ureter is intubated by previous retrograde or by antegrade splintage, using a guide wire or ureteral catheter. The incision of the UPJ is then made under visual control until the perirenal fat is reached (extravasation of contrast medium seen under fluoroscopic control; Figs. 4.**21b,c,d**). The incision can either be made with the rigid knife (according to an internal urethrotomy) or by a flexible knife that is guided over the ureteral wire.

Postoperatively, a ureteral stent is left in place for 2−3 weeks, until fluoroscopic control no longer shows evidence of extravasation.

Stenosis of the caliceal neck is preferably dilated using the telescope bougie, since incision with the knife may result in substantial parenchymal bleeding. If incision of the caliceal neck is performed, the course of the adjacent vessels must be kept in mind (ventral and dorsal to the caliceal neck; Janetschek, 1988).

4.8 Risks and Complications

The nature of percutaneous surgery involves a number of complications that may occur at all levels of the procedure. The intervention is not easy from a technical point of view, thus the rate of complications drops with increasing experience of the operator.

4.8.1 Perforation

Perforation of the RCS can occur at any time during the intervention. Smaller lesions (caused by puncture needle or by the guide wire) are negligible and do not require discontinuation of surgery.

With major defects of the RCS (caused by metal bougie or by nephroscope), the intervention should only be continued if it can be completed quickly. The low-pressure irrigation system is helpful to minimize extravasation. After surgery, it is important to ensure good drainage of the RCS by a large-sized nephrostomy catheter.

If multiple punctures (and perforations) do not lead to a definitive percutaneous access to the RCS, the ureteral catheter remains in the renal pelvis to ensure at least a minimal drainage. The clinical course of the patient will show whether or not the drainage is sufficient. Surgical intervention is only required if the patient exhibits relevant clinical symptoms, such as fever and pain.

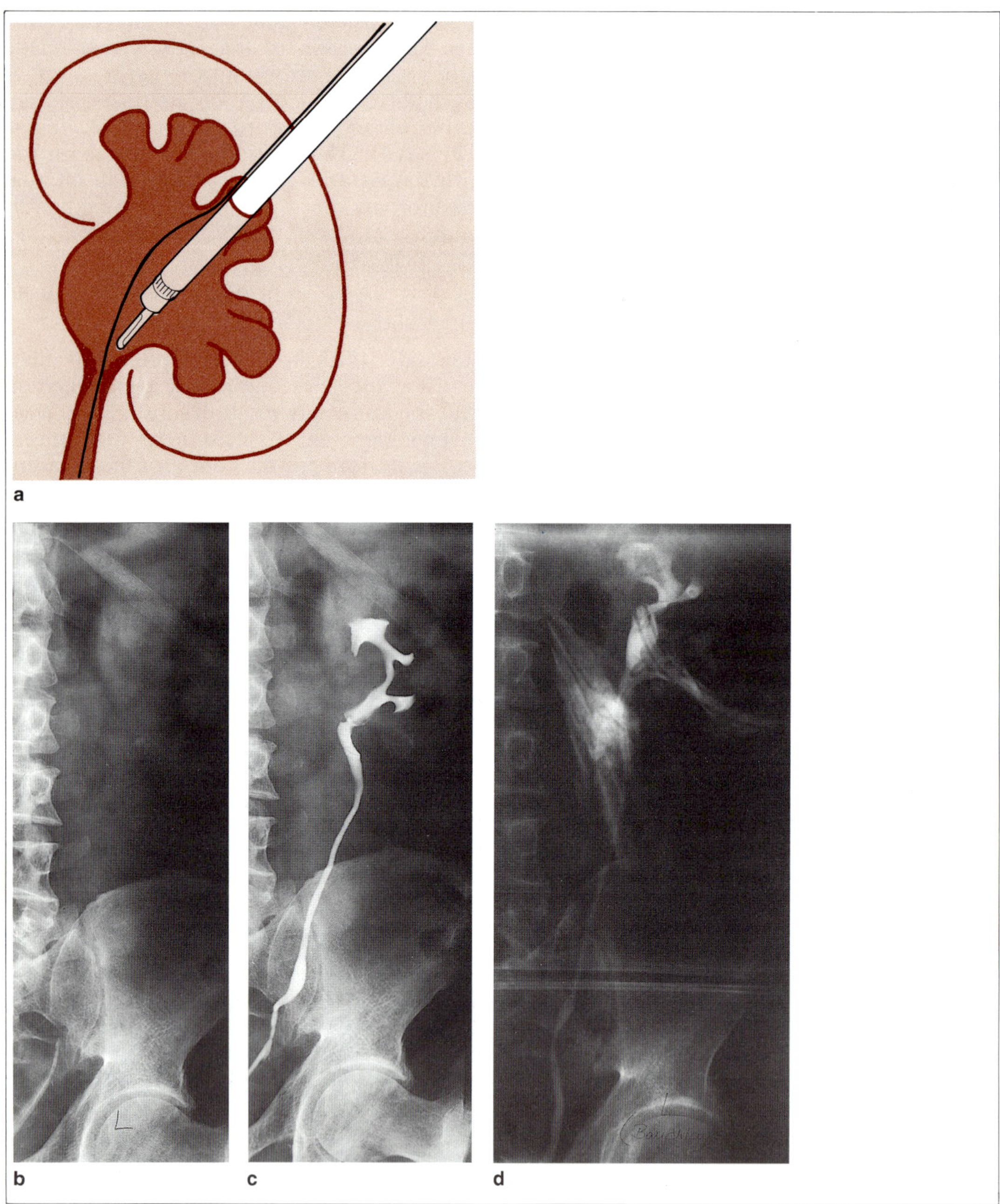

Fig. 4.**21**

a   Percutaneous incision of UPJ with rigid, cold knife

b−d Contrast medium extravasation, ureteric splint, and nephrostomy tube after percutaneous incision of a secondary UPJ stenosis

4.8.2 Hemorrhage

Bleeding of varying degrees may occur after puncture, incision, or dilatation of skin, fatty tissue, muscles, and renal parenchyma. The telescope bougie, nephroscope, and nephrostomy catheter normally produce sufficient compression to control such bleeding.

Mucosal lesions or parenchymal lacerations (caused by forced maneuvers with the rigid nephroscope) are a source of bleeding during stone manipulation. Massive hemorrhage requires discontinuation of percutaneous surgery if stone elimination will not be terminated within a short time. The nephrostomy catheter is inserted and clamped for 2–4 hours in order to stop the bleeding by tamponage.

Persistent bleeding only occurs in rare cases. Following transfemoral angiography, a superselective embolization should be attempted if the bleeding vessel can be indentified (Fig. 4.**22**). Only if this procedure is unsuccessful must nephrectomy be considered as the ultimate solution.

4.8.3 Infection and Septicemia

Percutaneous manipulation of infected stones may produce a massive absorption of bacteria into the blood vessels. Hence, sufficient antibiotic levels are required at the time of surgery to prevent the sequelae of septicemia. Fever in the postoperative course, which occurs, de-

pending on stone composition, in up to 50% of the patients (Snyder, 1987), is not a serious problem as long as sufficient diuresis and continuous drainage of the operative kidney is provided. However, the latter conditions cannot always be met, since postoperative bleeding sometimes requires clamping of the nephrostomy catheter. If this fatal combination of postoperative hemorrhage and infection occurs, the hazards of bleeding must be weighed against those of septicemia, and the treatment decisions made accordingly.

4.8.4 Pneumothorax and Hydrothorax

These complications may occur in conjunction with an intercostal puncture of the upper part of the RCS. Depending on the extent and clinical duration, suction drainage is indicated.

4.8.5 Lesions of Other Adjacent Organs

This complication can safely be prevented by ultrasound-guided puncture of the kidney. If it occurs despite this prevention, the indication for a surgical intervention must be made according to the clinical symptoms.

4.9 Follow-Up

At the end of the operation, X-ray control (hard copy) is obligatory. If complete stone removal is documented, the procedure is ter-

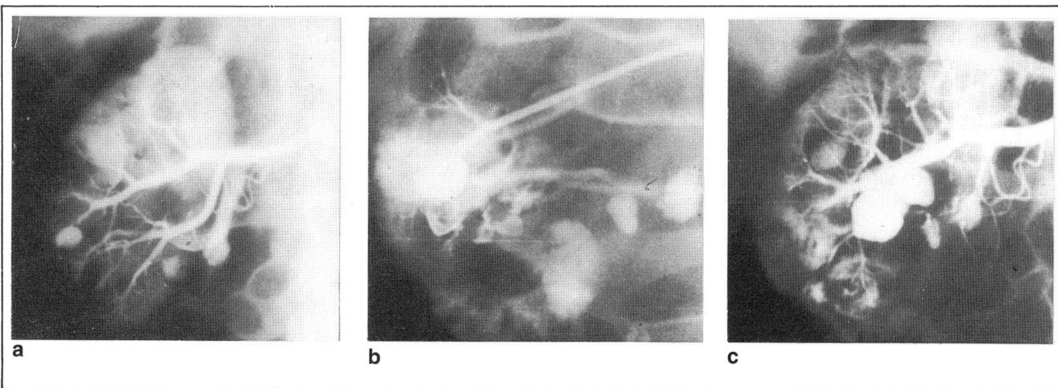

Fig. 4.22 Superselective embolization in the case of bleeding aneurysm of an arcuata artery after PCNL
a Representation of aneurysm
b Superselective exploration and embolization by Ethibloc
c After embolization, aneurysm no longer shows up

minated and a nephrostomy tube is placed. The nephrostomy tube is inserted through the nephroscope or the Amplatz sheath (Fig. 4.**23**). The tube should be as large in size as possible. To avoid dislocation of the tube, a balloon-catheter with a disconnectable adapting system is advantageous.

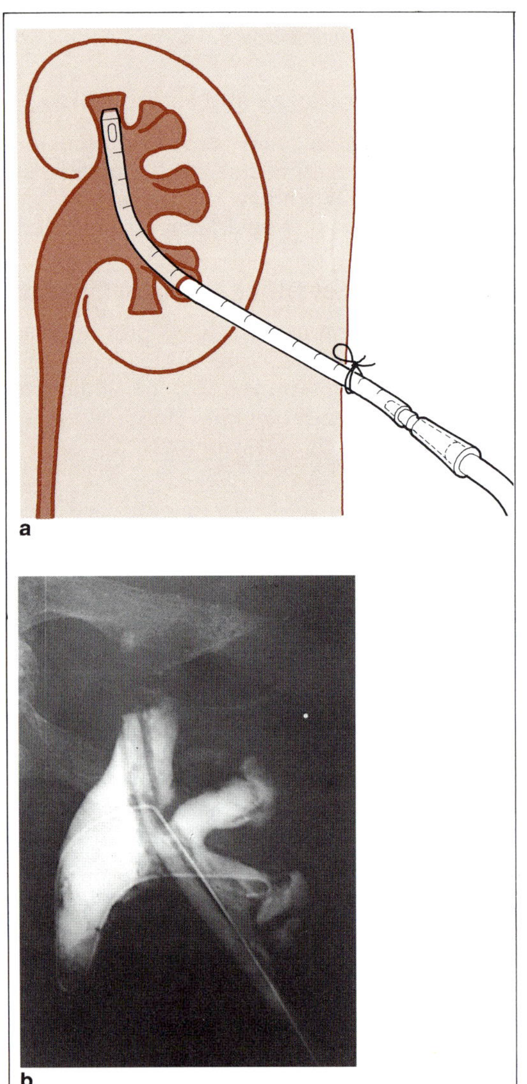

Fig. 4.**23**
a   Optimum position of fistula catheter with long intrarenal part (low risk of dislocation)
b   Immediate postoperative check, renal fistula catheter and guide wire in situ

Bladder and ureteral catheters are removed immediately after termination of the operation (exception: ureteral catheter may be required for drainage of the kidney; see "Complications").

It the plain X-ray shows evidence of residual fragments, an immediate "second look" is indicated to determine whether these fragments can be removed via the tract in use. If this is not the case, the aforementioned rules for the removal of residual fragments must be applied.

In the further postoperative course, fluid (parenterally or, from the second day on, orally supplied) and diuretics are generously administered in order to provide good "irrigation" of the operative kidney. Treatment with antibiotics should be continued (depending on the patients temperature and clinical symptoms) for at least one day after surgery.

Definite documentation of residual fragments or stone freedom by plain X-ray and nephrostomogram is then made two to four days postoperatively (depending on the degree of residual hematuria).

In the case of residual fragments, it must be decided whether a second look, ESWL, or other procedures (see above) provide the best chance to remove these fragments.

If the kidney is stone-free and the nephrostomogram shows free passage of the contrast medium to the bladder, the nephrostomy is clamped for 12 hours and then removed if no symptoms have occurred.

Patients that are discharged from the hospital with residual fragments should be closely followed by ultrasound and X-ray examinations. If the residual fragments do not pass within three months, further treatment should be considered depending on the clinical symptoms.

If complete stone elimination has been clearly documented, follow-up examinations can be restricted to ultrasound scanning once a year and appropriate stone prophylaxis.

4.10 Results

The results in terms of stone freedom depend largely on the patient selection and the experience of the operator. With a widening of the

ESWL indications, more and more "difficult" stones are left for percutaneous surgery, which then must often be used in combination with other procedures. Nevertheless, success rates, even for complicated stones, of as much as 90% (Lingeman, 1987) have been reported. However, it seems that an aggressive percutaneous approach using several tracts along with meticulous secondary endoscopic stone removal are prerequisites for complete clearance of a stone-bearing kidney. With the conventional combination of "one-track" PCNL and ESWL, only 55%−60% of patients can be rendered stone-free (Eisenberger, 1987; Miller, 1989).

Like the successrate, the complication rate depends largely on the operator's experience and the patient selection. Recently reported comparably high complication rates (Snider, 1987) particularly reflect the latter. Complication rates are summarized in Table 4.**1**.

Table 4.**1** **Complications of PCNL (own data, large stones and staghorn stones, N = 73)**

− Hemorrhage: transfusion		10%
embolization		1%
nephrectomy		2%
− Fever		32%
− Septicimia		3%
− Hydrothorax		2%
− Deterioration of renal function		3%

5 Ureteroscopy (URS)

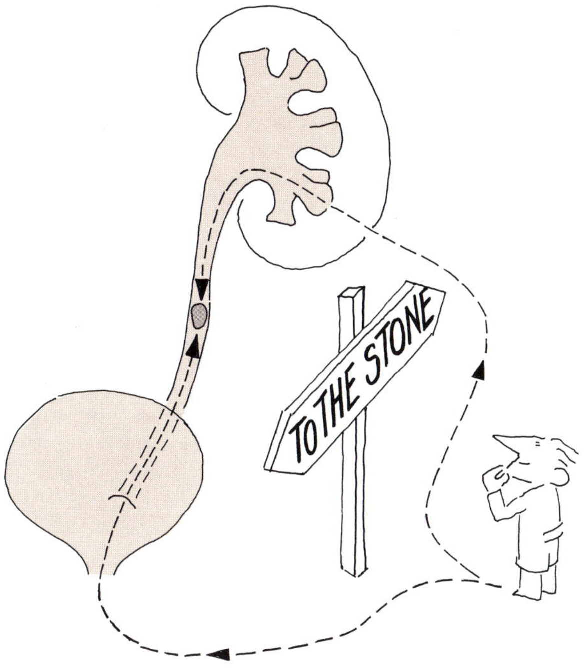

5.1 Retrograde URS

5.1.1 Patient Selection

- Absolute contraindications: untreated bleeding disorder
- Relative contraindications: pregnancy, untreated UTI, untreated tuberculosis
- Higher degree of difficulty: ureteral strictures (cicatrized, inflammatory) ureteral kinking, condition after ureteral reimplantation, condition after radiation in the small pelvis, ureterocele, adenoma of the prostate, urethral stricture

5.1.2 Indications

1. Ureteral calculi (following unsuccessful ESWL)
2. Persistent "Steinstrasse" after ESWL
3. Endoureteral diagnostic (filling defects on the IVP or retrograde pyelogram; follow-up in cases of conservatively treated urothelial tumors)
4. Endoureteral therapy (resection and laser therapy of superficial urothelial tumors; incision or dilatation of ureteral strictures)

5.1.3 Patient Preparation

For the urologist, excretory urography, urine analysis, urine culture, and clotting values are mandatory. Any further examinations (chest X-ray, ECG, further laboratory data) depend on the individual requirements set by the anesthesiologist involved. Further preparation of the patient is similar to that prior to percutaneous surgery (see Chapter 4).

5.1.4 Patient Information

The following complications may occur with retrograde URS:

- ureteral perforation (5%−20%), necessitating consecutive ureteral stenting;

Definition

Endoscopic exploration of the ureter for diagnostic or therapeutic purposes. Access to the ureter is established either transurethrally (retrograde URS) or percutaneously (antegrade URS).

– ureteral avulsion (0.3%), necessitating open surgical reconstruction;
– ureteral stenosis (1%–2%);
– vesicoureteral reflux (1%–2%).

The rate of complications is dependent upon the experience of the operator, as is the success rate. For distal ureteral calculi successful stone removal can be expected in more than 90% of the cases. This rate drops down to about 60% for removal of proximal ureteral calculi. The patient must be informed that acute complications of URS may require emergency surgery. Furthermore, it is advisable to preoperatively discuss with the patient what can be done in the case of a failed ureteroscopic approach:

– Perform ureterolithotomy to complete the stone removal in one session under any circumstances; or
– attempt another endoscopic approach in another, postponed session.

5.1.5 Anesthesia

Retrograde URS is routinely performed under regional (epidural catheter) or general anesthesia. General anesthesia should be preferred when time-consuming stone manipulations are to be expected (e.g., large, impacted calculi). Recently, first reports have been given on ureteroscopy under analgosedation only (Vögeli 1989). Although for a definitive assessment a broader experience has to be gained with this setting, the introduction of semirigid miniscopes holds promise for "anesthesia-free" ureteroscopy, at least for manipulations in the distal ureter.

5.1.6 Preoperative Adjuvant Measures

The patient is positioned in the lithotomy position on an urologic X-ray table (alternative: operating table plus C-arm). The patient's contralateral leg is abducted as far as possible to facilitate insertion of the ureteroscope sheath into the ureteral orifice and the distal ureter (Fig. 5.**1**).

For explorative cystoscopy, a cystoscope sheath the size of at least 21 Fr should be used. Following cystoscopy, the lens of the cystoscope can be removed and the ureteroscope can be passed through the cystoscope sheath. The cystoscope sheath provides drainage of the bladder during intravesical and intraureteral manipulation.

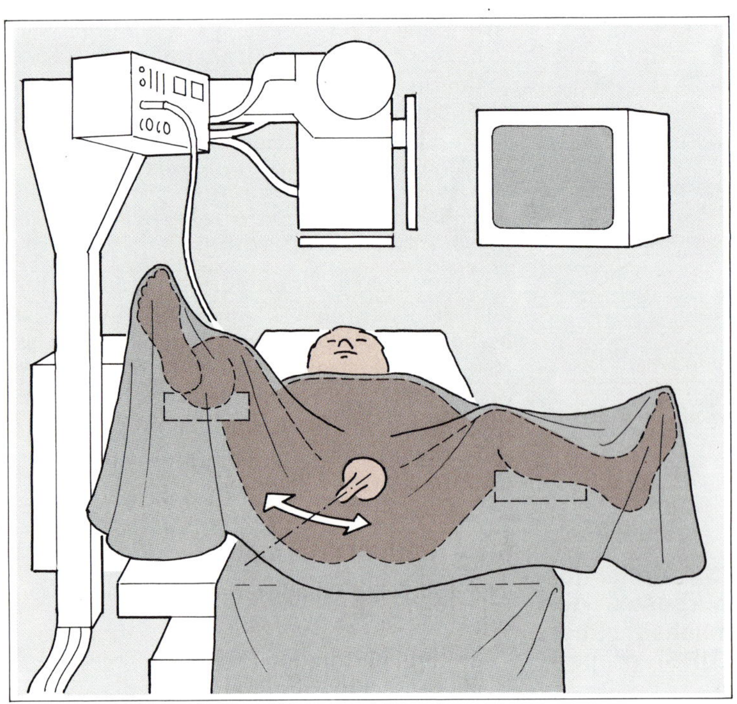

Fig. 5.1 **Asymmetric lithotomy position** for retrograde URS

Before starting with URS, a retrograde pyelogram is made to document the preoperative status of the ureter.

5.1.7 Technique and Strategy

5.1.7.1 Dilatation of the orifice. After endoscopically identifying the relevant ureteral orifice, it must be decided whether or not dilatation of the orifice is expected to be necessary. Miniscopes of 7–8 Fr diameter can virtually always pass the orifice without dilatation, whereas 11 or 12 Fr ureterscopes require preliminary dilatation in about 50% of the cases.

The following dilators are available:

– flexible olive-shaped bougies (9–15 Fr);
– Teflon bougies with a conical tip (7–15 Fr);
– Teflon telescope bougies (up to 15 Fr);
– cylindric or spherical dilatation catheters.

To meet the varying anatomical conditions, all types of dilators should be available at the beginning of the operation.

A further alternative for the dilatation of the ureteral orifice has recently been reported. Using intermittent pressure irrigation (Ureteromat, Storz Company), the orifice can be hydraulically dilated using the working channel of the ureteroscope. First reports on this technique (Perez-Castro, 1986; Eshghi, 1988) are promising; dilatation is safe, efficient, and reliable, and only about 1%–2% of the patients need additional dilating procedures. Moreover, the whole procedure of ureteroscopy is becoming substantially faster, since the same endoscopic instrument can be used throughout the procedure. The only concern raised against hydraulic dilatation is that the high pressure (up to 180 mmHg) and the high flow rate (up to 400 ml/sec) within the collecting system may cause pyelorenal reflux, and the subsequent absorption of irrigant and bacteria into the vasculature (Lyon, 1988). The actual adverse side-effects of these high-pressure forces is still the subject of discussion. Preliminary experimental data suggest that no harm is caused as long these forces are only applied within the bladder of the extreme lower ureter for the short process of dilatation (Eshghi, 1988).

If conventional dilatation is performed, placement of a guide wire in the ureter — preferably advanced beyond the stone — always makes the procedure safer and easier, no matter what sort of dilators are used (Fig. 5.2). With the guide wire in place, the dilatation process can be monitored fluoroscopically. This speeds up the dilatation considerably, particularly when dilators are used that must be inserted and removed one by one. If insertion of a guide wire is impossible (intramural stone), dilatation must be made very carefully under endoscopic vision. Particularly in this situation, any undue force should be avoided in order to prevent perforation of the intramural ureter with the nonguided bougie.

For a consecutive smooth passage of the ureteroscope, dilatation should not be limited to the orifice; rather, the whole intramural ureter should be dilated. Depending on the size of the ureteroscope, dilatation up to 13–14 Fr is sufficient.

5.1.7.2 Ureteroscopy. Depending on the purpose of the endoscopic operation, various instruments are available (Fig. 5.3).

Rigid ureteroscopes. The rigid ureteroscopes come with sizes from 9–13 Fr and with lengths of 30 or 40 cm; straight or oblique working channels make the crucial difference. For rigid auxiliary tools such as the ultrasound probe, the resectoscope loop, the cold knife, and the

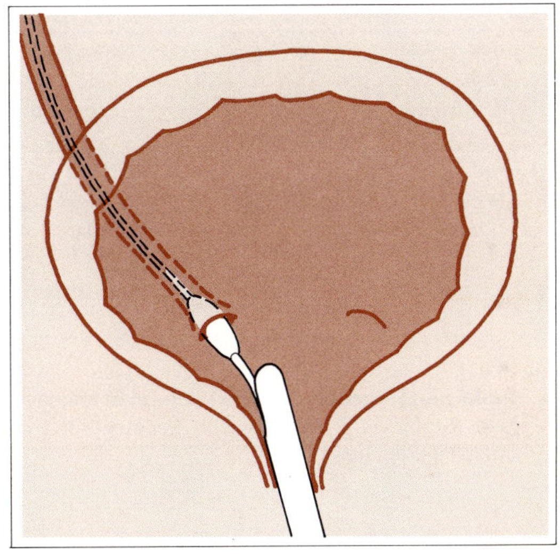

Fig. 5.2 **Dilatation of the orifice and intramural ureter** using flexible olive-shaped bougies. Guide wire in the ureter

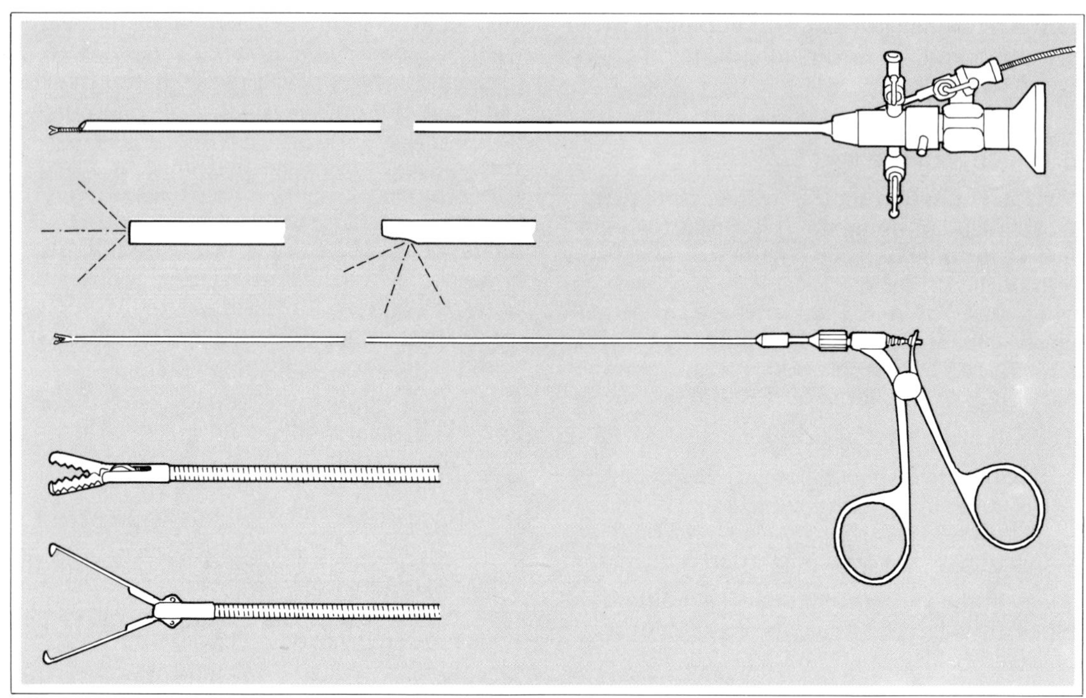

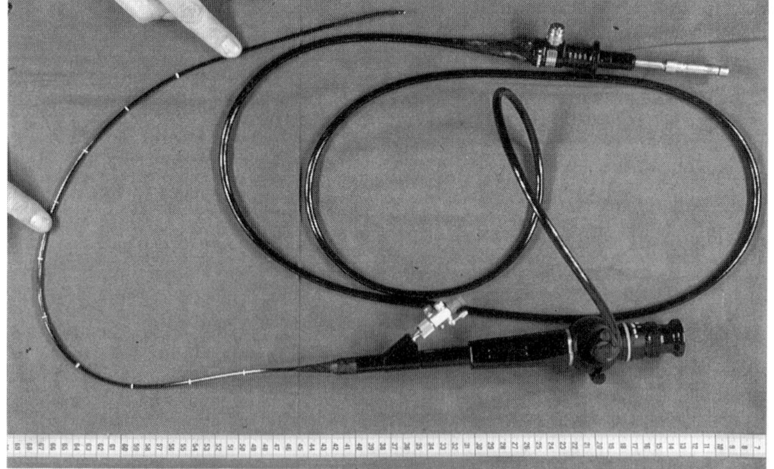

Fig. 5.**3**

a **Rigid ureteroscope** (11.5 Fr) with exchangeable lens (Storz); rigid forceps with various forms of grasping branches

b **Flexible ureteroscope** (10.5 Fr) with steerable tip (Olympus)

rigid forceps, the straight working channel (necessitating an offset or oblique lens) is mandatory. As the endoscopic orientation is easier with the straight lens, a system with interchangeable telescopes is naturally advantageous. On the other hand, these systems need more space, requiring at least an outer diameter of 11.5 Fr. The alternative is an instrument with an integrated telescope (straight or offset lens), requiring only a 9.5–10.5 Fr outer diameter of the sheath.

For manipulations within the ureter, a 0° or 5° telescope is used. For further diagnostic purposes (inspection of the RCS) a 70° lens is available (Fig. 5.**4**).

Semirigid ureteroscopes. Recently, 7–8 Fr semirigid ureteroscopes have been presented

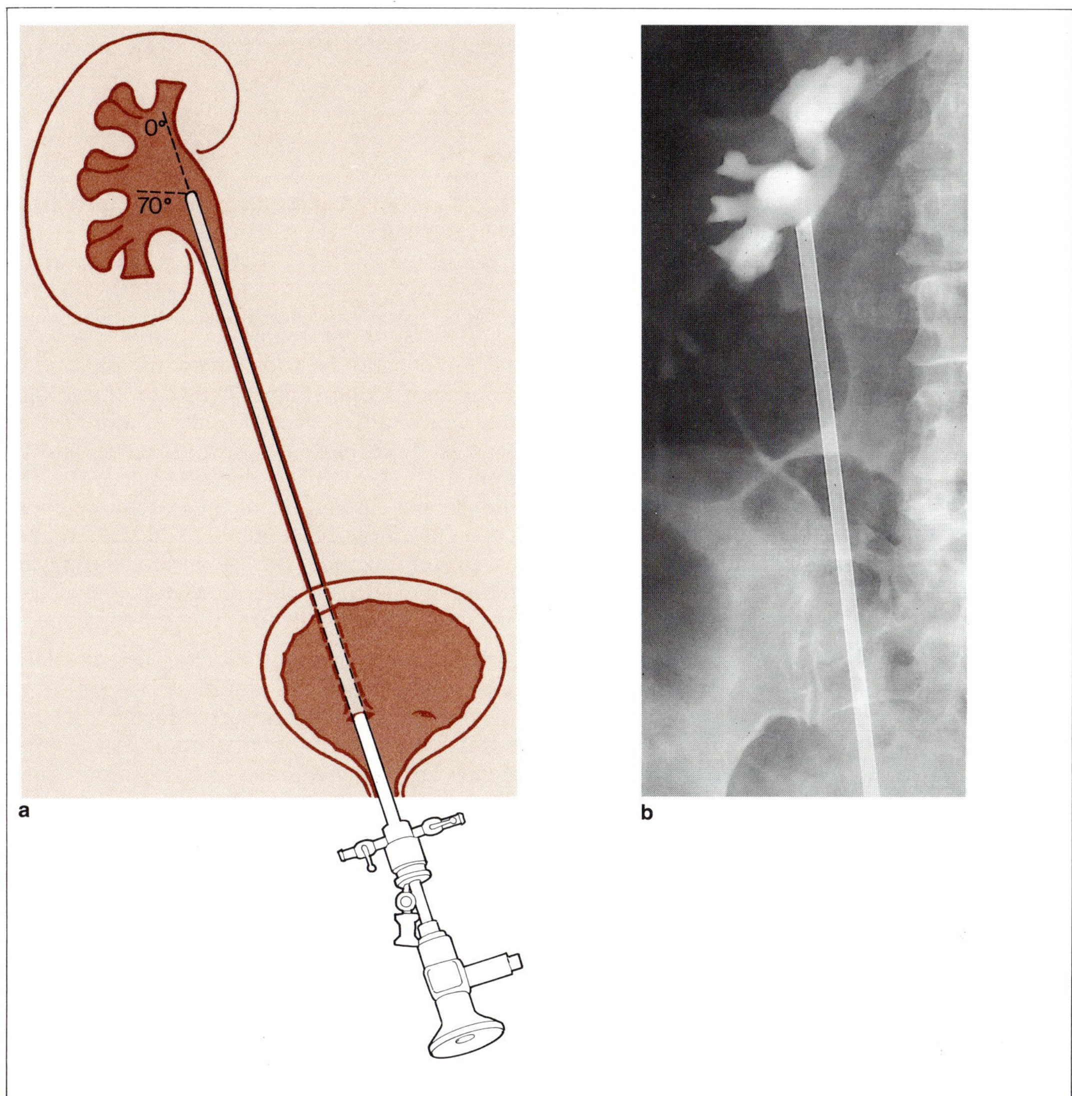

Fig. 5.**4a, b Retrograde exploration of the upper urinary tract.** For inspection of the RCS, a 0° and a 70° telescope is available

(Dretler, 1988) in association with laser lithotripsy. Reportedly, this endoscopes have some striking advantages, for example

– due to the small sheath diameter, virtually every ureter can be negotiated without preliminary dilation procedures;
– due to the fiberoptic system, the instrument can be bent without compromising the field of vision.

Further experience of other operators must be awaited before a definitive assessment of this system is possible.

Flexible ureteroscopes. Flexible ureteroscopes are available with a steerable (8.5–10.5 Fr) or nonsteerable (6–8 Fr) tip. For better maneuverability, the steerable tip is obviously preferable. However, the problem with the 10.5 Fr flexible scope is that introduction through the orifice and the intramural ureter may be difficult or impossible, since the force applied at the end of the scope to move it forward is not sufficiently translated to the tip of the instrument. Another problem of the flexible scopes in general is that if any manipulation must be carried out with auxiliary tools (laser lithotripsy, EHL) "three hands" are necessary to handle the endoscope and the auxiliary instrument.

For stone manipulations, mainly rigid instruments are currently used since they bring about the utilization of various efficient auxiliary tools. Flexible ureteroscopes are still limited to diagnostic purposes. However this may change if the technical problems and the costs of laser lithotripsy are improved in the future.

According to the aforementioned reasons, the following practical hints refer primarily to the use of conventional rigid ureteroscopes.

When introducing the endoscope, the beveled tip of the sheath is rotated 80° as it passes the ostium and then gently twisted back again (Fig. 5.**5**). The further instrument passage up the ureter is performed under endoscopic vision and continuous irrigation until the stone is visualized. A guide wire or a ureteral catheter in place facilitates orientation in the bladder, passage of the orifice, and advancement up the ureter (Fig. 5.**6**).

Technical problems and their solution. Narrowing of the ureter. At any level of the ureter

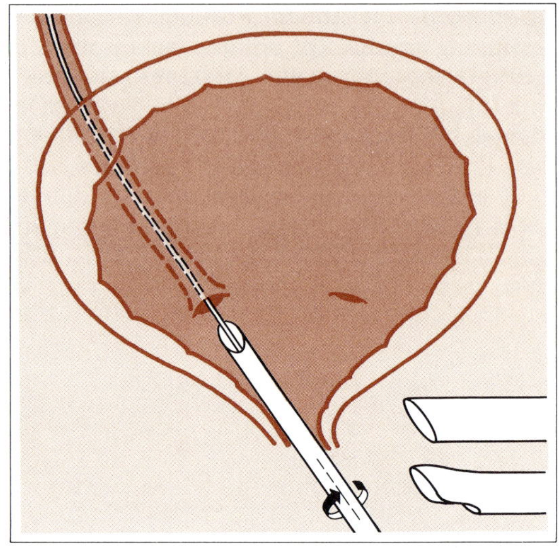

Fig. 5.**5** **Insertion of the ureteroscope into the ureter by rotation**

the lumen may be too narrow for passage of the ureteroscope (Fig. 5.**7**) due to physiologic anatomical differences or other conditions (see page 109). In these cases, no force should be applied to overcome the obstacle with the endoscope. Dilatation of the narrow segment can be attempted in a manner similar to that of the ureteral orifice. For dilatations during the course of URS, a balloon dilator is available that can be passed through the ureteroscope.

If the balloon does not effect sufficient dilatation, a wire-guided dilatation using conical or olive-shaped bougies under fluoroscopic control is sometimes more efficient and successful. However, this technique is much more time-consuming because the ureteroscope has to be completely removed and then reinserted after dilatation.

In rare cases, the narrowing cannot be overcome by any dilatation technique whatsoever (fixation of the ureter by fibrous stenosis). In this situation, too, any undue force is to be avoided. Instead, the endoscopic procedure should be discontinued and an alternative way of treatment considered. Depending on the stone site, the amount of obstruction, and the consent of the patient, either antegrade URS, open surgery, or a percutaneous nephrostomy are the available alternatives.

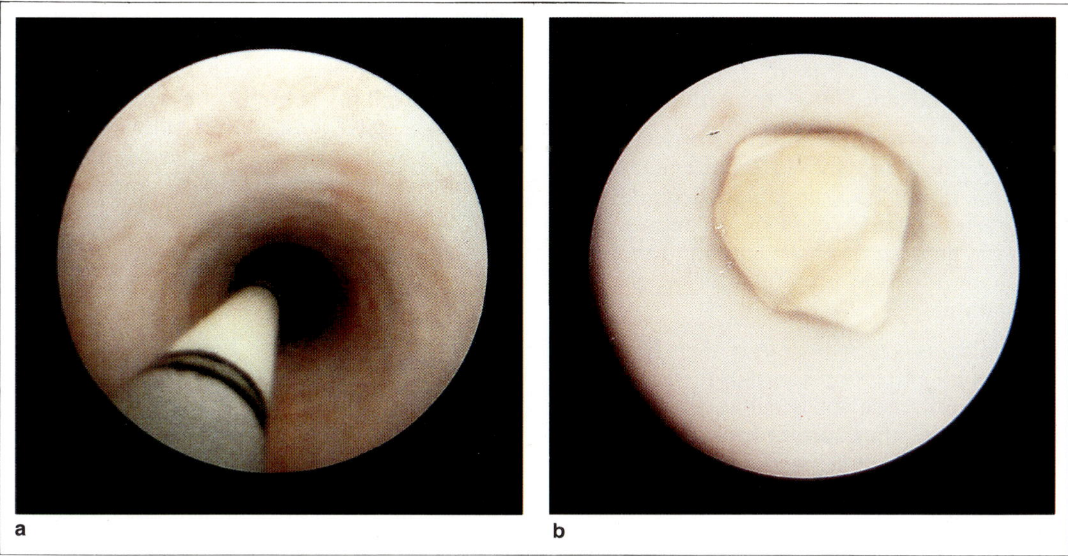

Fig. 5.6

a **Endoscopic image of the ureter;** ureteral catheter as guide splint in situ

b **Visualization of the stone**

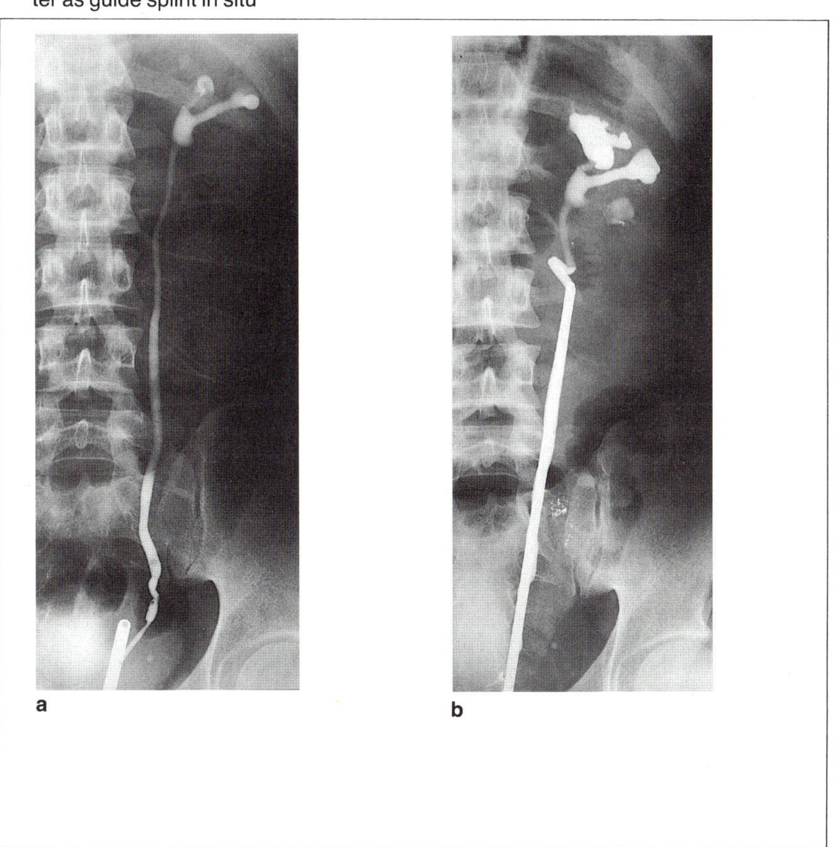

Fig. 5.**7 a, b** **Narrow proximal ureter.** Passage of the ureteroscope beyond this point is impossible. Any attempt to advance the instrument further (**b**) results in kinking of the ureter (danger of avulsion of the ureter!)

Kinking of the ureter. A tortuous ureter can be overcome by insertion of a ureteral catheter that straightens the lumen. The ureteroscope can then be advanced over the catheter.

5.1.7.3 Stone manipulation. The decision of whether the stone should be extracted as a whole or rather be fragmented first, depends on the site and the size of the calculus as well as on the amount of obstruction and the reactive changes of the ureteral wall (edema, inflammation).

If the calculus is mobile or only slightly impacted and total extraction through the orifice and the distal ureter seems feasible with regard to the stone size, the Dormia basket is the most efficient tool at hand (Fig. 5.**8**).

Technically, the most difficult part of stone basketing is to engage the stone safely within the wires of the basket. For this purpose, the closed Dormia basket is passed beyond the stone and then opened and carefully withdrawn. When the wires are at the level of the stone, they are gently twisted in both directions until the stone is engaged. Continuous visual control is essential when the Dormia basket is closed in order to prevent engagement of the ureteral wall. For a clear vision, intermittent pressure irrigation may be necessary; this can be achieved by the use of a transfusion cuff.

When the stone is safely engaged and mobile, the entire instrument assembly is slowly pulled back, again under continuous irrigation and endoscopic control. When the ureteral orifice is reached, a resistance must usually be overcome in order to manipulate the stone into the bladder. While any force should be avoided during passage of the Dormia basket through the mobile part of the ureter a "little" force can be applied to overcome the resistance at the ureteral orifice, since it is at this level that the ureter is firmly embedded within the bladder wall.

Stone extraction with forceps is only feasible for small, mobile calculi since the pressure of the forceps branches is normally too weak to mobilize impacted calculi. Likewise, forceps extraction may be useful for mobile fragments of a "Steinstrasse" after ESWL and for the fragments produced by USL.

Impacted calculi, causing an edematous reaction of the ureteral wall in the vicinity of the stone, are better approached by lithotripsy. This is preferably done with the ultrasound probe, due to a lesser risk of damaging the ureteral wall in comparison with EHL. An attempt to pass these stones with the Dormia basket is likely to result in a perforation of the edematous ureter. Likewise, large calculi, which cannot be maneuvered through the ureter or the ureteral orifice without considerable force, should be fragmented and then extracted in several steps.

As previously mentioned, the technique most widely used for endoureteral stone disintegration is USL (Fig. 5.**9**). The same hardware as for percutaneous lithotripsy can be used, with the probe length and diameter adjusted to the size of the ureteroscope.

The use of USL under fluoroscopic control is now considered obsolete, as the oblique or offset telescope enables continuous visual control of the procedure.

With the hollow ultrasound probe, small stone particles are immediately removed during the lithotripsy process by suction through the probe. Accidental contact of the probe tip with the ureteral wall is harmless unless it repeatedly occurs at the same spot (risk of mucosal injury) or if the probe tip is firmly pressed against the wall (risk of perforation).

If USL is applied continuously for several minutes, the probe may become hot. Thus, only limited (one minute) applications with short breaks should be performed in order to avoid the risk of thermal damage to the ureteral wall.

If severely impacted ureteral calculi are to be dealt with, USL should merely be used to disimpact the stone rather than to remove it completely. Prolonged maneuvers at the site of an edematous ureteral wall enhance the risk of perforation as well as the long-term risk of secondary stenosis. In these situations, a ureteral stent should be placed following disimpaction of the stone; in addition the patient should be treated by ESWL or a second endoscopic approach in another session at a later date.

Fig. 5.**8a—c Endoscopic extraction of a ureter** ▶
stone using the Dormia basket

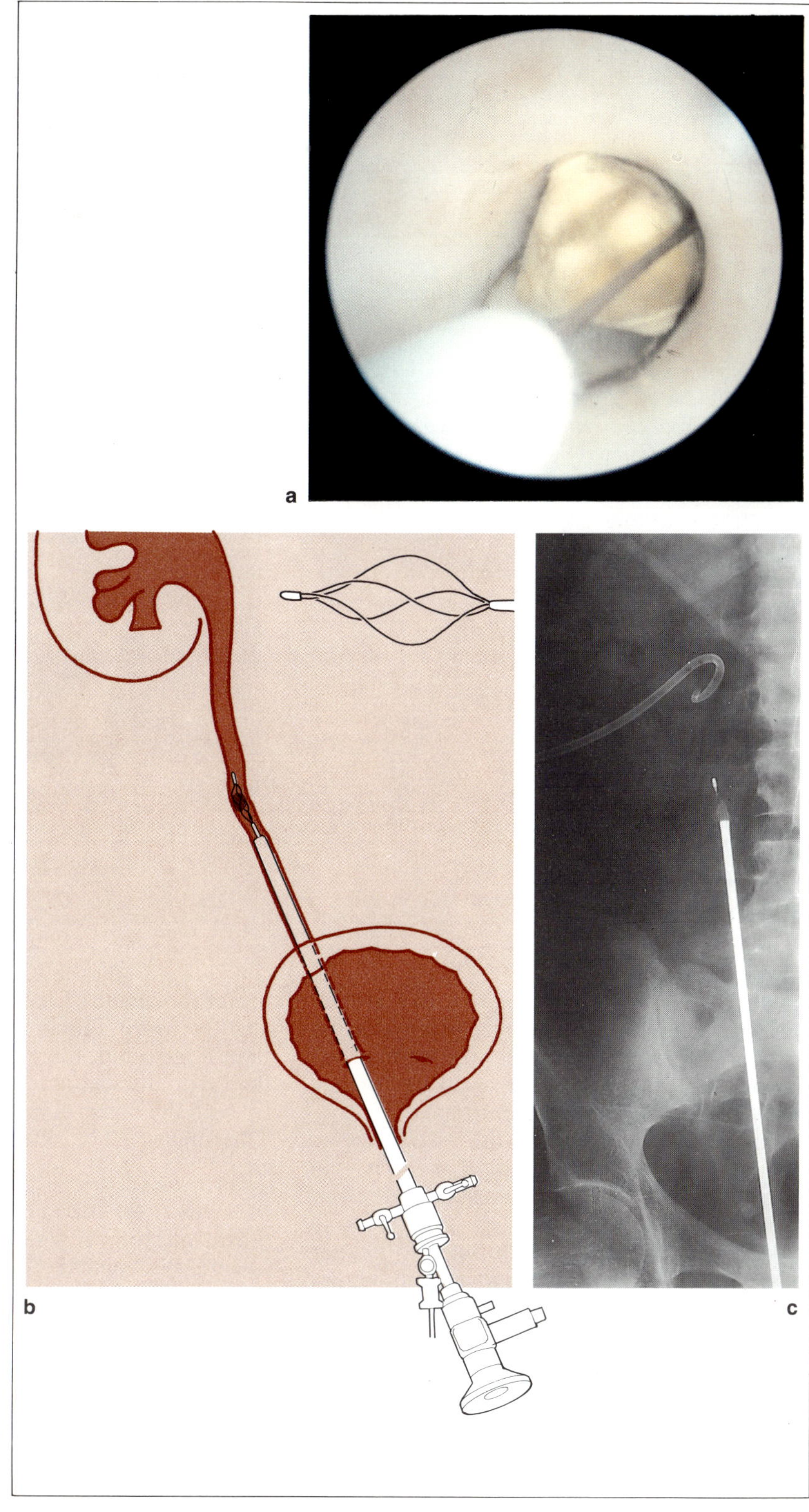

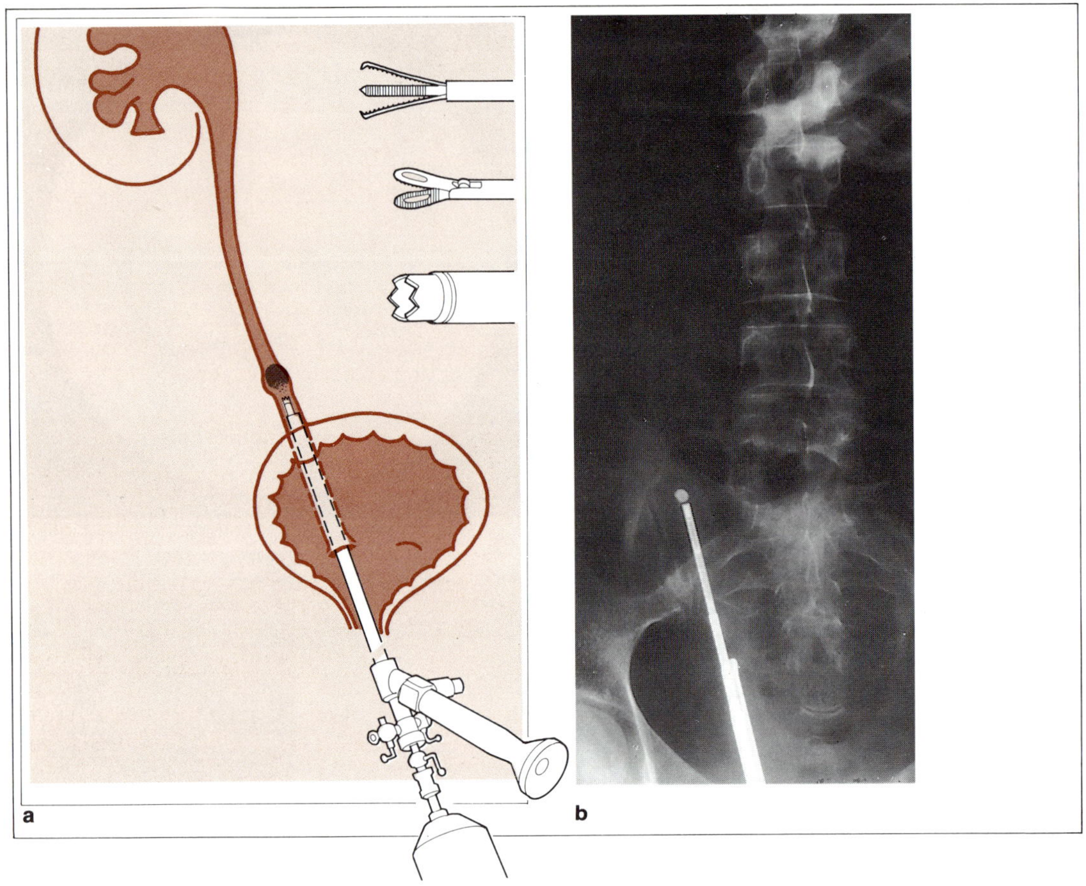

Fig. 5.**9a,b**   **Endoureteral USL**

The same rule can be applied for an impacted "Steinstrasse". At first, larger fragments are further disintegrated with the ultrasound probe until they can be removed by forceps. This procedure is repeated until the stone fragments can be passed with the instrument or with a guide wire. A ureteral stent is then placed and the procedure terminated. Complete removal of all stone fragments is not only tedious and time-consuming but also dangerous. Prolonged transuretheral manipulation imposes the risk of both long-term urethral and ureteral stenoses. Once the stone fragments of a "Steinstrasse" are disimpacted, the residual concretions may pass spontaneously without any problems.

More recently, EHL has been used by several authors (Willscher, 1988) for fragmentation of ureteral calculi. Electrohydraulic energy is slightly more efficient and therefore faster than ultrasound, but it has the clear disadvantage that any contact of the discharging probe tip with the ureteral wall results in perforation. This makes EHL obviously more hazardous than USL.

Moreover, no suction is provided for the removal of stone fragments, which must all be secondarily removed by forceps. Hence, the authors hold that the advantages of EHL do not outweigh its drawbacks.

The final goal of utilizing a small, flexible probe for endoureteral lithotripsy may be better realized by laser technology in the near future. To date, the device with the best documented clinical results is the pulsed dye-laser

(Dretler 1986, 1988; Watson 1983, 1987). The dye-laser allows the use of a fiber of only 200 µm, and it provides sufficient energy and an appropriate wave length to disintegrate the majority of calculi. Only very hard stones (calcium oxalate monohydrate, cystine) may resist fragmentation by laser lithotripsy (Dretler, 1988).

The *Nd:YAG* laser has also proved its stone-fragmenting abilities in a clinical setting. However, this laser still needs at least a 600 µm fiber, which diminishes its usefulness particularly in conjunction with flexible scopes; if the steerable scope-tip is deflected more than 60°, the fiber breaks.

The common problem of all laser devices currently in clinical use for lithotripsy is the comparably high price, on the one hand, and the comparably low technical reliability, on the other hand. However, since there is intensive research in this field (see Chapter 8), further developments and improvements can be expected.

5.2 Antegrade URS

The higher the stone is located within the ureter, the greater the amount of problems that may arise from retrograde URS:

- While the pelvic part of the ureter can be reached with the ureteroscope in virtually every patient, passage of the instrument proximal to the iliac vessels may be impossible (due to the anatomical conditions) in up to 30% of the cases (Segura, 1984).
- Due to the long endoureteral way, injuries of the ureteral mucosa are more likely to be caused by the ureteroscope itself, particularly when stone manipulation is time-consuming and stone fragments have to be removed repeatedly by pulling out the entire instrument assembly.

The fact that the success rate for ureteroscopic stone removal in the upper ureter is significantly lower than in the distal ureter also reflects the aforementioned problems. Therefore, antegrade URS has its place in the algorithm for the management of ureteral calculi. If a transurethral endoscopic approach is unsuccessful, antegrade URS may be the last option available to avoid open surgery.

Preparing and informing the patient, anesthesia, and equipment are similar to PCNL and retrograde URS. In addition to the percutaneous armamentarium, a rigid ureteroscope (with a straight working channel for USL) can be used.

Since there is a varying angle between the percutaneous tract and the course of the upper ureter, the use of flexible endoscopes greatly facilitates antegrade endoscopic exploration. However, the problems of stone manipulation in conjunction with flexible scopes (see Chapter 4) must be kept in mind.

Since antegrade URS is mainly indicated when a stone in the upper ureter either cannot be mobilized for consecutive ESWL or cannot be managed transurethrally with the ureteroscope, the preliminary retrograde procedure should be terminated by placing a ureteral balloon catheter immediately below the stone. Percutaneous access to the renal collecting system is then installed via a lower or middle calyx. The rest of the procedure parallels that for percutaneous removal of renal calculi.

After dilatation of the tract and identification of the UPJ via nephroscopy, the ureteroscope is introduced through the nephroscope or Amplatz sheath. If a rigid ureteroscope is used, the kidney must be tilted by the nephroscope sheath until direct access to the ureter can be established (Fig. 5.**10**). Access to the ureter is facilitated by prior insertion of a guide wire.

In some cases (previous surgery, anatomical variations), the kidney may not be mobile enough to intubate the ureter with the rigid instument. In these cases, the exclusive use of the flexible nephroscope or ureteroscope allows access to the upper ureter. The problem of efficient stone manipulation in association with flexible scopes has already been mentioned (see above).

The same rules can be applied for antegrade endoureteral stone manipulation as for retrograde URS. Since the proximal ureter may be dilated, depending upon the degree of obstruction, total stone extraction may be easier than via the retrograde approach.

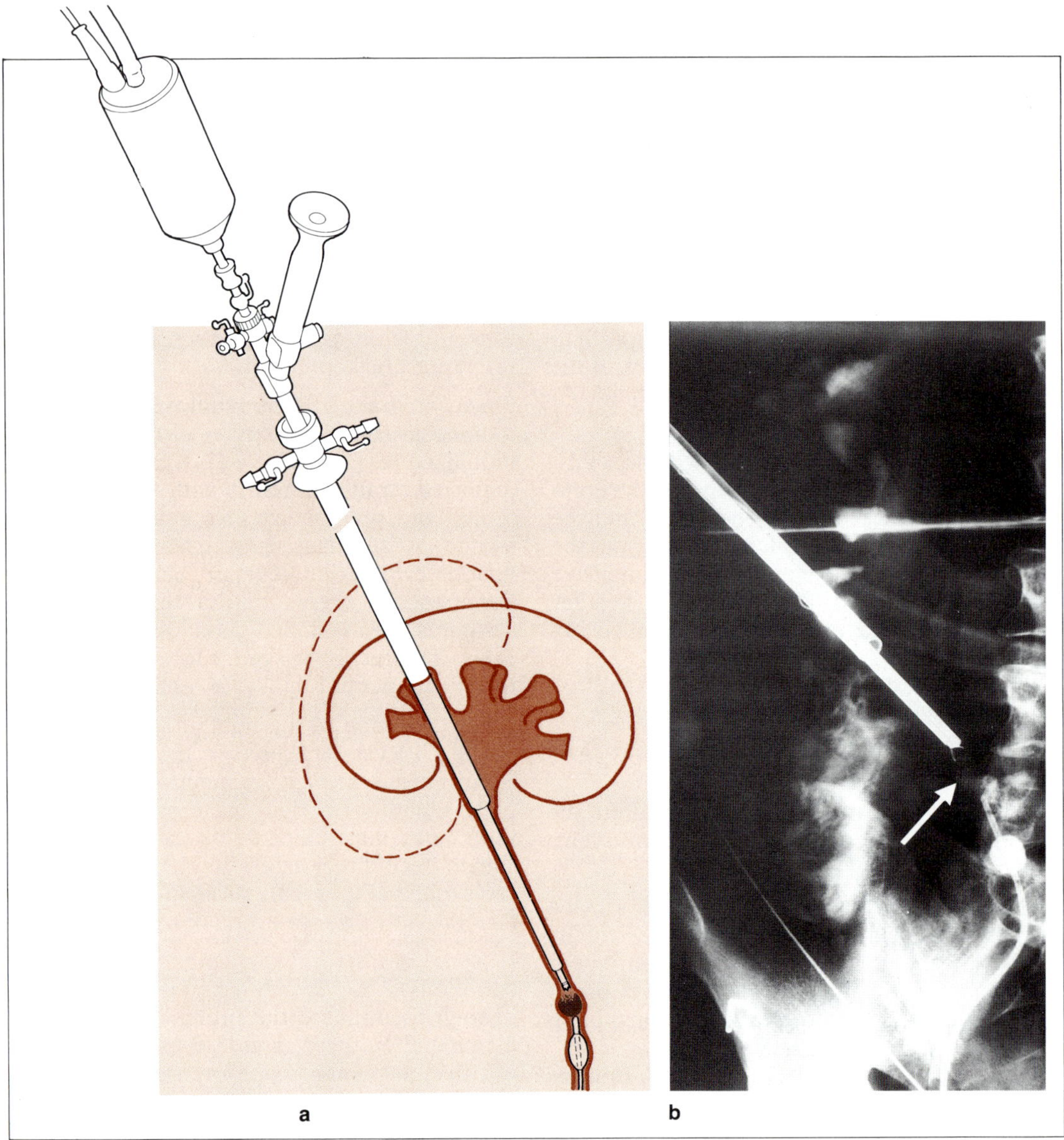

Fig. 5.10

a **Tilting of the kidney** using the nephroscope sheath facilitates insertion of the rigid sheath into the upper ureter

b **Antegrade stone extraction** from the proximal ureter using grasping forceps

5.3 **Risks and Complications**
(Table 5.**1**)

The following types of ureteral damage of varying degrees can arise at any level (dilatation, ureteroscopy, stone manipulation) of the procedure:

- superficial tears of the ureteral mucosa
- tears of the complete ureteral wall
- perforation
- avulsion of the ureter
- instrument breaking
- impacted Dormia basket

If a lesion of the ureter is suspected, the diagnosis should be confirmed by injection of dye via the ureteroscope. The management of ureteral injuries depends on the site and grade of the damage, and encompasses endourological as well as open surgical procedures.

Stenting of the ureter is sufficient in the case of

- perforation *after* stone extraction;
- superficial tears of the ureteral mucosa;
- short tears of the ureteral wall.

Percutaneous nephrostomy is indicated, if

- the ureteral stent does not ensure sufficient drainage of the kidney;
- a ureteral stent cannot be placed due to technical reasons;
- ureteral injury occurs before the stone is reached and no ureteral stent can be passed beyond the site of the stone.

Ureterolithotomy is performed

- after single or repeated unsuccessful URS (depending on the consent of the patient);
- in the case of an impacted Dormia basket.

Furthermore, open surgery is required when complete avulsion of the ureter has occurred. The actual technique for reconstruction depends upon the site of the injury, as follows:

- ureteral reimplantation (distal ureter)

Table 5.1   Complications of ureteroscopy (own data, N = 93)

– Perforation: ureteral stent	17	%
surgery	1	%
– Fever	5	%
– Stenosis: endourological therapy	1,5	%
surgery	0,5	%

- end-to-end anastomosis (middle ureter)
- ureteral pelvic anastomosis (upper ureter)

Late complications after ureteroscopy are

- stenosis of the ureter;
- vesicoureteral reflux (Table 5.**1**; for management see "follow-up").

5.4 **Follow-Up**

A ureteral stent is routinely placed after every ureteroscopic manipulation since obstruction of the ipsilateral kidney is likely to occur, owing to the postprocedural swelling of the ureteral mucosa. Moreover, contamination of the upper tract by the endoscopic manipulation must be expected, making free drainage of the kidney even more essential.

This rule should only be abandoned in the case of a very fast and easy procedure (i.e., no dilatation of the orifice, total stone extraction, or rapid stone disintegration with extraction of a few fragments).

The stent should be left in place for a period of at least 48 hours (after an uncomplicated procedure), and up to four weeks when injuries of the ureter have occurred (see "Complications").

Immediately after removal of the ureteral stent, sonographic evaluation of the ipsilateral kidney is a routine procedure performed to indicate any residual obstruction.

In case of residual hydronephrosis, the patient should be followed with further (weekly) sonographic checks. An IVP should be taken after six weeks, at the latest, in order to document the stone status, function of the kidney, and the ureteral passage.

If ureteral obstruction continues to be evident for more than three months, it must be considered to be irreversible. Depending on the degree of the obstruction, further examinations (diuretic sonography, percutaneous nephrostomy, antegrade or retrograde pyelography, Whittaker-test) are necessary in order to determine whether reconstructive surgery is indicated.

Strictures of the ureter are comparably rare but well-documented sequelae of URS (Stackl, 1986; Lytton, 1986; Kramolowsky, 1987, O'Brien, 1988). Depending on the site

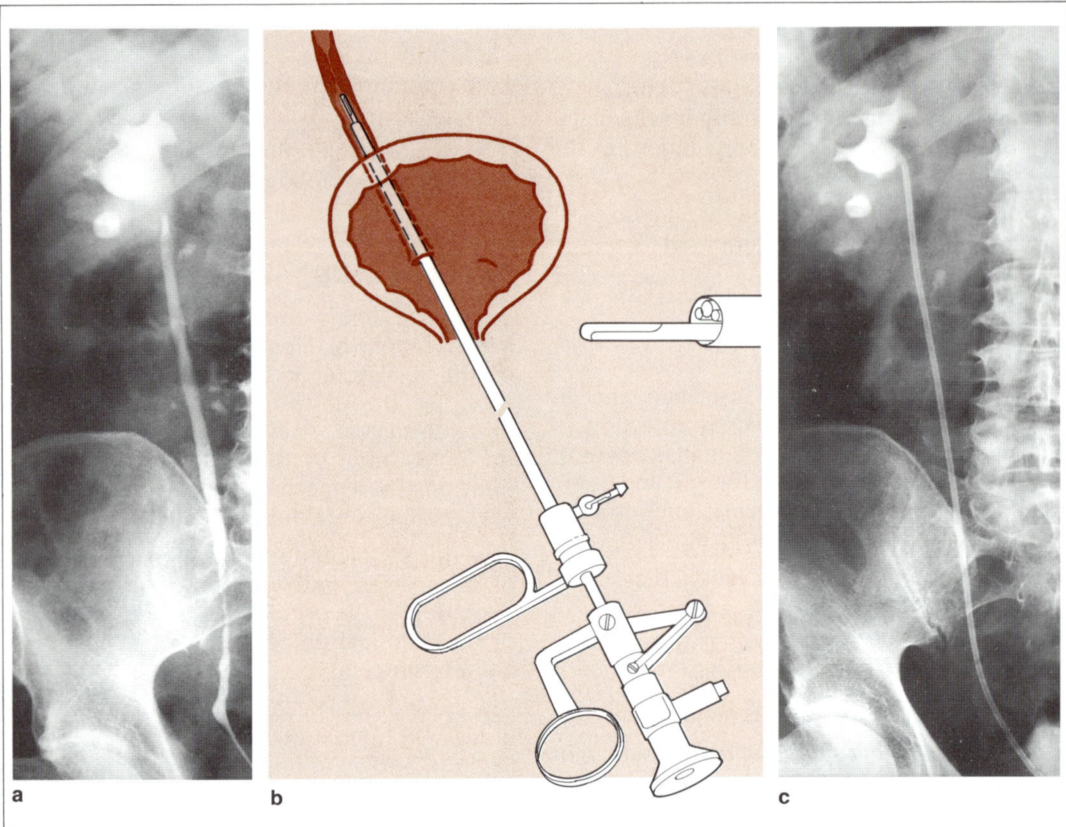

Fig. 5.**11a−c Endoscopic incision of a cicatrized stenosis (arrow) of the distal ureter** using the cold knife

and the length of the stricture, an endourological attempt can be made for reconstruction; when the narrowing has been negotiated with a guide wire, the stricture can either be incised under endoscopic guidance with the ureteroscope (Fig. 5.**11**) or dilated with an angioplasty balloon catheter. After these endoureteral procedures, a stent should be left indwelling for another four to six weeks.

If an endourological approach has failed to solve the problem, open surgery is necessary. The procedure of choice depends on the site of the stenosis; Psoas-hitch reimplantation (distal ureter), end-to-end anastomosis (middle ureter) and ureteral pelvic anastomosis (upper ureter) are the available options.

5.5 Results

All authors invariably report on a steep learning curve in conjunction with URS. This means that the success rate largely depends on the experience of the operator (Weinber, 1986). Once experience with more than 50−100 cases has been gained, virtually every calculus can be removed from the distal ureter, while the success rate for retrograde removal of proximal calculi can be expected to be only around 60%. If a complete armamentarium is at hand, antegrade URS is successful in more than 95% of the cases. Thus open surgery is still required for the removal of ureteral calculi in only 1%−2% of patients.

6 Open Surgery

Increasing experience with the endourologic technologies has made it possible to treat about 99% of all stone patients without the need for open surgery.

As a consequence, the following are the few indications remaining for an open approach to urinary calculi:

- ureteral calculi following unsuccessful URS or damage of the ureter in the course of URS (see Chapter 5)
- stones in conjunction with a stenosis of the UPJ, if the operator tends to perform open pyeloplasty rather than an endourologic incision of the stenosis (see Chapter 4)
- staghorn calculi in children, when multiple sessions (also requiring multiple general anesthesia) must be anticipated with the endourologic approach
- staghorn calculi with a predominantly peripheral stone burden in a deformed RCS (multiple caliceal neck stenosis; see, Chapter 3).

Because the authors still prefer open pyeloplasty to endourological incision in cases of congenital stenoses of the UPJ, the removal of a calculi in conjunction with this condition occurs from time to time; this also encompasses nephrotomies when caliceal calculi cannot be removed via the open renal pelvis.

The same holds for ureterolithomy, which is occassionally necessary when URS is unsuccessful.

6.1 Surgical Nephrotomy

Incision of the renal parenchyma for stone removal may become necessary when a UPJ stenosis associated with caliceal stones is surgically approached, or when the caliceal branches of a staghorn stone cannot be removed via the renal pelvis. In these situations, radial nephrotomies are the most "kidney preserv-ing" access to a renal calyx. Due to technical advancements, these nephrotomies can now be performed without clamping and cooling of the kidney in the majority of the cases.

The course of the peripheral vessels on the kidney surface can be mapped with the Doppler probe (Fig. 6.1), thus avoiding major bleeding, when the parenchyma is opened. Furthermore, the calyx stone can be located by use of a special 5 or 7 MHz ultrasound transducer (Fig. 6.1) whereby the exact direction from the kidney's surface to the calyx is simultaneously defined.

However, since vascular damage may occur in rare cases despite Doppler localization, the pedicle of the kidney should always be prepared for clamping, and crushed ice should be available to cool the renal surface.

Animal experiments (Fitzpatrick, 1980) and clinical trials (Türoff and Riedmüller, 1982; 1983) have shown that the radial nephrotomy technique keeps impairment of renal function at a minimum.

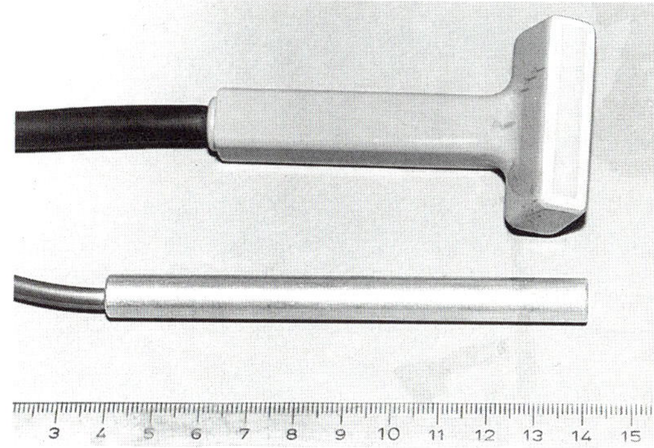

Fig. 6.1 **Ultrasound probe** (B mode, 5 or 7 MHz) for intraoperative stone location (top). Doppler probe (bottom) for vascular location in the renal parenchyma

6.2 Ureterolithotomy

The standard approach to the upper ureter is via a flank incision; approach to the lower ureter is via a pararectal incision. As ureterolithotomy is almost always performed secondary to a failed ureteroscopic approach, ureteral stenting is obligatory when the stone is removed. The stent is left in place for two to three weeks, with further follow-up paralleling that after URS (see Chapter 5).

6.3 Pyeloplasty

Operation guides are referred to for the many different techniques of open pyeloplasty. The standard technique used in our institution is the dismembered pyeloplasty (i.e., Anderson-Hynes or V-Y-procedure). With this technique, a wide access to the renal pelvis is provided and, in conjunction with a completely mobilized kidney, stone removal from the renal calyces is normally easy via the pelvic access. If an intrarenal, not grossly dilated pelvis has to be dealt with, the transpelvic caliceal access may be difficult or impossible. In these cases, nephrotomies are carried out according to the aforementioned principles.

7 Comparison of Second-Generation Lithotriptors

7.1 Introduction

Ten years after the first clinical application of ESWL by Chaussy et al. in 1980, technical evolution has resulted in the introduction of more than 20 "second-generation lithotriptors" (Table 7.1).

The development of second generation lithotriptors mainly concentrated on the utilization of different principles of shock wave generation, focusing, coupling, and localization system, with the aim of achieving the "golden standard of the Dornier HM3". The following was considered by the manufacturers during the development of the machines:

- the same range or even an extention of indications achieveable with the Dornier HM3
- pain-free application using minimal or no analgesia
- considerable cost reduction compared with the purchase price and operating expense of the Dornier HM3

Among the clinically used lithotriptors, seven machines have sparked interest since they proved to be successful in substantial clinical trials (Table 7.2). However, these studies are not completely comparable owing to the different range of indications and patient selection criteria of the machines. Therefore, a protocol has been designed comparing second-generation lithotriptors in practical use and using in vitro studies (Table 7.3).* The following issues were compared:

- shock wave efficacy (using two in vitro models)

---

* We would like to acknowledge those urologic departments that participated in this study and also thank the lithotriptor manufacturers for their assistance.

- pain during treatment (self-trial)
- handling of the lithotriptor in clinical ESWL

7.2 Materials and Methods
7.2.1 Shock Wave Efficiency

Physical characterization of shock waves is problematic because there are no standardized hydrophones available for measurements of shock wave characteristics (i.e., rise time of the shock wave front, duration of impulses, peak pressure). Therefore, the results differ significantly when different probes are used. For this reason, two stone models were used for in vitro studies to determine the "punch" of each machine. To begin with, the authors counted the number of impulses necessary for complete, fine disintegration of standardized 1.2 cm chalk cubes at the mean treatment energy of each lithotriptor. In addition, they used a standardized piece of plaster (3.5 × 3.5 × 1.5 cm), to which 100 shock waves were applied, using various shock wave energies. In this model, the volume of the cavity produced by the different shock wave sources was measured.

An interesting study has recently been published by Coleman and Saunders comparing the acoustic field of the same lithotriptors tested in the authors' study. Therefore, some of their results are included in the tables (i.e., acoustic energy per impulse, pressure at skin); significant correlations were found.

7.2.2 Classification of Pain

The sensation of pain induced by the different lithotriptors was tested in a self-trial treating the kidney and bladder at increasing levels up to the mean treatment energy used clinically. The pain was classified in accordance with the following dolor scale: 1 = absolutely pain-free; 2 = uncomfortable but tolerable sensation at

Table 7.1   Characteristics of second-generation lithotriptors

	Shock Wave Generation	Focusing (aperture)	Coupling	Locating	Clinical Use Since
Dornier:					
HM3	Underwater electrode (80 nF)	Semiellipsoid (15 cm)	Complete water bath	2 under-couch X-ray tubes	1980
HM3, modified	Underwater electrode (40 nF)	Semiellipsoid (17 cm)	Complete water bath	2 under-couch X-ray tubes	1986
HM4	Underwater electrode (40 nF)	Semiellipsoid (17 cm)	Water cushion	2 under-couch X-ray tubes	1986
MPL 9000	Underwater electrode (80 nF)	Semiellipsoid (22 cm)	Water cushion	1 lateral ultrasound + 1 coaxial ultrasound	1987
MFL 5000	Underwater electrode (40 nF)	Semiellipsoid (17 cm)	Water cushion	1 rotating under-couch tube	1988
Compact	Electromagnetic element	Acoustic lens (14 cm)	Water cushion	1 lateral ultrasound	1989
Technomed:					
Sonolith 3000	Underwater electrode (50,000 shocks per electrode set)	Semiellipsoid (22 cm/16 cm)	Partial water bath	1 lateral ultrasound + 1 coaxial ultrasound (1988)	1985
Siemens:					
Lithostar	Electromagnetic element	Acoustic lens (12 cm)	Water cushion	2 over-couch X-ray tubes	1986
Wolf:					
Piezolith 2300	3000 piezoelectric elements	Spherical alignment (50 cm)	Partial water bath	2 coaxial ultrasound scanners	1987
EDAP:					
LT01	320 piezoelectric elements	Spherical (54 cm)	Water cushion	1 coaxial ultrasound scanner	1986
Yachiyoda:					
Extracorporeal Microexplosion Lithotriptor	Lead azide pellet	Semiellipsoid	Complete water bath	1 rotating C-arm/ X-ray	1986
Medstone:					
1050	Underwater electrode	Semiellipsoid (14 cm)	Water cushion	1 rotating over-couch tube	1987
Northgate:					
SD-3	Underwater electrode	Semiellipsoid	Water cushion	Coaxial ultrasound	1987
Nitech:					
Lithotriptor	Underwater electrode	Semiellipsoid	Water cushion	Coaxial ultrasound	1987
John Hopkins:					
Lithotriptor	Underwater electrode	Semiellipsoid	Water cushion	Coaxial ultrasound	1987
Direx:					
Tripter X1	Underwater electrode	Semiellipsoid (20 cm)	Water cushion	Adaptable to X-ray or ultrasound	1987

Table 7.1   Characteristics of second-generation lithotriptors (continued)

	Shock Wave Generation	Focusing (aperture)	Coupling	Locating	Clinical Use Since
Biolithos:					
Mark III	Underwater electrode	Semiellipsoid	Water cushion	2 under-couch X-ray tubes	1989
Lithoring:					
Multi One	Underwater electrode	Semiellipsoid (25 cm)	Water cushion	1 rotating X-ray tube	1989

Table 7.2   Clinical results of new lithotriptors

	Dornier HM3	Dornier HM3, modified	Dornier HM4*	Dornier MPL 9000	Technomed Sonolith	Siemens Lithostar	Wolf Piezolith	EDAP LT01
	(N = 3,700)	(N = 334)	(N = 130)	(N = 104)	(N = 270)	(N = 628)	(N = 378)	(N = 370)
Stone location (%):								
Calix	50.0	39.6	54.6	69.0	60.5	52.1	56.9	64.0
Pelvis	28.0	26.9	19.2	24.0	34.1	26.0	15.9	37.0
Branched	5.0	2.4	3.8	3.0	2.3	1.0	4.2	—
Ureter	17.0	31.0	29.4	2.0	3.1	20.9	23.0	9.0
Upper	14.0	20.3	26.0	1.0	3.1	14.1	11.4	5.3
Middle	—	6.6	—	—	—	—	5.0	—
Lower	3.0	4.2	3.4	1.0	—	6.8	6.6	4.7
Mean size (mm)	13	12	11	12	13	14	13	13
Treatment data:								
Number of impulses	1,268	1,997	1,117	1,500	1,750	1,260	2,855	3,300
Successful disintegration (%)	97.0	99.2	99.9	91.0	95.0	97.0	94.5	87.0
Auxilliary measures (%)								
Before ESWL	10.0	21.6	6.0	11.0	14.5	27.0	14.8	3.9
After ESWL	14.0	5.1	10.4	3.0	6.9	6.9	14.37	3,9
2nd or 3rd session	14.0	13.6	8.0	18.0	13.0	11.4	45.0	13.0
Treatment time (min)	33	30	45	45	40	60	49	44
Perirenal hematoma (%)	0.3	0.2	—	—	0.4	0.3	—	0.6
Stone-free after 3 months (%)	73.0	75.0	60.0	75.0	81.0	69.0	72.0	61.0

* 80 nF generator

Table 7.3 Tested lithotriptors

Lithotriptor	Stone Center
Dornier:	
HM3	Orange County Kidney Stone Center, Ireland
	Hôpital Edward Herriot, Lyon, France
HM3+	Katharinen Hospital, Stuttgart, FRG
HM4	Munich University Clinic, Grosshadern, FRG
	Tübingen University Clinic, FRG
MPL 9000	Katharinen Hospital, Stuttgart, FRG
Technomed:	
Sonolith 2000 and 3000	Hôpital Edward Herriot, Lyon, France
	American Hospital, Paris, France
Wolf:	
Piezolith 2200 and 2300	Kreiskrankenhaus Kempten, FRG
Siemens:	
Lithostar	Mainz University Clinic, FRG
	Mannheim University Clinic, FRG
EDAP:	
LT01	Clinique Porte de Choisy, Paris, France

the surface of the skin; 3 = slight superficial pain, intolerable over 100 shocks; 4 = slight visceral pain, intolerable over 10 shocks; and 5 = severe, intolerable pain.

7.2.3 Handling the Lithotriptor

After introduction by the local urologist, several (3 to 15) ESWL treatments were performed in a clinical setting. The following criteria were taken into consideration: (1) Spatial requirements of the machine; (2) preparation time for treatment; (3) layout and flexibility of the different panels; (4) the training period (learning curve) required for operating the lithotriptor; and (5) the advantages of special features of each machine such as respiratory triggering, auto-focus, multifunctional table, variation of shock wave energy and frequency, and adaptable C-arm.

7.3 Technical Data of Lithotriptors

7.3.1 Shock Wave Operation and Coupling

Dornier first-generation and second-generation lithotriptors still use the underwater electrode for shock wave generation (Table 7.**4**). In contrast, shock waves are generated by the

Table 7.4 Shock wave (SW) generation and coupling of tested lithotriptors

	Coupling	SW Generation
Dornier HM3	Water bath	Electrode
Dornier HM4 and MPL 9000	Water cushion	Electrode
MFL 5000	Water cushion	Electrode
Lithostar	Water cushion	Electromagnetic element
Sonolith 2000	Partial water bath	Long-term electrode
Piezolith 2300	Partial water bath	Piezoelectric
EDAP LT01	Water cushion	Piezoelectric

Lithostar with the aid of an electromagnetic element. The Piezolith 2300 and the EDAP LT01 produce shock waves with the aid of piezoelectric elements focused by spherical alignment of the energy sources. The Wolf

Piezolith 2300 and the EDAP LT01 contain 3000 and 320 shock wave elements, respectively. The Sonolith has a long-term electrode that allows 100 treatments per electrode. The majority of second-generation lithotriptors have a water cushion for shock wave coupling. Only the Sonolith 3000 and Piezolith 2300 use a partial water bath.

7.3.2 Locating Systems

Several different types of locating systems are integrated in the various machines. Generally, the locating systems are divided into those using fluoroscopy and those using ultrasound (Table 7.5). The Dornier HM4 has two under-couch tubes; the Lithostar has two over-couch tubes. Only one rotating under-couch tube is installed in the new multifunctional Dornier MFL 5000 (Fig. 7.1), which, theoretically, might be preferred to over-couch systems because of the lower radiation exposure for both the patient and the operator.

Other lithotriptors use ultrasound for stone localization. The Piezolith and EDAP LT01 use coaxial ultrasound systems. The Sonolith has a lateral probe; a coaxial probe is planned for real-time scanning. Both systems — coaxial and lateral — are realized in the MPL 9000.

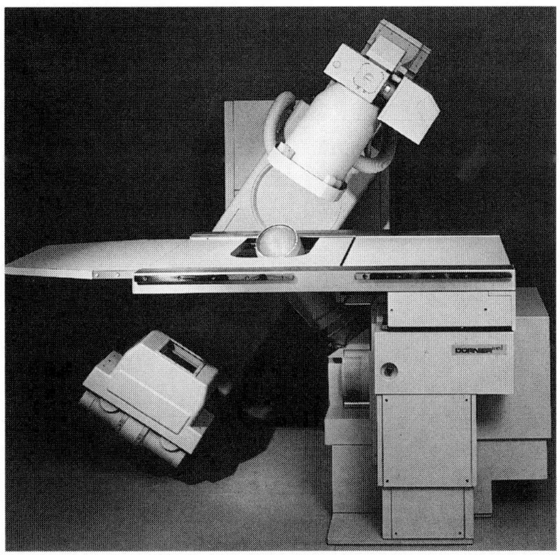

Fig. 7.1 **Multifunctional lithotriptor Dornier MFL 5000**

7.4 Results

7.4.1 In Vitro Efficacy of Lithotriptors

Model 1 (disintegration of chalk cube). Table 7.6 demonstrates that all second-generation lithotriptors allowing pain-free treatment or

Table 7.5 **Locating systems and problems of tested lithotriptors**

	Locating System	Problems
Dornier HM3+ and HM4	2 under-couch tubes	Stones close to vertebral column Slightly opaque calculi
Lithostar	2 over-couch tubes	
Dornier MFL 5000	1 under-couch tube	
Piezolith 2300	Ultrasound (2 coaxial probes)	Midureteral calculi Multiple stones (e.g., after PCNL)
EDAP LT01	Ultrasound coaxial	
Sonolith 3000	Ultrasound lateral	
Dornier MPL 9000	Ultrasound lateral and coaxial	

Table 7.6 Second-generation lithotriptors. Shock wave efficacy using stone model (1.2 cm chalk cube) at mean treatment energy

Lithotriptor	Energy setting	Impulses	Focal size (cm)*	Acoustic energy** in focal zone (mJ)
Dornier HM3	20 kV	80− 100	10.0 × 1.6	90
Dornier HM3+ and HM4	20 kV	350− 400	4.0 × 7.5	No measurements
MPL 9000	18 kV	480− 560	3.4 × 3.5	No measurements
Sonolith	13 kV	320− 380	5.5 × 1.5	30
Lithostar	19 kV	420− 470	9.5 × 0.9	17
Piezolith	IV	830− 850	1.2 × 0.2	2
EDAP LT01	10%	1,500−3,000***	2.3 × 0.5	3

  * Data provided by different companies
 ** Measurements by Coleman and Saunders, 1989
*** Data of the prototype (model 1) after revision, and of model 65

treatment under intravenous analgesia required a higher number of shock waves for disintegration of the piece of chalk compared with the standard Dornier HM3. Furthermore, these results correlate reciprocally with the focal size. Focal size is considerably smaller in lithotriptors with a large aperture, particularly in those machines using piezoceramic elements for shock wave generation.

The small focal size of the shock wave may be the reason why a higher number of shock waves is required with some types of lithotriptors. These data correlate with clinical experience showing that piezosystems require a significantly higher number of shocks for de-finitive stone disintegration than machines with electrohydraulic or electromagnetic shock wave sources (Table 7.**3**).

On the other hand, such a small focal size may allow fine, punctuate fragmentation (i.e., for treatment of staghorns). Figure 7.**2a** depicts a cavity produced by the Piezolith 2300. Except for the EDAP LT01 and the Dornier MPL 9000, such cavities have not been achieved with shock waves generated by other second-generation lithotriptors.

Model 2 (cavity in plaster cube per 100 shocks). Figure 7.**3a** demonstrates the low range of energy of the piezoceramic system and the wide range of energy provided by the Dornier electrode, particularly by the MPL 9000. Model 2 also reflects the focal sice in that even on maximal energy, the cavity produced by 100 impulses using the piezoceramic system is small. On the other hand, except with the MPL 9000, which provides a small focal size owing to the aperture of the ellipsoid, such a small cavity was never produced by the electrohydraulic or electromagnetic systems (Fig. 7.**4**) tested in this study.

Clinically, evaluations are necessary for determining whether the wide range of energy demonstrated by the MPL 9000 in the authors' in vitro studies is advantageous. Theoretically, in the majority of cases, pain-free treatment can be performed at low energy levels (14−16 kV). Additionally, there is the possibility of

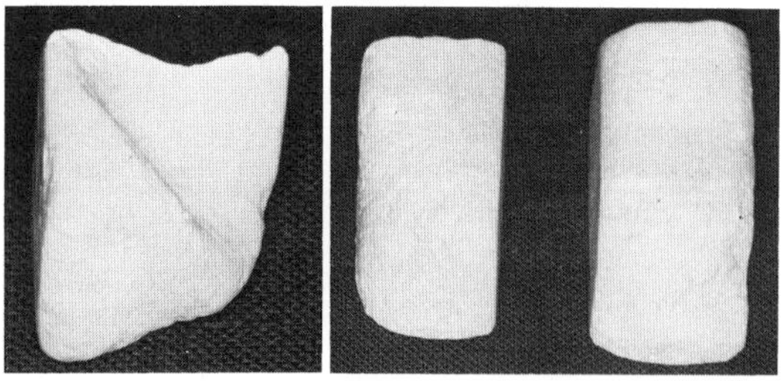

a   b

Fig. 7.2 Cavities in a cube of chalk produced by 75 shock waves
a *Piezolith:* Small punctuate cavity due to small focal zone
b *HM3:* Broad and homogeneous disintegration of the chalk due to large focal zone

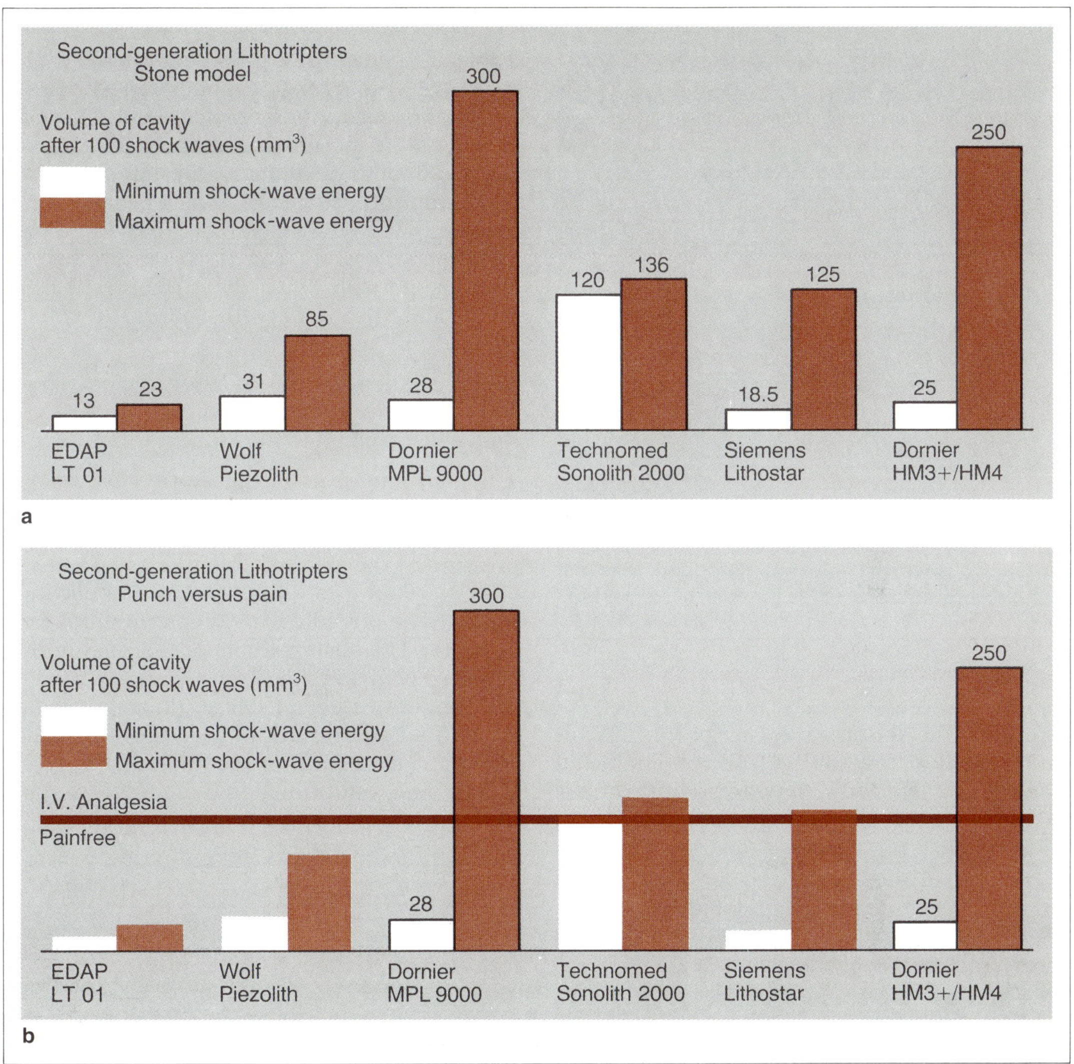

Fig. 7.3 Volume of cavity (mm³) of plaster piece after 100 shock waves with the second-generation lithotriptors tested

a Small range of piezoceramic systems (EDAP LT01, Piezolith) compared with electrohydraulic systems (Dornier MPL 9000, HM3 +, and HM4)

b Correlation of disintegration volume and necessitation of anesthesia. Independent of the lithotriptor, shock wave application became intolerable at energy settings producing a cavity larger than 80 mm³

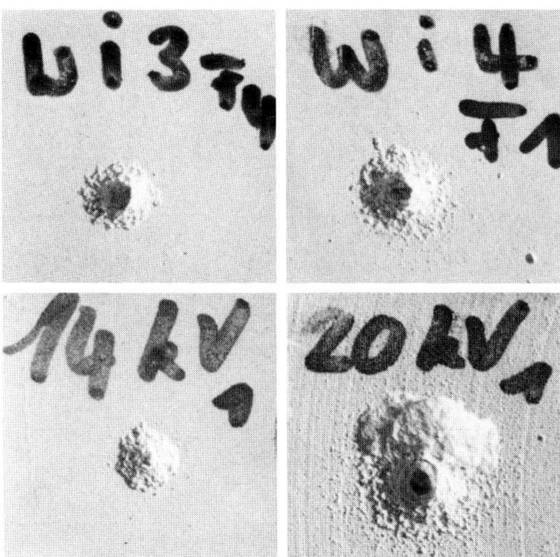

Fig. 7.4 Cavity created in plaster (model 2) after 100 shock waves at minimal (left) and maximal (right) energy settings a Wolf Piezolith **b** Dornier MPL 9000

increasing the shock wave energy for difficult cases such as cystine calculi or impacted stones. In such cases, however, intravenous analgesia is necessary during treatment.

7.4.2 Pain Evaluation

Table 7.**7** illustrates that "tolerable" (dolor scale 2 to 3) shock wave application with lower levels of generator voltage (12−15 kV) is possible with the modified Dornier HM3, Dornier HM4, Sonolith 3000 and Lithostar. Slight visceral pain (dolor scale 4), which became intolerable above 100 shocks, was experienced with higher energies. In contrast, pain-free treatment is possible with the Piezolith, EDAP LT01, and MPL 9000 (with a generator voltage of 14−17 kV).

When applied to the bladder region, shock wave lithotripsy was considerably less painful than when applied to the kidney.

The pain sensation during shock wave release corresponds closely to the size of the aperture of the focusing system and the measurement of pressure at the skin by Coleman and Saunders (1989). Pain-free shock wave application seems to be possible with an aperture of 21 cm or more. The best example of the relationship between pain and aperture is demonstrated by the Siemens Lithostar. Here, the pain produced with an aperture of only 11 cm was tolerable. The importance of the integration of such a unit into multifunctional fluoroscopic and urologic tables must be considered.

Table 7.7 Pain measurement in self-trial

Lithotriptor	Dolor rating	Aperture (cm)	Pressure at skin (mPa)*
Dornier:			
HM3	Intolerable (5)	15	20.0
HM3 modified	Tolerable (2−4)	17	No measurements
HM4	Tolerable (2−4)	17	No measurements
MPL 9000	Pain-free (1−2)	22	No measurements
Siemens:			
Lithostar	Tolerable (2−4)	12	6.4
Technomed:			
Sonolith 3000	Tolerable (2−4)	16**	3.5
EDAP:			
LT01	Pain-free (1−2)	54	1.3
Wolf:			
Piezolith	Pain-free (1)	50	0.6

* Coleman and Saunders, 1989
** New ellipsoid with 22 cm aperture

Furthermore, an interesting correlation was observed between the pain experienced with each lithotriptor and the disintegrative efficacy in the stone model (Fig. 7.**3b**). Shock wave application proved painful when the cavity produced by 100 impulses was larger than 80 mm^3.

7.4.3 Handling the Lithotriptor

The following is a summary of the main features of the different machines.

Dornier HM4 (Fig. 7.**5**). Owing to computerization of the panel, treatment with the Dornier HM4 is more complex than with the HM3; flexibility is also restricted. With the new system, for example, shock wave release, fluoroscopy, and positioning of the patient cannot be carried out at the same time. The computer system is also incompatible with IBM personal computers; therefore the recorded data cannot be easily transferred to a personal computer for statistical use. The design of the four handswitches for shock wave release, patient positioning, fluoroscopy, and respiratory triggering seems to be exaggerated. It would have been better to include at least two of these functions on the panel. The special video monitor for controlling coupling is an expensive solution to the problem.

Summarizing, the spatial requirement of the Dornier HM4 is considerable (40−45 m^2). This machine provides a wide range of energy owing to the electrohydraulic generation. Pain-free application is possible up to 16 kV, but intravenous analgesia is applied in the majority of clinical cases. There is a short learning curve owing to the two fluoroscopic systems and a wide range of indications for in situ ESWL. Despite the expensive X-ray system, the Dornier HM4 is not a multifunctional table.

Siemens Lithostar (Fig. 7.**6**). The Lithostar has a compact ESWL panel, but the X-ray functions are not included; in addition a second board is necessary for fluoroscopy. The computer-assisted operating system proved ineffective in some cases. An experienced operator is the cheapest and most effective means of stone localization.

The quality of the fluoroscopic image on the anteroposterior monitor during treatment is influenced by superpositioning of the water bag. Thus, focusing of slightly opaque or of smaller calculi may be problematic and time-consuming. The X-ray system guarantees a short learning curve.

Summarizing, the spatial requirement of the Lithostar is considerable (40−45 m^2). It provided a medium range of energy in the in vitro study. Pain-free application is possible up to 16

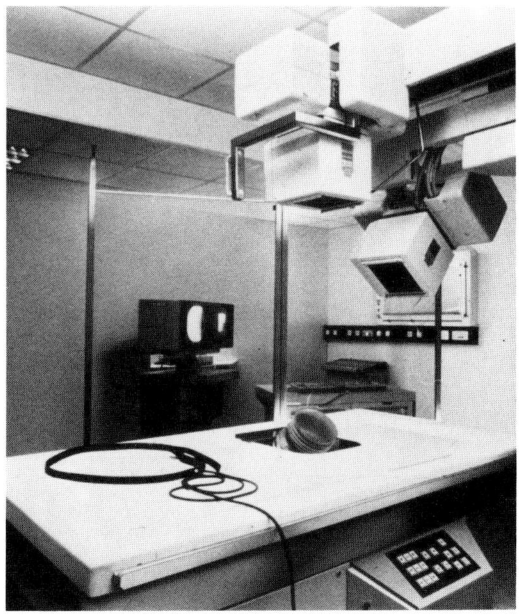

Fig. 7.**5** **Dornier HM4**

Fig. 7.**6** **Siemens Lithostar**

kV, but intravenous analgesia is given to the majority of patients as sufficient stone disintegration can only be achieved at higher energy level (18–19 kV). Fluoroscopic stone localization allows for a wide range of indications. The main advantage of this lithotriptor is the multifunctional urologic table. The multifunctional utility is ideal if an IVP, KUB, percutaneous nephrostomy, or PCNL is to be performed. However, in the case of retrograde maneuvers such as URS or even a simple retrograde pyelogram, the nonmotorized mobility of the X-ray film cassettes necessitates a comprehensive manual procedure (i.e., positioning the patient under the anteroposterior tube, moving the cassette below the patient, pressing the "backing" button, taking the X-ray, moving the cassette car to the top of the machine, and then moving the patient back to the original position).

Technomed Sonolith (Fig. 7.**7**). The IBM-compatible computer system of the Sonolith consists of a color monitor and a small panel with only five functional keys. The software program is easily adaptable. Its special design allows 100 treatments to be performed with one electrode. The locating arm is adaptable to most ultrasound devices, but, unfortunately, this arm cannot be locked. As a result, real-time monitoring during treatment — the main advantage of ultrasound — is not possible. For this reason, a coaxial ultrasound probe is integrated in the new Sonolith 3000 model.

Another disadvantage of this machine, as compared with other lithotriptors, is the absence in the panel of the possibility of easy, continuous graduation of shock wave energy; the generator voltage can only be altered after removal of the lateral covering.

Summarizing, the Sonolith 3000 has a small spatial requirement (25–30 m^2). The new generator provides a medium range of energy, but only allows pain-free ESWL up to a specific energy level. Clinically, intravenous analgesia was used in the majority of cases. The range of indications is restricted by the ultrasound stone localization system. The introduction of the Sonolith 3000, utilizing a flat position of the patient, made localization easy; the treatment of distal ureteral and gallbladder stones has also been made possible. The learning curve appears to be shorter with the lateral ultrasound scanner than with the coaxial systems of other machines. Owing to the different deviation of ultrasound and shock wave, it must be emphasized that the relatively large focal zone (55 × 15 mm) compensates for the inaccuracy of the lateral ultrasound localization.

EDAP LT01 (Fig. 7.**8**). Both panels of the EDAP LT01 are rather complicated when compared with the other lithotriptors (exept the Dornier HM4). However, many functions are integrated, including continous graduation of energy (0%–100%) and frequency (1.25–100 Hz). Unfortunately, impulse registration is not included in the panel. The use of frequencies higher than 2.5 Hz seems to be less effective and more traumatic, causing increasing cavitation (Vallancien et al., 1988). The computer software and hardware (monitor)

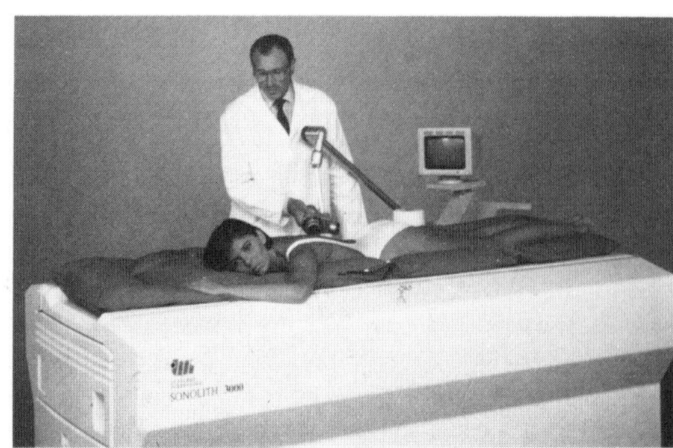

Fig. 7.**7**   **Technomed Sonolith 3000**

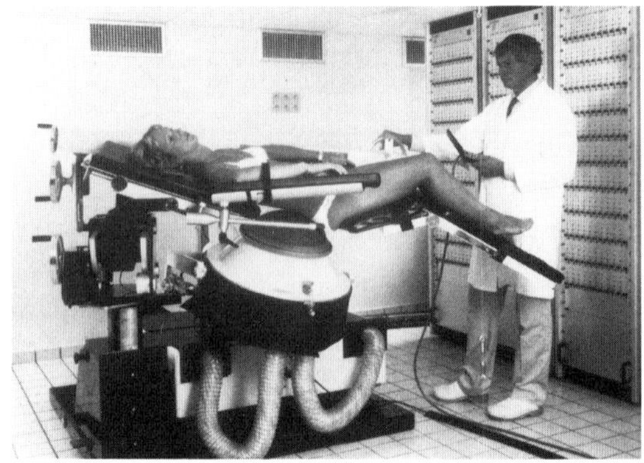

Fig. 7.**8**   **EDAP LT01**

are less sophisticated than that of the Sonolith 3000. An interesting feature is the "shot control", which only releases shock waves if the stone is in the focus. Clinically, this feature was only rarely used.

The most interesting feature of the EDAP machine is the mobile ESWL head with energy source and ultrasound system, allowing stone localization without moving the patient. This adds to the comfort of the patient. This principle of moving the energy source instead of the patient seems to be beneficial. Additonally, a C-arm can be used for roentenologic assessment of results but not for stone localization.

Summarizing, the EDAP LT01 has a medium spatial requirement (30−35 m^2). The lithotriptor allows pain-free application, and the energy range per shock wave is minimal. The range of indications for in situ treatment is limited by ultrasound stone localization. In addition the learning curve is longer.

Wolf Piezolith 2300 (Fig. 7.**9**). The Piezolith 2300 has a compact panel with an integrated system. The functions of ESWL are minimized to four degrees of patient movement, four levels of shock wave energy, and four frequencies (1−4 Hz). This proves advantageous with respect to the training period for handling the lithotriptor. Owing to the two coaxial ultrasound devices for stone localization, the learning curve is considerable, prolonging treatment time at the beginning. The localization of problematic calculi such as ureteral stones is

particularly difficult and time-consuming. Moreover, the modified second ultrasound probe seems to be overdesigned.

Summarizing, the Piezolith only has a small spatial requirement (25−30 m^2) since the generator and the water system are integrated in the machine. Sufficient punch is achieved, but the range of shock wave energy is limited. This corresponds to the significant increase in the number of shock waves for satisfactory stone disintegration in clinical trials. Although this machine allows pain-free ESWL treatment, the range of indications for in situ treatment is restricted by the ultrasound system.

MPL 9000 (Fig. 7.**10**). The Dornier MPL 9000 has a compact panel with an integrated ultrasound system. The computer program is a definite improvement over the Dornier HM4. However, it is still not IBM-compatible. Despite various functions for moving the patient and the energy source, localization of difficult calculi is time- consuming and requires a longer training phase. With small patients in particular (i.e., upper ureteral stones), positioning on the shock wave head may prove uncomfortable. This lithotriptor has the advantage of an additional lateral, lockable ultrasound scanner, which can be effectively utilized, in combination with the computerized localization system ("autofocus"), for the localization of difficult calculi.

Summarizing, the MPL 9000 has a medium spatial requirement (30−35 m^2). In the authors' in vitro studies, it provided the widest

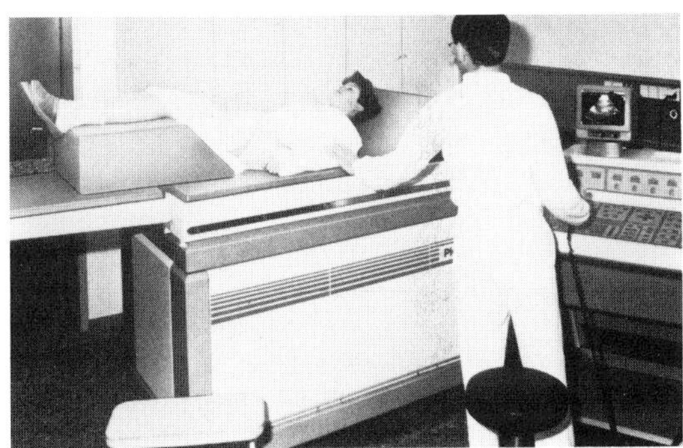

Fig. 7.**9**   **Wolf Piezolith 2300**

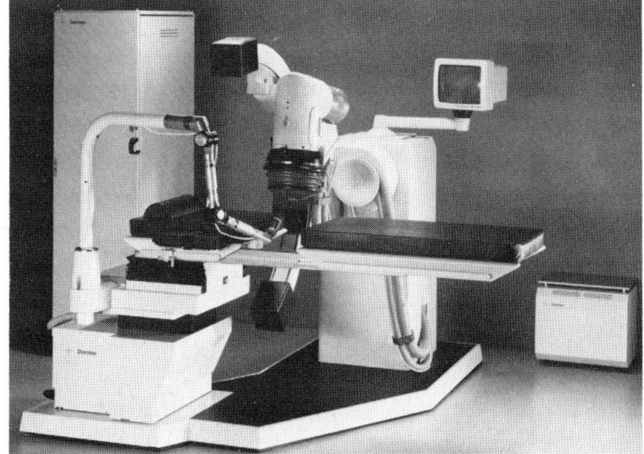

Fig. 7.**10**   **Dornier MPL 9000**

range of energy of all tested lithotriptors. Pain-free ESWL is possible at lower generator voltage (14−17 kV), which is employed in the majority of clinical cases. Treatment under intravenous analgesia can be performed for calculi necessitating higher generator voltage. There is a restricted range of indications of in situ treatment, despite the use of two ultrasound scanners, and a long learning curve for stone localization. To date, the MPL 9000 is the most widely-used lithotriptor for the treatment of biliary calculi.

7.5 Conclusion

With respect to *all* different criteria, none of the lithotriptors tested proved to be superior. Thus, the advantages and disadvantages of each machine must be taken into account.

The introduction of second generation lithotriptors with different principles of shock wave generation, focusing, coupling, and stone localization has lead to a new technical design of the lithotriptor and to a new ESWL treatment strategy based on this design.

7.5.1 Lithotriptor Hardware

Chiefly, there are two types of hardware. First, there is a *multifunctional table* (i.e., Dornier MFL 5000, Siemens Lithostar), which is used for urological purposes only. This table mainly consists of a high-standard fluoroscopic unit (X-ray table) with an integrated shock wave unit (electrohydraulic, electromagnetic) with the necessary small aperture (up to 17 cm). In the meantime additional ultrasonic stone localization system (i.e., lateral or co-axial scanner) has been integrated into these lithotriptors. The flexibility of the multifunctional table and easier handling of fluoroscopic stone localization as compared to ultrasound are the reasons why most urologists prefer to use these space-consuming, expensive machines.

Second, is the *interdisciplinary multipurpose lithotriptor* (i.e., Dornier MPL 9000, Sonolith 3000, Wolf Piezolith 2300), which utilizes ultrasound for stone localization only. The aperture of the shock wave source is not limited as with the fluoroscopic multifunctional table. In addition, the large aperture size of such machines enables pain-free application. This lithotriptor is most suitable for ESWL alone, but it may also be utilized for the interdisciplinary treatment of both urinary and biliary calculi. These machines are less expensive, but it must be stressed that, despite increasing experience with ultrasonic stone localization, about 20%−30% of the calculi (i.e., midureteral, bile duct) cannot be treated in situ.

7.5.2 Lithotriptor Software

Since the introduction of piezoelectric ESWL system, treatment is mainly based on two different *software concepts*. First, there is the *piezoelectric system* (i.e., Wolf Piezolith, EDAP LT01), with a large shock wave source aperture (50 cm) that results in a small focal size; this necessitates a high number of impulses for satisfactory stone disintegration, as well as further treatment sessions (Table 7.**2**). However, this system enables possible pain-free treatment; in addition the piezoceramic elements are long-lasting.

Second, is the *electrohydraulic system* (i.e., Dornier HM3, MPL 9000, Sonolith 3000), which provides a wide range of energy; therefore, a lower number of impulses are required for stone disintegration. The aim is to reduce the number of further treatment sessions to a minimum. The disadvantage of this more efficient lithotriptor is that intravenous analgesia is necessary with high-energy treatment. Furthermore, the electrodes are less durable (3000−4000 impulses per electrode).

The *electromagnetic element* of the Siemens Lithostar ranges between these two latter systems and provides a medium range of energy. The durability of this element is approximately 100 000 impulses per element. Further, improved development of the electromagnetic system may make it an important shock wave source of the future (see Chapter 8).

It is difficult and, to a certain extent, almost impossible to compare the different types of lithotriptors. For this reason, only the advantages and disadvantages of these machines have been compared. It must be emphasized that these machines proved to be clinically effective. In the meantime, the lithotriptors tested have been improved still further and new technical concepts have been introduced. Therefore, the analysis of the hardware and software may become outdated in the near future (see Chapter 8).

8 Stone Therapy — Trends and Future Aspects

8.1 Endourology

8.1.1 Endoscopes

In general, the *rigid instruments* used for PCNL and URS have been well-adapted to these procedures. This applies particularly to the optical quality, handling, and utilization of secondary instruments.

The *Amplatz sheath* is an efficient tool for reducing the time-consuming period of retrieval of stone fragments after EHL or USL during *percutaneous treatment* of larger stones. Using a canine kidney. Wepp and colleagues showed that there was no difference in scar formation when the percutaneous tract was only 24 Fr or even 36 Fr. The *combination of ultrasound and fluoroscopy* has lead to a further decrease of complications of kidney puncture (i.e., colon perforation, pneumothorax, hydrothorax).

There is a trend in *URS* towards reducing the size of the instruments employed (7.2−9.5 Fr). Using a pig model, Watson and colleagues experimentally demonstrated that the larger the endoscope, the greater the extent of damage to the ureteral wall. Smaller ureteroscopes have the advantage of better handling (i.e., dilatation of the orifice is not necessary, and passage inside the ureter is easy). The problem at present is that, apart from the Dormia basket, no other reliable auxiliary instrument (i.e., forceps) is available for primary extraction of the stone. However, major advances have been made in the field of *endoscopic stone disintegration,* and further development is expected (Fuchs et al. 1990).

8.1.2 Intracorporeal Lithotripsy

Laser lithotripsy. Extensive research has been conducted to evaluate the possibilities of laser lithotripsy with various laser system (Fair, 1978; Pensel, 1981; Watson 1983, 1987; Reichel, 1983; Hofmann, 1988; Miller, 1989;

Rassweiler, 1989; Weber, 1989). In vitro studies showed the principle capability of the various system to disintegrate most urinary stones sufficiently; in vivo studies on different animal models demonstrated their safety for human medicine. In particular, there was no major damage to the ureter that would not be expected after ureteroscopic treatment or retrograde manipulation alone.

Three systems are currently used under clinical conditions. The flash-lamp pumped and Q-switched *Nd:YAG laser* is a solid state system that emits very short, highly energetic pulses in the nanosecond range. It uses 300 to 600 μm fibers that must either be equipped with a coupling device or melted to a bulb at the tip. The shock wave is created at the outside of the stone with the energy focused at a distance of 3−4 mm in front of the fiber (Fig. 8.**1**). The advantage of this system is that it is relatively cheap, technically reliable, and has a good fragmentation capacity. The major disadvantage are caused by the problem of coupling the high energy pulses into the fiber and onto the stone (Rassweiler, 1989). The coupling devices

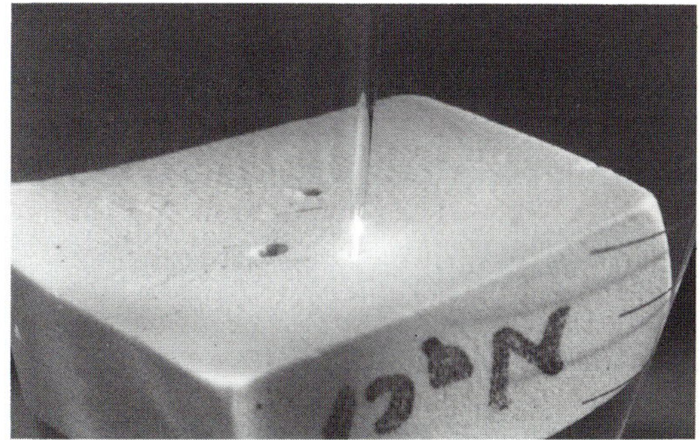

Fig. 8.**1**   Laser-induced (Q-switched Nd: YAG) breakdown approximately 3 mm from the cone-shaped tip of a fiber 600 μm quartz leads to fragmentation of a test stone *without* touching the plaster cube

further increase the size of the fiber, which necessitates the use of larger instruments. The highly energetic pulses can cause damage to the fiber itself, so that a relatively frequent change of the fiber may be necessary.

The flash-lamp pumped and Q-switched *dye-laser* is tunable with the use of different dyes, but mainly used at a 504 nm wavelength (Cumarin green). It proceduces comparatively lower energy pulses with a duration of 1 ms that still give good fragmentation rates and enable the use of small 200 to 300 μm fibers, thus facilitating its use in small (6–7.5 Fr) endoscopes (miniscopes) for ureteric endoscopy. Its disadvantages are the relatively high price, as well as some technical problems related to the use and change of the laser dye.

The recently introduced pulsed and Q-switched *Alexandrite laser* is an uncomplicated and relatively cheap solid state system emitting pulses in the 150 to 800 ns range into a 200 to 300 μm fiber; it has good stone fragmentation, and there are no detrimental effects to the urinary tract when applied directly to the ureteric and bladder wall (Weber, 1989). Thus, this laser system holds the promise of combining the advantages of the two previously existing systems while at the same time avoiding their disadvantages (Fig. 8.**2**).

The development of laser system that have good fragmentation capacity while using very fine fibers is the dominant, but not the only, aspect in the future of intracorporeal lithotripsy. The other important point is the ongoing improvement of semirigid and flexible endoscopes for the ureter. With these endoscopes of 7 Fr or less, a much less traumatizing approach to ureteric stones has become possible; even first experiences under local anesthesia have been gained. Although ESWL is the standard treatment of choice for ureteric calculi today, the use of laser lithotripsy via miniscopes may change this approach in the future. With the increasing distribution of solely ultrasound-equipped ESWL devices that give no access to the ureter, an alternative method to treat these stones has become essential. While at present most centers with these lithotriptors would have to manipulate the ureteric stone back into the renal pelvis by retrograde manipulation with a ureteric catheter ("push and smash"), in the future they would be able to accomplish stone disintegration with an endo-

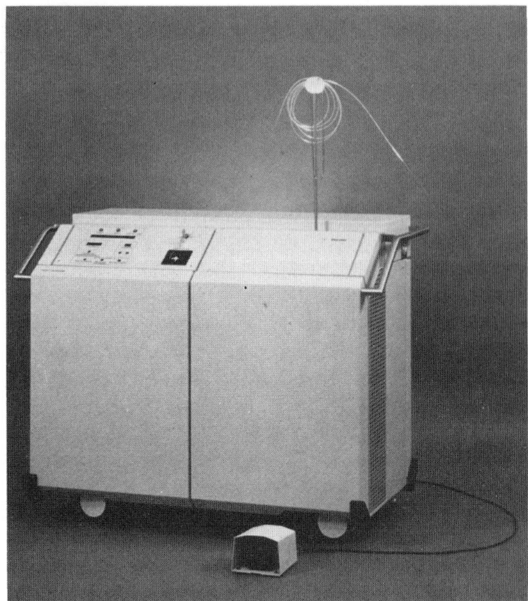

Fig. **82**   The Alexandrite-laser (Dornier).

scope of the same size at the same time ("smash and go"). This could very well make ureteric stone treatment an office procedure again or at least give some of the stone treatment back to smaller centers. One combination device of an ultrasonically guided electromagnetic ESWL and a pulsed dye-laser has already been released; there are certainly more to follow.

Since the drawbacks (anesthesia, ureteral trauma) that may be encountered even when using flexible endoscopes and miniscopes have not been completely overcome yet, other investigators have focused on methods to avoid ureteric endoscopy during laser lithotripsy altogether (Coptcoat, 1987; Schmeller, 1989). Under fluoroscopic guidance, the laser fiber is advanced through the ureter onto the stone; with the aid of a radiopaque fiber tip, stone disintegration is performed under X-ray control. To improve disintegration results and to minimize detrimental effects for the ureter, feedback systems are currently being developed (Muschter, 1989). The rationale of the feedback system is that the laser will not deliver a "complete" pulse into the fiber if the feedback system does not indicate that the fiber tip is in contact with the stone. While a ureteric endoscopy is not necessary for this procedure, a major disadvantage of this concept is that the fragmentation effect is difficult or impossible to quantify.

The development of steerable, flexible ureteroscopes of 6 or 7 Fr may further improve the possibilities of nontraumatizing laser lithotripsy in the ureter; however the use of the semirigid miniscopes currently seems to be more favorable since it usually allows a faster and easier access to ureteric stones than the flexible scopes.

Electrohydraulic lithotripsy (EHL). The development of ultra-fine probes for EHL (≤3Fr) may be able to compete with the different laser system for lithotripsy if the potential damage to the urinary tract by EHL can be more securely avoided. A possible solution to this problem is the use of a *shielded electrohydraulic probe* (Fig. 8.**3**) with a metal cap at the end of the tip to reduce the well-known side effect of EHL on the ureteral wall (Bhutta and Dretler, 1989). This 3 Fr probe could be easily attached to any EHL generator and, therefore, possibly be a cost-effective alternative to laser lithotripsy.

8.1.3 Stents

There has been a great increase in the use of *Double-J stents* as an auxiliary measure prior to using ESWL, ever since the first reports of Griffith and Libby (1985) that indicated that a significant reduction of the side-effects of ESWL in cases with large stone burdens could be achieved with ureteral stents. This lead to a further extension of the range of indications for ESWL monotherapy, which also includes staghorn calculi. However, it must be emphasized that the combination of PCNL and ESWL is most often applied, particularly in cases with a large stone burden and a dilated collecting system.

Indwelling stents have proved to be a very useful addition to ESWL for the following reasons:

- prevent descention of a ureteral stone after retrograde mobilization
- an obstructing ureteral stone can be bypassed
- urine drainage is guaranteed in the case of a symptomatic "Steinstrasse"

The following special devices have been designed for these often complicated maneuvers (Fig. 8.**4**):

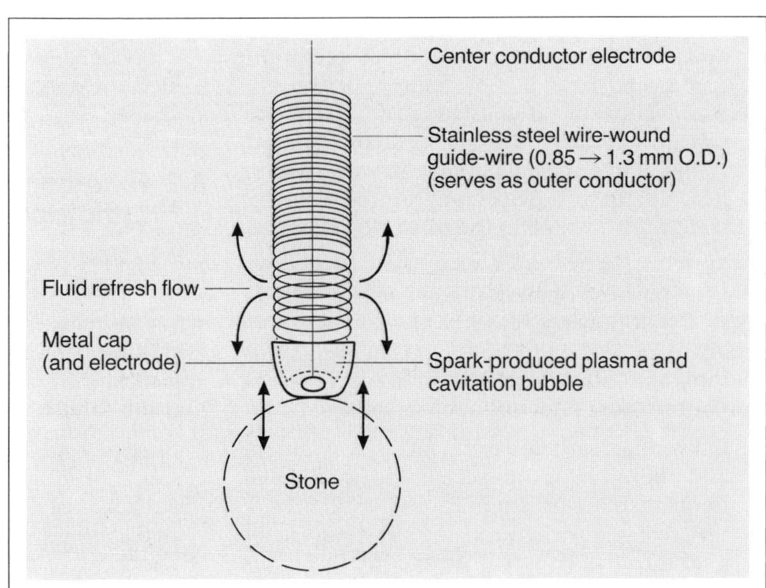

Fig. 8.**3** **Schematic drawing of prototype spring and cap-shielded electrohydraulic device** (from Bhutta et al., 1989)

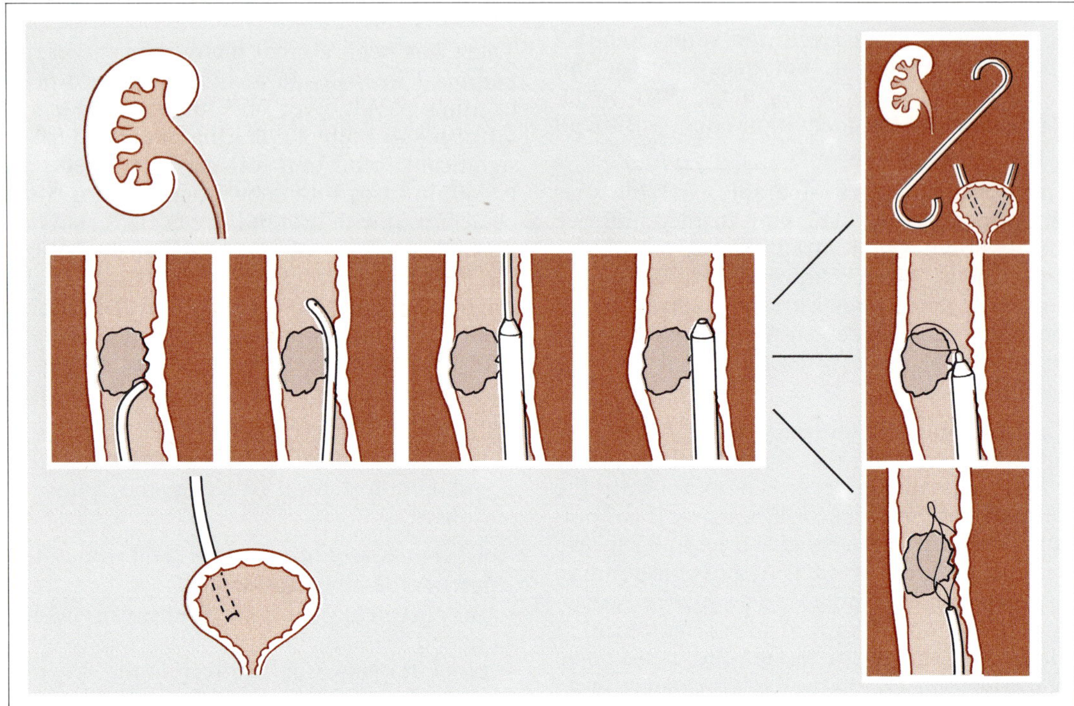

Fig. 8.**4   The use of a coaxial stent-dilator set for placement of indwelling ureteral stents.** The 4 Fr Tiemann-tipped catheter bypasses the obstructing stone. A dilator sheath (8 Fr) is then moved forward in coaxial position. Finally, a Double-J stent can be positioned via an angiographic guide wire or a loop directly inside the sheath

- a disconnectable stent with a guideable tip and special coupling nipple integrated in the guide wire (Brandl and Chaussy, 1989)
- a coaxial stent set consisting of a Tiemann-tipped catheter (4 Fr), a dilator sheath (8 Fr), and a special guide wire with rigid or flexible tip for placement of the ureteral stent after bypassing the obstacle (Rassweiler and Tschada, 1990)

For the purpose of guaranteeing urinary drainage, the following reasons have lead to an *increase in the application of internal stents* before and after ESWL and a decrease in temporary percutaneous nephrostomies:

- indwelling catheters are more convenient and therefore more acceptable to the patients than nephrostomies
- on acute obstruction, the ureteral stent guarantees adequate drainage in most cases (Tschada et al., 1988)

- dilatation of the orifice and ureter facilitate secondary ureteroscopic maneuvers (i.e., stone extraction, removal of the "Steinstrasse"

8.2 Extracorporeal Shock Wave Lithotripsy (ESWL)

8.2.1 Optimal Use of the Dornier HM3 Lithotriptor

After a phase of stabilization, the Dornier HM3 lithotriptor was tested in additional trials and technically modified to enable more effective and safer ESWL in the following ways:

- *Special positioning techniques* for a wider range of indications for in situ ESWL, that is, horizontal position (gluteal shock wave application) or sitting position (perineal shock wave application) for distal ureteral stones, or prone position for the treatment of concrements in the midureter (at the sacroiliac joint).

- *Considerable reduction of the radiation load (exposure)* of the patient by standardized methods of stone localization. This is accomplished mainly by prepositioning without X-ray, in accordance with the coordinates displayed on the machine or the skeleton shown on the KUB before treatment. Primarily, short-time fluoroscopy is used with early collimation and fewer photographs are taken with the high-current fluoroscopy technique ("quick pics"). Furthermore, X-rays can even be taken in the bath tub with the aid of a special holding device for the X-ray cassettes.

- *Special shock wave focusing techniques,* that is, cranial focusing (Fig. 8.**5a**) for large obstructive ureteral calculi in a dilated ureter for fragmentation at the interphase urine to stone at the top of the calculus. In the case of multistage ESWL of staghorn stones after treatment of the pelvic area, the treatment proceeds from cranial to caudal in order to avoid stone fragments dropping into the lower stone-filled calix group, which could prolong spontaneous passing (Fig. 8.**5b**).

- *Stone-specific shock wave energy,* that is, low generator voltage for calcium oxalate dihydrate or struvite stones to avoid scattering of larger fragments in the collecting system and to avoid further impulses. Initially, high generator voltage is applied for hard stones (e.g., cystine, calcium oxalate monohydrate, or cholesterol) and impacted calculi (ureter or bile duct). The energy can be reduced as soon as the stone begins to break up.

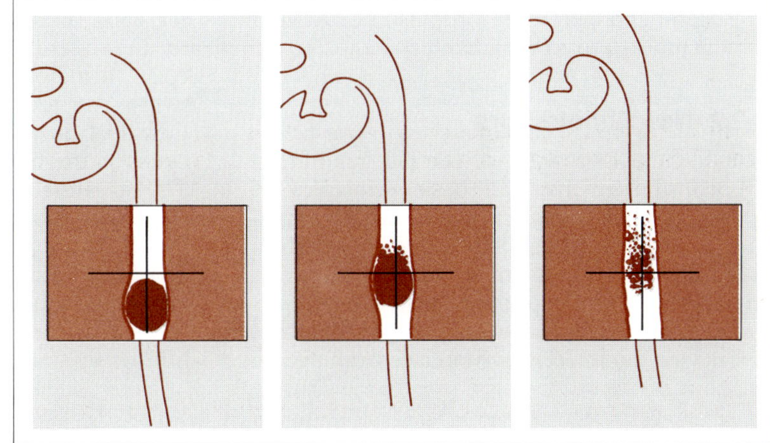

a

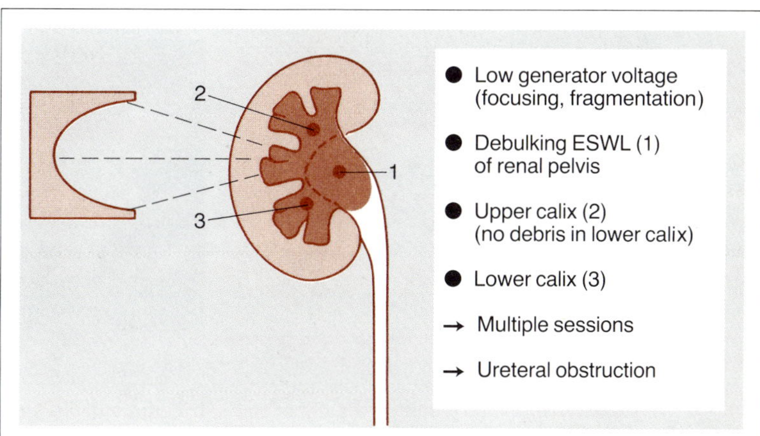

b

Fig. 8.**5 Focusing techniques for ESWL a** Cranial focusing for impacted ureteral stones **b** Multistage ESWL for staghorn calculi

– *Measurement of CT density* did not prove to be very helpful in ESWL of urinary calculi (except for the diagnosis or urate and cystine stones), owing to the high percentage of stones of mixed composition (Fig. 8.**6**). In contrast, this procedure proved to be effective for the differentiation of pigmental calculi from cholesterol stones in ESWL of biliary calculi. Pigmental calculi are not suitable for oral chemolysis and should be excluded from ESWL. Pure cholesterol stones have a CT density of less than 60 Houndsfield units.

– Subsequent to the installation of a *lower voltage generator* (40 nF vs 80 nF) and an ellipsoid with a larger aperture (17 cm vs 15 cm), treatment under intravenous analgesia or even without anesthesia can be carried out, thus guaranteeing a higher patient throughput on the machine.

Most of these issues refer to ESWL treatment in general and can, therefore, also be adapted to new lithotriptors (see Chapters 3 and 7).

8.2.2 New Lithotriptors

The technical progress of second generation lithotriptors involved all basic principles of ESWL such as shock wave generation, focusing, energy coupling, and stone localization (see Chapter 7). In the meantime, with respect to general clinical experience with second generation lithotriptors, the results of the first series (see Table 7.**1**) have been reproduced by other centers on most of the machines. The successful stone disintegration rate ranges between 80% and 95%. Unfortunately, this sometimes includes a considerable retreatment rate (Wolf Piezolith 2300 = 45%). Some common principles could be implemented in future lithotriptors, despite the various technical concepts (Table 8.**1**).

1. *Shock wave generation*
   Electromagnetic elements may be preferred as a shock wave source in the future, as they are more durable than electrodes, enable continuous graduation of shock wave energy, and provide sufficient shock wave pressure, even with a smaller aperture of the focusing system. They can, therefore, be integrated in multifunctional tables. The shape of the electromagnetic membrane can be modified, and it enables different focusing-principles.
   Because the *electrodes* must be changed after each treatment, causing inconvenience to the operator and higher maintenance costs, a major disadvantage is posed. The twin-pulse technique compensates for the time lost during renewal of the electrodes between treatments.
   The greatest disadvantage of *piezoelectric elements,* despite technical improvement (Wolf Piezolith 2500), is the restricted energy of each element, affording a large aperture of the focusing system. An adjustable frequency scale is of minor importance for lithotripsy since high frequencies (>2.5 Hz)

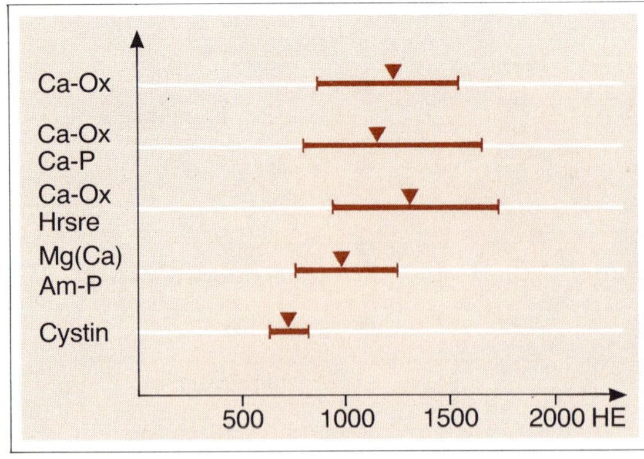

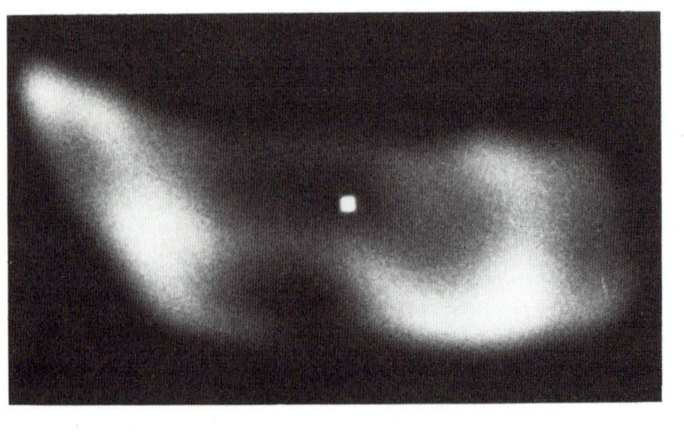

Fig. 8.**6** **CT density of urinary calculi a** Only exact discrimination of cystine (and urate) stones is possible

b Large struvite stone with marked inhomogeneity of radiodensity

Table 8.1   Advantages and disadvantages of the different principles of shock wave (SW) generation

SW generation	Advantage	Disadvantage
Electrode	Wide range of energy Twin-pulse technique Flexible size of aperture (15–26 cm)	Short lifespan (3,000–4,000 SW) Renewal expensive Minimal energy necessary for discharge
Piezoelectric elements	Very long lifespan (> 1,000,000 SW) Variation of frequency (1–100 Hz) Target control	Limited range of energy Large aperture necessary (> 40 cm)

Electromagnetic elements	Wide range and continuous graduation of
	  energy
	Flexible size of aperture
	Long lifespan (200,000–400,000 SW)
	Multiple focusing principles
	  – membrane + acoustic lens
	  – cylinder + paraboloid
	  – spherical shape
		Metal membrane must still be changed

are less effective and cause severe tissue damage. A theoretically possible "hit control", which converts the echo-signal of the stone recorded by one of the piezoelectric elements, has not yet been realized in clinical lithotriptors.

An *electromagnetic cylinder for shock wave generation together with a paraboloid metal reflector* (Fig. 8.**7b**) is an interesting modification of an electromagnetic element. As a self-focusing system without an energy-absorbing acoustic lens, it produces a high range of shock wave pressure. Contrary to the electrohydraulic system, the cylinder allows the coaxial integration of an ultrasound probe that does not lie in the blast path.

No advantage is gained from other modifications to shock wave generation, such as pulsed laser or microexplosion with lead acetate pellets; these can be disregarded in the future.

2. *Shock wave coupling*

As with the shock wave source, there are still some technical alternatives. However, the coupling of shock wave energy will only be carried out via a *water cushion and ultrasonic gel* in all future lithotriptors. Only one of the new machines still has a partial water bath (Sonolith 3000). Owing to the membrane of the water cushion, the attenuation of shock wave energy amounts to approximately 15% in comparison to a water bath;

this can be easily compensated by an increase in generator voltage. The results are an enormous reduction in the size of lithotriptors and more favorable maintenance costs (Fig. 8.**7b**).

3. *Positioning*

Because of the water cushion, the energy source can be included in an ordinary treatment table. As a result, special positioning techniques (i.e., sitting position for distal ureteral stones) have become less important. The patient must be in a flat, supine position, as for a normal IVP, if *fluoroscopic stone localization* is used for renal and upper calculi. A flat, prone position is recommended for midureteral and lower ureteral stones. An oblique position of the patient is favorable for the *purely ultrasonic localization* of upper ureteral stones, while a prone position with a semi-filled bladder is preferred for patients with distal ureteral stones.

4. *Stone localization*

Many of the new lithotriptors utilize ultrasound for stone localization. The reasons for this are (1) the large aperture of the focusing system prevented easy-integration of the X-ray; (2) cost reduction; and (3) to enable the treatment of gallbladder stones.

A major advantage of *ultrasound* is the real-time monitoring that excludes radiation exposure during treatment and enables "auto-

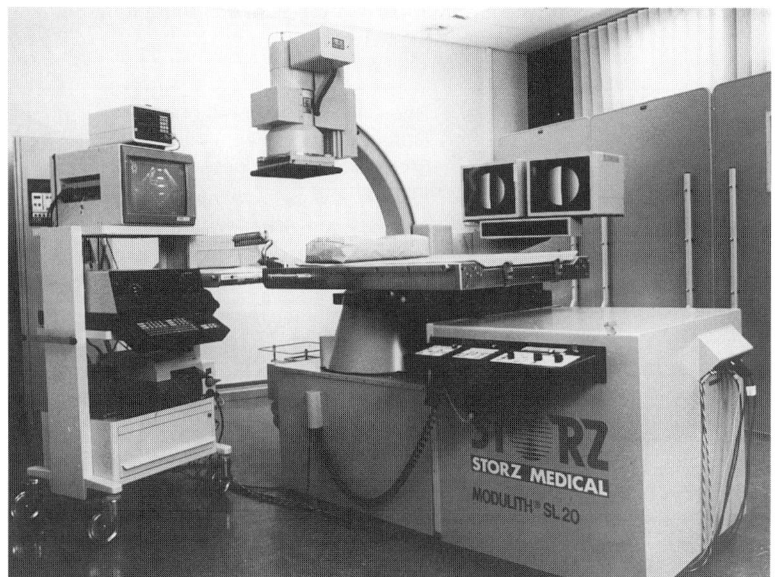

a

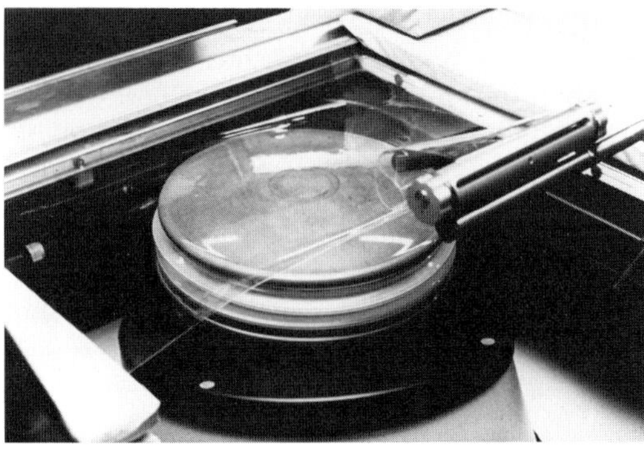

b

Fig. 8.**7** **Storz Modulith SL 20 a** Compact lithotriptor with integrated C-arm and coaxial ultrasound scanner **b** Shock wave source consisting of an electromagnetic cylinder, parabolic reflector, water cushion, and in-line ultrasound. Patient is positioned on an impedance-adapted foil ("acoustic cradle")

focusing" of the stone by the patient's own breathing. This regulation of the patient's breathing is much more effective and far cheaper than a computerized respiratory gating or even a "hit control" by a piezo-electric element. Despite the low cost and wider range of indications for ESWL (i.e., radiolucent calculi, biliary stones), ultrasound also has some disadvantages.

Ultrasonic localization of calculi in the mid-ureter is almost impossible, and multiple stones can be problematic. The lengthly learning curve is another disadvantage. Even a sonographically-experienced urologist requires considerable time to distinguish betweeen actual fragmentation of secon-

dary artifacts and intrarenal gas formation such as air bubbles released by shock waves or cavitation (Fig. 8.**8**).

Fluoroscopic stone localization is much safer, since the chance of missing radiopaque calculi is minimal. This results in a shorter learning curve. Furthermore, fluoroscopy guarantees a wide range of indications for in situ treatment and enables multifunctional use of X-rays (diagnostic, endourologic). Fluoroscopic localization of stones close to the vertebral column and of radiolucent calculi is especially difficult. The adequate treatment of gallbladder stones, in particular, is not possible.

The highest demand on future interdisci-

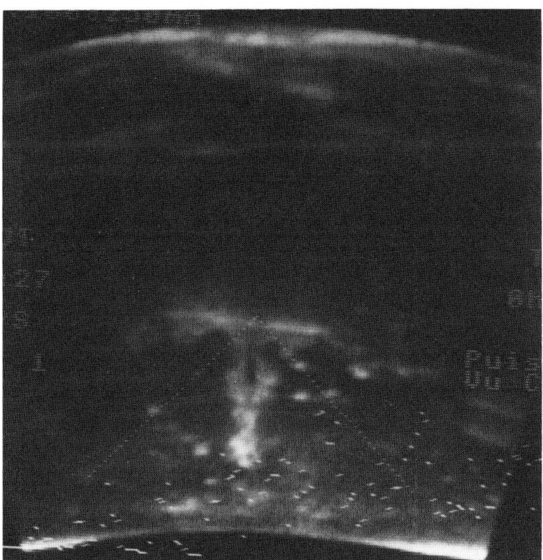

Fig. 8.**8 Hyperechogenic reflex pattern of a test stone (EDAP LT01) on ultrasound scan during shock wave exposure.** Air bubbles due to shockwaves release and/or cavitation make exact discrimination of fragmentation impossible because of similar reflex patterns

plinary lithotriptors ("third generation lithotriptors") is the *combination of ultrasound and fluoroscopy* (Table 8.**2**). The following are the present technical alternatives to this localization method (Table 8.**3**):

a. In-line ultrasound probe with integrated C-arm for fluoroscopic localization
 – using a virtual focus (F_v) and moving the patient on the shock wave source: Storz Modulith SL20 (Fig. 8.**7**), Diasonics Therasonic Lithotriptor (Fig. 8.**9**);
 – parallel to ultrasound, with oblique coupling of the shock wave source: Dornier MPL 9000-x (Fig. 8.**10**);
 – using an in-line C-arm integrated in the shock wave source: Wolf Piezolith 2500 (Fig. 8.**11**).
b. One rotating X-ray tube with an integrated lateral computer-assisted ultrasound scanner: Dornier MFL 5000-u (Fig. 8.**12**), Medstone 1000-s.
c. Two fixed X-ray tubes with two independent shock wave sources and an overhead module consisting of a third shock wave source with coaxial ultrasound probe: Siemens Lithostar Plus (Fig. 8.**13**).

Table 8.**2 Demands and characteristics of third generation lithotriptors**

Demand	Characteristic
Biliary and urinary calculi	Fluoroscopy and ultrasound
Better efficacy than Dornier HM3	Wide energy range of shock wave source
Anesthesia-free treatment (maximum IV analgesia)	Large aperture of focusing system
Multifunctional use of table	Integrated fluoro-table for endoscopy
Economical machine	Low costs and maintenance

The compact form of a unit utilizing a *virtual focus (F_v)*, enabling easy handling and multifunctional use of the lithotriptor, is very advantageous. Unfortunately, real-time fluoroscopy during treatment is not possible. It must be stressed that, owing to accurate mechanical design and calibration, exact focusing is possible unless the patient is moved on the shock wave source after fluoroscopy.

Simultaneous fluoroscopy and ultrasound can be carried out by *parallel use of a C-arm*. The combination of two C-arms (shock wave head and fluoroscopy), however, makes handling of the device somewhat complicated.

Integration of the fluoroscopic system in the large aperture of the shock wave generator provides an interesting and compact lithotriptor design. On the other hand, this type of machine cannot be used for multifunctional purposes.

Both basically X-ray-guided system provide the widest spectrum for multifunctional use. The implementation of a *lateral computer-assisted ultrasound probe* permits easy handling, but focusing is restricted by the following:

– deviation of lateral ultrasound owing to diffraction and declination amount to approximately 5 mm on x-and y-axis (Folberth 1989)
– the computer-assisted positioning of the

Table 8.3　Third-generation lithotriptors: Comparison of the main technical concepts combining ultrasound and fluoroscopy for stone localization

Localization concept	Multifunctional use	Simultaneous X-ray and ultrasound	Real-time fluoroscopy	Handling	Machine	Reliability of focusing
1. In-line ultrasound with integrated C-arm						
– External fluoroscopy with virtual focus (Modulith SL20)	++	No	No	Easy	Compact	+++
– Parallel fluoroscopy (MPL 9000-x)	++	Yes	Yes	Easy*	Complex,	+++
– In-line fluoroscopy (Piezolith 2500)	+	No	difficult**	Easy***	Compact	+++
2. One rotating X-ray tube with lateral ultrasound (MFL 5000-u)	+++	Yes	Yes	Easy	Expensive (space required, computer-assisted ultrasound)	++
3. Two X-ray converters plus independent shock wave head with coaxial ultrasound (Lithostar plus)	+++	No	Yes	Easy	Expensive (3 shock wave sources)	+++

  * But X-ray C-arm has to be adapted prior to treatment
  ** Fluoroscopy in water with deflated balloon of X-ray tube
*** But inflation and deflation of the balloon of X-ray tube recessory for fluoroscopy and ESWL respectively (like at Dornier HM3)

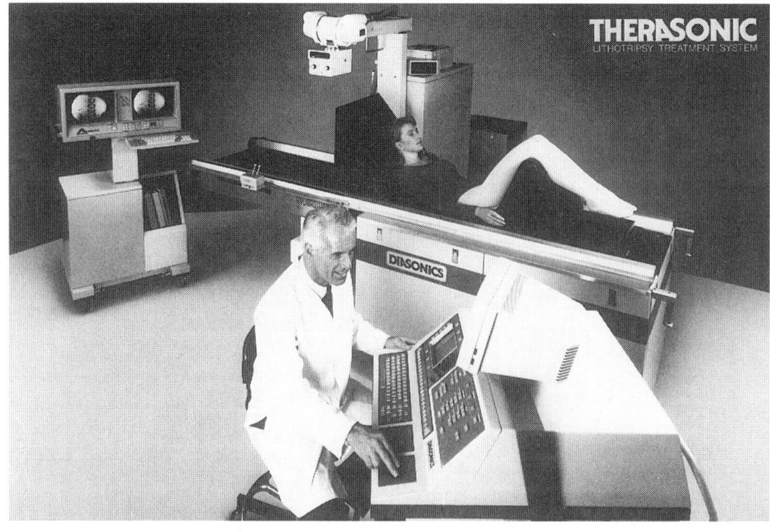

Fig. 8.9　**Therasonic lithotriptor with an integrated X-ray table, coaxial ultrasound, and a piezoelectric energy source**

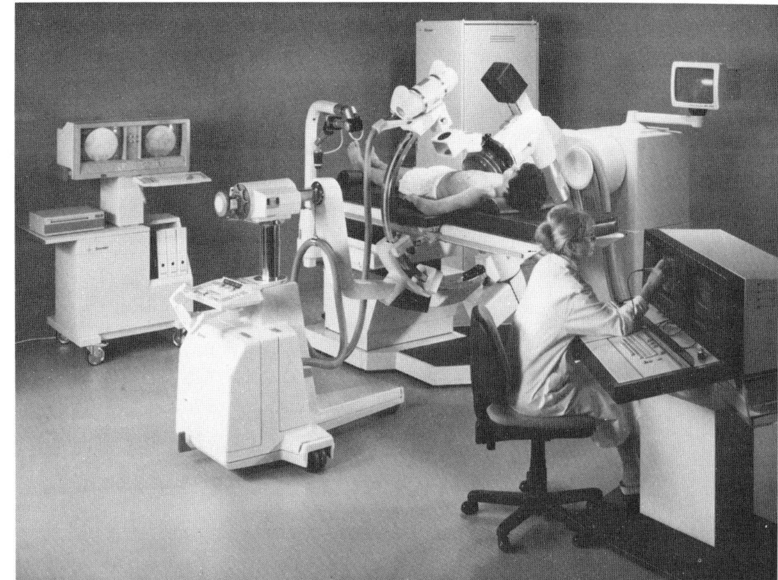

Fig. 8.**10** **Dornier MPL 9000-x.** Multi-purpose lithotripter with mobile X-ray C-arm, in-line and lateral ultrasound scanner. Automatic positioning capability in X-ray and US-mode. Electrohydraulic energy source with metall ellipsoid and water cushion. Lateral shockwave coupling.

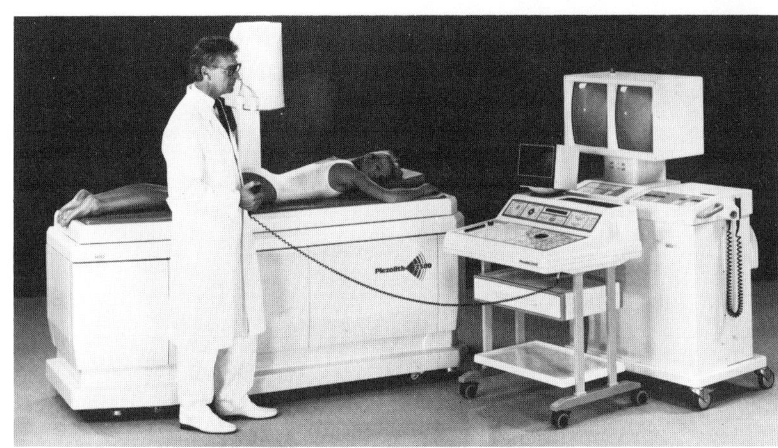

Fig. 8.**11** **Wolf Piezolith 2500: in-line ultrasound and in-line fluoroscopy for stone localization.** Energy source consists of piezoelectric elements and a water cushion

patient after ultrasonic determination of the stone coordinates is not precise enough

Alternatively, the installation of an *independent ultrasonic-guided overhead module* is an expensive solution. Almost all types of stones can be treated on such a machine, but there is no provision for the simultaneous use of ultrasound and fluoroscopy. The most appropriate concept for interdisciplinary lithotripsy will be determined in the future.

8.2.3 Choice of Lithotriptor

The rapid development of new lithotriptors has initiated a worldwide boom of these machines, mainly in the *United States and West Germany,* and has lead to an affluence of stone machines. Twenty-two urologic ESWL centers were installed in 1986; this number was considered sufficient for the FRG. At present there are more than 75 lithotriptors being utilized for interdisciplinary ESWL, and still further installations are planned. In the USA, there

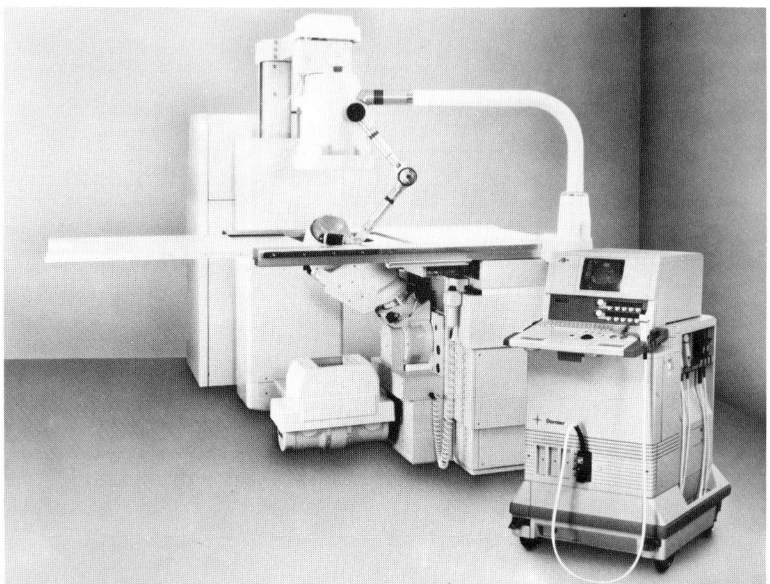

Fig. 8.**12** **Dornier MFL 5000-u.** Multifunctional Lithotripter with rotating X-ray tube and lateral ultrasound scanner. Computer assisted positioning in X-ray and ultrasound mode. Electrode and water cushion

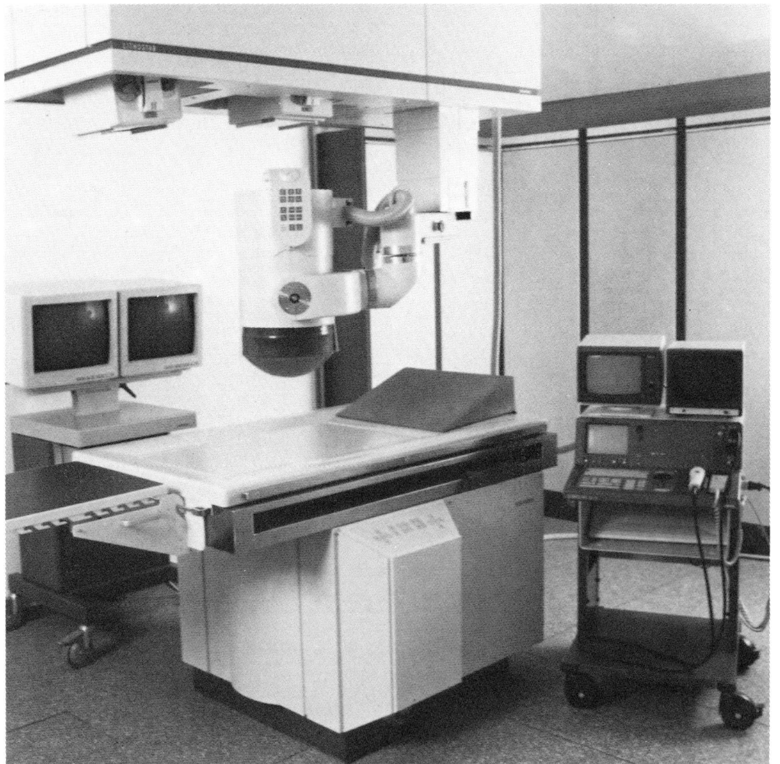

Fig. 8.**13** **Siemens Lithostar Plus: standard lithotriptor with two shock wave heads and two overcouch X-ray systems.** Independent overhead module with coaxial ultrasound scanner, mobile acoustic lens, and water cushion

are more than 25 stone machines being used in Los Angeles alone. This increase in stone centers has lead to a marked change of the clientele undergoing ESWL. In 1984, ureteral stones were treated in only 15% of all ESWL patients, whereas in 1989 ureteral calculi were treated in 45% of ESWL cases.

The trend to decentralize ESWL will continue in the future. As a result, an increasing number of urologists will treat a decreasing number of stones. This could affect the quality of treatment of the following reasons:

- an increase in the use of *mobile lithotriptors* (Fig. 8.**14**), making the necessary re-treatment on the following day difficult
- *outpatient treatment of ESWL,* which complicates follow-up

Moreover, as a result of this trend towards decentralization, urologists will no longer be classified into two groups (i.e., those with and those without lithotriptor).

In *developing countries* (e.g., India, South America, Africa), ESWL use has just started; in addition, a very large number of patients require stone treatment. Thus, especially in

these countries, ESWL and endourology will be the chief means of stone management. Financial problems will limit the number of lithotriptors in these countries for the next few years.

For these reasons, it is obvious that no specific choice of lithotriptor can be made. The following are the important factors to be considered:

1. The *size of the unit* allowing for
   - the number of patients;
   - the financial support; and
   - choice of urological or interdisciplinary stone center.
2. The *distribution of calculi,* that is,
   - localization (renal vs ureteral); and
   - size of stones.
3. *Experience of the urologist* with
   - ESWL; and
   - ultrasound.

Small urological units can choose from three alternatives: (1) a "low-cost lithotriptor" (Fig. 8.**15**, 8.**16**) based mainly on ultrasonic stone localization; (2) a more expensive multifunctional table based on fluoroscopy that could

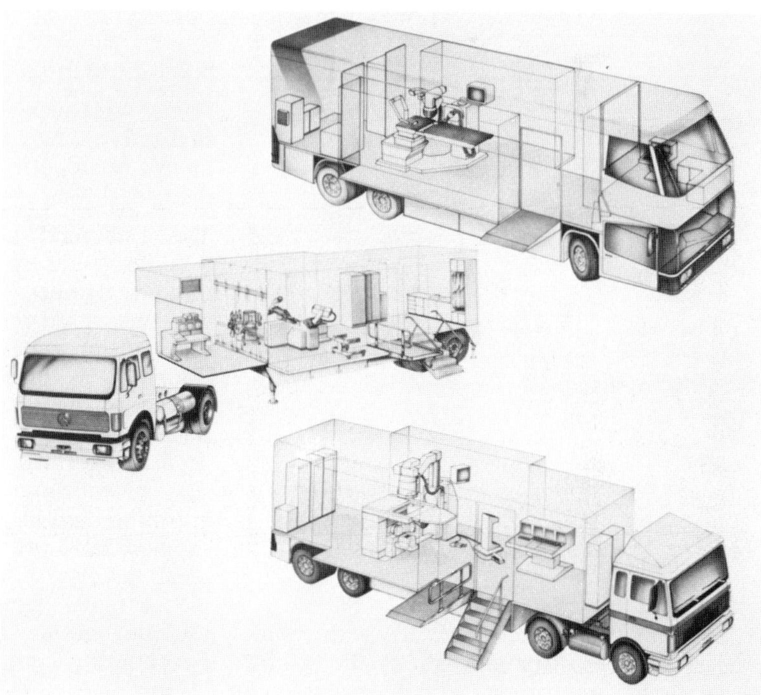

Fig. 8.**14** **Mobile lithotripters.** Here Dornier MPL 9000, HM4, and MFL 5000.

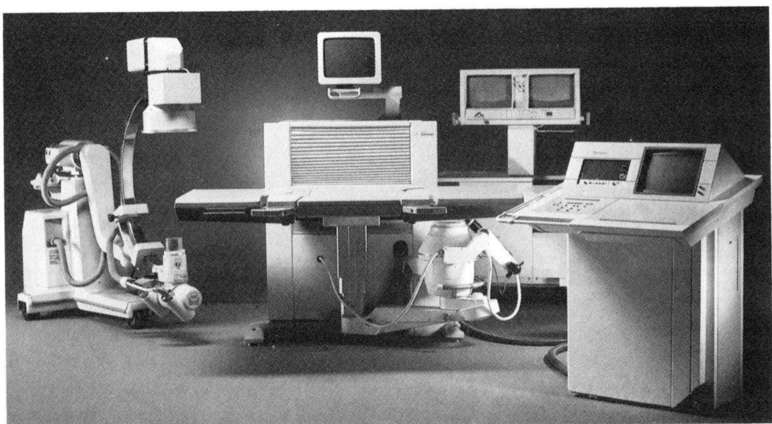

Fig. 8.**15** **Dornier Compact.** "Low-cost lithotriptor" with an electromagnetic shock wave source and lateral ultrasound scanner for stone localization. C-arm not integrated for stone localization

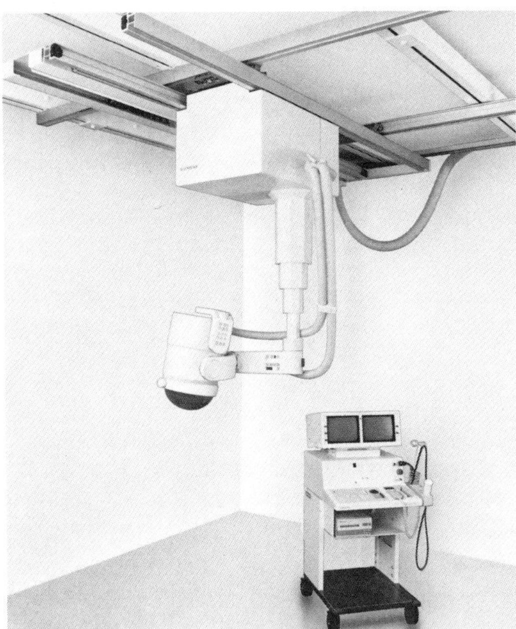

Fig. 8.**16** **Siemens Lithostar Ultra.** "Low-cost lithotriptor" consisting solely of overhead module providing only ultrasonic localization

also be used for other urological purposes; and (3) a mobile lithotriptor with the afore mentioned disadvantages.

The aim of *larger urological units* with a substantial number of patients should be a third generation lithotriptor encompassing all

ESWL requirements. If necessary, interdisciplinary lithotripsy would then also be possible.

A third generation lithotriptor should also be the first choice of an *interdisciplinary stone center*. However, if a standard lithotriptor with fluoroscopic stone localization (i.e., Dornier HM3, MFL 5000, or Siemens Lithostar) already exists, an ultrasound-based stone machine could be a good addition. Seven to 10 patients per day must be treated at such "two-machine stone centers" in order to make both lithotriptors worthwhile.

8.2.4 Fourth-Generation Lithotriptor

Some futuristic ideas have been conceptionally realized in the "Lithomed" system (Fig. 8.**17**) aiming at an optimal working station for stone disease.

The "Lithomed" system has been developed as a design study by students in the course of a diploma project. Free of economic and production-related restrictions, it basically represents an integrated, multipurpose, multifunctional "work station" for any kind of stone treatment. Any parts of the system — central patients table, control monitors, keyboards, shock wave generator, laser lithotriptor, ultrasound localization system, anesthesia unit — are integrated in a global room concept. "Lithomed" also provides some interesting technical details: shock waves are provided by piezoceramic elements that are not focused by the conventional hemispherical arrangement, but rather by computer-calculated consecutive "firing" of the single elements. Thus, mechani-

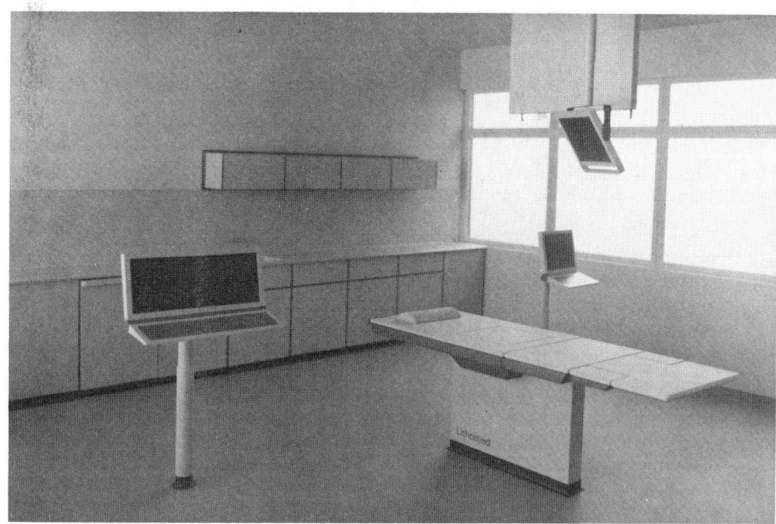

Fig. 8.**17** **Fourth-generation lithotriptor** (Rahe and Vedder, 1989).

cal movements of the shock wave source are unnecessary. All tools for intracorporeal laser lithotripsy (fibers), anesthesia (e.g., tubes, EKG cables) and stone localization (ultrasound scanner) are released from an overhead module for direct application at the patient, whereas the "energy" sources (e.g., laser lithotriptor, anesthesiological gas supply) are built into the furniture system of the room. Integrated control terminals for the operator as well as the for the anesthesist show the current ultrasound picture plus the relevant personal and medical data of the patient.

8.2.5 Comparison of Lithotriptors

The introduction of new lithotriptors has made comparison of the different machines necessary. Whereas the technical differentiation of the lithotriptors (i.e., shock wave generation, focusing, coupling, and localization) is simple classification of the disintegrative efficacy still remains problematic. The development of new shock wave sources, in particular, requires a *standardized classification* to determine the range of shock wave pressure (or generator voltage) for safe clinical use.

This can be done by

– physical measurements;
– stone models;
– animal studies.

Physical measurements. Ideally, shock wave generators should be classified with acoustic measurements. Theoretically, they can be defined by (Fig. 8.**18**)

– the rise time (T_r);
– peak positive pressure ($\hat{P}_{max}$);
– peak negative pressure (P^-_{max});
– duration of impulse (T);
– spectrum of frequencies (f);
– size of focal area (A);
– acoustic energy of every impulse (E_s).

At present, there are *no standardized hydrophones* available. Accurate measurement requires a durable and sensitive pressure probe with adequate rapid response time to record the fast rising peak pressures. Previously, shock wave measurement was carried out with a narrow band width of PCB probes and was, therefore, less accurate (i.e., Finlayson et al., 1986). The use of a broad band PVDF needle probe ensures more reliable data (Fig. 8.**19**). Recently, Coleman et al. demonstrated significant differences (i.e., frequency response) between needle probes, even between those from the same manufacturer, leading to varying statistics in the focal zone. As Coleman and Saunders have shown, this unreliable measurement method is of minor importance when different shock wave sources are tested utilizing the *same* hydrophone. Nevertheless, it is understood that a significant comparison of

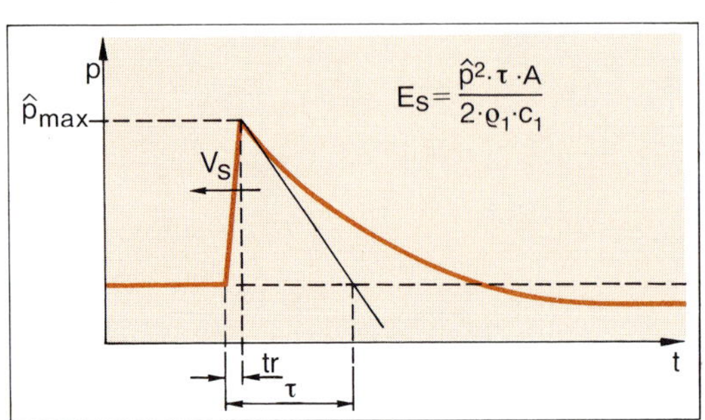

Fig. 8.**18 Theoretic profile of a shockwave.** E_s = acoustic energy of impule; $\hat{P}_{max}$ = peak pressure; T = pulse length; A = focal area; G_1 = specific density of medium; C_1 = sound velocity of medium

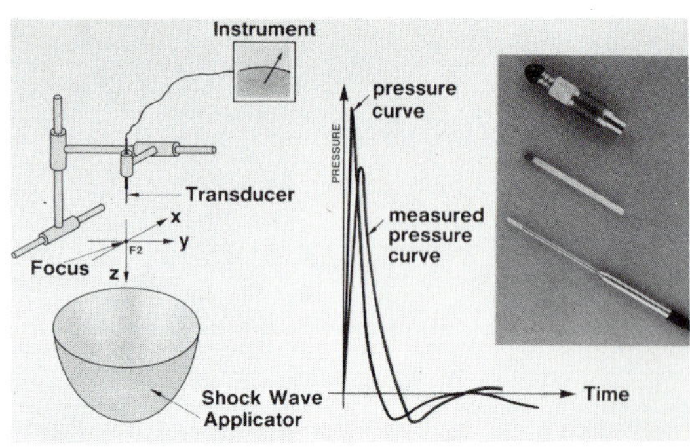

Fig. 8.**19 Measurement of shockwave profile.** Difference between theoretic and measured pressure curve. PCB- versus PVDF-needle hydrophone (lower probe)

lithotriptors can only be made with a reliable, well-defined measurement standard of shock waves. It is possible that the laser hydrophone (see Chapter 3) will become such a standard instrument.

Stone models. The problem of physical classification of shock waves is the main reason why the exact impact of each of the different parameters for stone disintegration with minimum tissue traumatization has still not been adequately defined and, as a result, is not yet completely understood. Standardized in vitro stone models have, therefore, become important for the classification and comparison of shock wave efficacy.

Stones, chalk pieces, plaster cubes, and pellets made of dental cement were utilized in preliminary studies to measure both the number of impulses for complete disintegration and the cavity produced after a defined number of shock waves (see Chapter 7). The possibility of determining a characteristic curve of impulses vs generator voltage for different shock wave sources (Fig. 8.**20**) was demonstrated. The movement of the curve (to the left or right) along the x-axis was caused by the hardness of the stone tested or by shock wave attenuation (use of a water cushion). These characteristic curves could be useful for

- determining the optimal generator voltage range for effective stone fragmentation;
- comparing the therapeutic broad band of different shock wave sources.

An easy check of the actual machine power can also be made, particularly in less successful clinical cases. Any decrease in disintegrative efficacy (i.e., owing to defect transducers) can be demonstrated on an standardized stone model by increasing the impulses for fragmentation.

Plaster cubes can also be used for the exact regulation of the focusing and localization system. It is important that a considerable deviation of shock wave focus and geometrical focus amounting to approximately 2–3 mm in the electrode ellipsoid system as well as in the electromagnetic membrane — acoustic lens device (Fig. 8.**21**) — is possible. This deviation is less important in shock wave sources with a large focal zone (12 or 9 mm, respectively, on x- and y-axis) than with a small focal area (3–5 mm, respectively, on x- and y-axis). In comparison to the geometrical focus determined by fluoroscopic localization, the focal zone of the shock wave can be depicted by means of a plaster cube; this makes time-consuming pressure measurements unnecessary.

Animal studies. At present, the degree of tissue trauma produced by shock waves cannot be predicted by physical measurements of in vitro stone models, since pertinent standards are still missing. It has been well documented that only focal and reversible intrarenal hematomas occur when a medium range of shock wave energy is applied (see Chapter 3). The introduction of shock wave sources that pro-

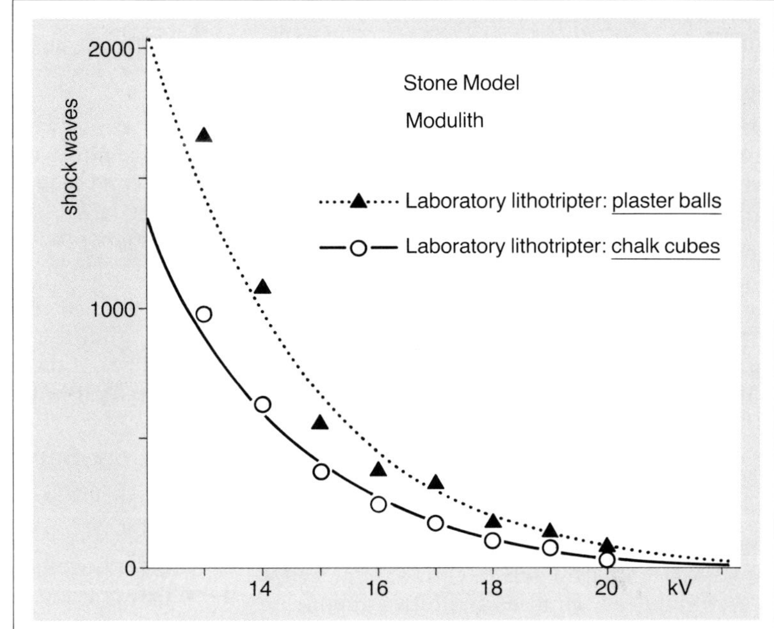

Fig. 8.**20   Various standardized, in vitro stone models characterizing a shock wave source** (Storz Modulith). In comparison with the chalk cubes, the harder plaster balls require approximately 2 kV more for the same degree of fragmentation (impulses)

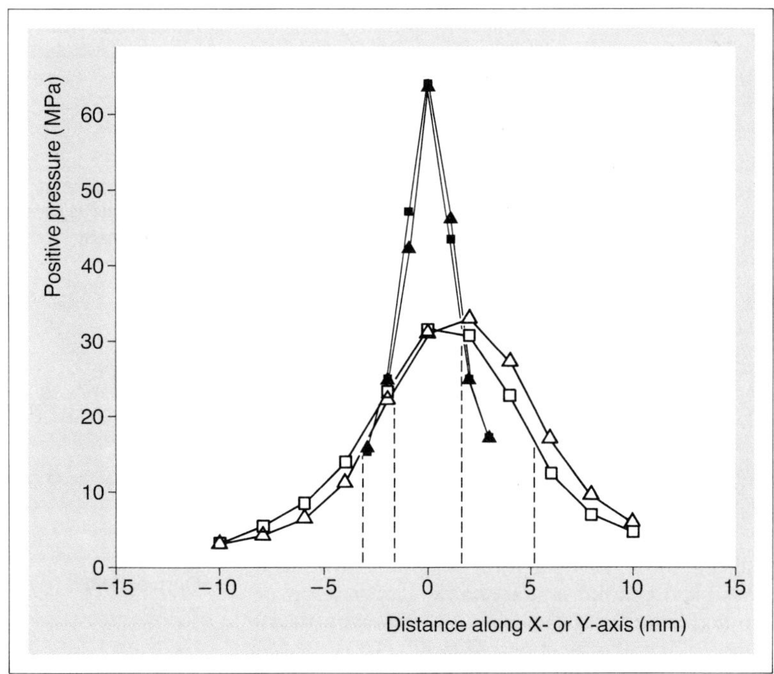

Fig. 8.**21   Deviation of shock wave focus in vitro from geometrical focus (Siemens Lithostar) on x- and y-axis.** Maximum pressure of the lithostar shock wave head approximately 3 mm from geometrical focus (Vergunst et al., 1989)

duce higher pressure levels (i.e., Storz Modulith SL20, Lithostar overhead, Dornier MPL 9000, Piezolith 2500) has made the characterization of renal trauma occurring with higher energy levels a matter of great importance if severe clinical complications are to be avoided.

Three animal models can be utilized (canine, New Zealand rabbit, and mini-pig), and at least two of these should be standardized with respect to the experimental design (e.g., number of shocks, localization, positioning) for future studies. Nevertheless, a well-defined standard of physical measurements should be achieved using standardized, reliable hydrophones. The correlation of this standard to in vitro and in vivo studies should finally make animal experiments unnecessary.

Clinical trials. Even though in vitro stone models have been correlated to clinical experience (i.e., number of impulses and retreatment rate vs number of shocks for disintegration of test stone), only clinical trials can estimate the exact capability of a lithotriptor. A prospective randomized phase III study at one center would be the best method of clinically comparing different stone machines. Unfortunately, very few centers have more than one lithotriptor. Diverse stone distribution and treatment strategies of each ESWL unit make a simple comparison of the available clinical data difficult.

Since phase III studies cannot be performed in most cases, the following represents a suitable method for comparing clinical results:

– definition of treatment strategy (i.e., in situ ESWL for ureteral calculi or "push and bang")
– determination of stone size, and localization and adjustment procedures before ESWL
– definition of success, that is, degree of disintegration and stone-free rate after 3–6 months

Taking these criteria into consideration, it is possible to make a reasonable comparison of clinical results obtained with different lithotriptors. The *"efficiency quotient"* (EQ) (Table 8.4) recently defined by Preminger and Clayman enables the determination of a specific figure expressing the clinical efficacy of a stone machine.

$$EQ = \frac{\%\ \text{of stone-free patients}}{100\% + \%\ \text{retreated patients} + \%\ \text{secondary procedures}}$$

It is interesting to compare the similarity of EQ for small stones between the most important second generation lithotriptors and the Dornier HM3. The EQ for larger calculi is much higher with the Dornier HM3 (Table 8.4).

Future clinical trials based on the afore mentioned criteria must confirm the theoretical advantages of the new (third generation) interdisciplinary lithotriptors in clinical practice.

8.2.6 Cost-Benefit Evaluation

The financial aspects of ESWL comprise the following three points:

– shorter hospitalization
– shorter period of indisposition

Table 8.**4** **Comparison of clinical results of the most important second generation lithotriptors using the efficiency quotient** (from Preminger and Clayman)

a) For stones less than 1 cm

	SFR	RE-TX	AUX	EQ
Dornier HM3	77%	5%	12%	0.66
Dornier HM4	85%	38%	4%	0.60
Direx	75%	24%	7%	0.57
EDAP	72%	29%	2%	0.55
Siemens	74%	7%	16%	0.60
Technomed	81%	13%	7%	0.68
Wolf	86%	16%	4%	0.72

b) For stones 1–2 cm

	SFR	RE-TX	AUX	EQ
Dornier HM3	75%	10%	11%	0.62
EDAP	64%	68%	6%	0.37
Siemens	65%	12%	12%	0.52
Wolf	69%	27%	2%	0.53

SFR   stone-free rate
RE-TX   retreatment rate
AUX   percentage of auxilliary measures
EQ   efficiency quotient

– reduction of stone-induced cases requiring dialysis

Previous calculations (Miller, 1984; Rassweiler, 1985) were made on the basis of a comparison between ESWL and open surgery. The calculation of the above parameters showed a net revenue of ca. $ 3600 per ESWL treatment. However, this figure is no longer valid.

Nowadays, more than 90% of patients could certainly be treated with endourological methods (PCNL, URS). Therefore, ESWL cost-benefit analysis must be based on a comparative study of the data relevant to endourological surgeries.

Here, contact-free kidney stone disintegration would presumably not shorten hospitalization or the period of indisposition. Furthermore, percutaneous surgery is a reno-protective method, which, like ESWL, can be repeated as often as necessary. Contact-free kidney stone disintegration does not provide any foreseeable financial advantages and does not reduce the number of stone-induced dialysis cases.

In comparison to endourological methods, the benefits of ESWL are the nonfinancial aspects: noninvasiveness with less postoperative morbidity and mortality and a reduced fear of surgery.

Current cost-benefit evaluations emphasize the importance of *reducing present costs of contact-free kidney stone disintegration.*

8.3 Further Applications of Shock Waves

Clinically, the most interesting extension of indications for ESWL is the treatment of *pancreatic duct and salivatory duct stones*, since extensive surgery can be avoided in both cases.

To date, the treatment of stones in the salivatory gland (i.e., submandibular, parotid gland) was performed by glandectomy, with the possibility of significant injury and postoperative complications (i.e., paresis of the facialis nerve). The most extended experience with salivatory lithotripsy has been gained with the Piezolith (Gundlach 1990) and the Modulith (Kater and Meyer 1990).

Another possible clinical application of shock waves is the treatment of *pseudoarthrosis.* In 1989, Valchanau et al. presented their first experience with 53 patients suffering from pseudoarthrosis of fractures over an average of 20 months. On shock wave treatment, the pseudoarthrosis was brought to a stand still for an average of 81 days. Shock wave therapy was successful in 88% of the patients. These results have been experimentally sustained by Haupt et al. (1990), who could demonstrated the positive effect of shock waves on the healing of a fracture.

Contrary to this, the *treatment of tumors with shock waves* is still at an early experimental phase. Here, the clinical relevance is still unknown, even though early investigations demonstrated the significant dose-dependent damage caused by high-energy shock waves (see Chapter 3). Only a temporary effect was determined in most studies; furthermore, very little information exists on the tumor-specific effect of shock waves. Shock waves will have to be modified for any future treatment of neoplasms. Whereas, in ESWL sources, shock waves have been developed with the aim of minimum tissue trauma in mind, maximum traumatization is the aim of tumor treatment. The increase in cavitation or the use of higher frequencies are important factors in this respect. In 1989, Peschke et al. demonstrated, on normal tissue, that 5 Hz impulses caused more distinct damage to Dunning Ly/Lu prostate carcinoma of the rat than 1 Hz did.

Owing to the essential difference of shock wave quality, all experimental studies concerning the treatment of tumor cells — including chemotherapy — are elementary. The same applies to the *shock wave treatment of benign prostatic hypertrophy* (Erlich et al., 1989).

Aiming at drug carriers with shock waves could be another interesting application. In 1989, Jones et al. loaded autologeous erythrocytes with H3-methotrexate and demonstrated a 107% increase of the cytotoxic drug in the shocked area. These findings could reduce the toxic side effects of cancer chemotherapy.

The afore mentioned methods are still far from clinical application.

References

Abomelha MS, Said MT, Otaibi KE. ESWL monotherapy in staghorn calculi. Wld Congress Endourol 1987;5:

Abrahams C, Lipson SB, Ross LS. The effects of shock wave lithotripsy (ESWL) on canine kidneys. J Urol 1988;139:324A.

Algood CB, Sood N, Fairchild T, Mayo M. Experimental study of ureteral calculus disease: effects of calculus size, obstruction and hydration. J Urol 1983;130:999–1004.

Alken P. Perkutane Nephrolithotomie. Urologe (A) 1984;23:20–4.

Alken P. The telescope dilatators. World J Urol 1985;3:7–10.

Alken P, Rassweiler J. Complications of ESWL. In: Proceedings of the Seventh World Congress on Endourology and ESWL, November 27–30, 1989, Kyoto, Japan (abstract L4).

Alken P, Hutschenreiter R, Guenther M, Marberger M. Percutaneous stone manipulation. J Urol 1981;125:463–6.

Alken P, Thüroff JW, Riedmiller H, Hohenfellner R. Doppler sonography and B-mode ultrasound scanning in renal stone surgery. Urology 1984;23:455–60.

Alken P, Hardemann S, Wilbert D, Thüroff J, Jacobi GH. Extracorporeal shock wave lithotripsy (ESWL): alternatives and adjuvant procedures. World J Urol 1985a;3:48–52.

Alken P, Thüroff J, Walz P, Hohenfellner R. Perkutane Nephrolithotomie. Dtsch Ärztebl 1985b;82:257–66.

Andrulakis P, Frangoulis E, Lefkidis C, Varkarais M, Delivelotis A. Kidney damage in recurrent renal lithiasis. Eur Urol 1982;8:261–4.

Baumgartner BR, Dickey KW, Ambrose SS, Walton KN, Nelson RC, Bernardino ME. Kidney changes after extracorporeal shock wave lithotripsy: appearance on MR imaging. Radiology 1987;163:531–4.

Baumüller A, Schmeller NT, Hofstetter AG. Perkutane Nephrolithotomie und Litholapaxie. Fortschr Med 1984;36:900–2.

Becht E, Moll V, Neisius D, Ziegler, M. Treatment of prevesical ureteral calculi by extracorporeal shock wave lithotripsy. J Urol 1988;139:916.

Becopoulos T, Karayanis A, Mandalaki T, Karafoulidou A, Markakis C. Extracorporeal lithotripsy in patients with hemophilia. Eur Urol 1988;14:343–5.

Begun FP, Lawson RK. Renal injury resulting from focused electrohydraulic shock waves. J Urol 1988;139:323A.

Berens ME, Schostock C, Hart L, Barshira Z, McCullough Dl. Effect of cell cycle and temperature on the antiproliferative effects of acoustic shock waves (SW) against human tumor cells. J Urol 1988;139:304A.

Berger RE. Transurethral ureteroscopy and nephroscopy in men and women using standard adult endoscopic equipment. J Urol 1983;129:581–3.

Bhatta KM, Rosen DI, Dretter SP. The electromagnetical impactor: animal studies and first clinical experience. J Endourol 1990;4:5–127 (Suppl.)

Bichler KH, Erdmann D, Schmitz-Moormann P, Halim S. Operatives Ureterorenoskop für Ultraschallanwendung und Steinextraktion. Urologe (A) 1984;23:99–104.

Blandy JP, Singh M. The case for a more aggressive approach to staghorn stones. J Urol 1976;115:505–6.

Bomanji J, Boddy SA, Britton KE, Nimmon CC, Whitfield HN. Radionuclide evaluation: pre- and postextracorporeal shock wave lithotripsy for renal calculi. J Nucl Med 1987;28:1284–9.

Boyce WH. Renal calculi. In: Glenn JF, Boyce WH, eds. Urologic surgery. 2nd ed. New York: Harper and Row, 1975.

Boyce WH, Elkins IB. Reconstructive renal surgery following anatrophic nephrolithotomy: follow-up of 100 consecutive cases. J Urol 1974;111:307–12.

Bowdon FP, Brunton JH. The deformation of solid by liquid impact and supersonic speeds. Proc R Soc A 1961;263:433–50.

Brandl H, Chaussy C, Thüroff J, Leser C. First results with the multifunctional lithotripter MFL 5000. In: Proceedings of the Seventh World Congress on Endourology and ESWL, November 27–30, 1989, Kyoto, Japan. 62 (abstract 02–2).

Brannen GE, Bush WH. Ultrasonic destruction of kidney stones. West Med 1984;140:227–32.

Brannen GE, Bush WH, Correa RJ, Gibsons RP, Elder JS. Kidney stone removal: percutaneous versus surgical lithotomy. J Urol 1985;133:6–12.

Bräuner T, Brümmer F, Hülser DF. Histopathology of shock wave treated tumor cell suspensions and multicell tumor spheroids. Ultrasound Med Biol 1989;15:451–60.

Brendel W. Stosswellen. Ein neues therapeutisches Prinzip der Medizin. Münchn Med Wochenschr 1984;126:1–3.

Brendel W, Conzen P, Goetz AE, Königsberger R. Experimentelle Tumortherapie mit Schockwellen. Erste Ergebnisse. In: Verhandlungsbericht, Vereinigung der Bayerischen Chirurgen, 64. Tagung vom 16.–18. Juli 1987, Bad Reichenhall.

Brendel W, Wilmer A, Delius M. Effekt von Stosswellen auf Tumorzellen in Suspension. In: Verhandlungsbericht, Vereinigung der Bayerischen Chirurgen, 64. Tagung vom 16.–18. Juli 1987, Bad Reichenhall.

Brendel W, Delius M, Goetz A. Effect of shock waves on the microvasculature. Progr Appl Microcirc 1987; 12:41–50.

Brewer SL, Atala AA, Ackerman DM, Steinbock GS. Shock wave lithotripsy damage in human cadaver kidneys. J Endourol 1988;2:333–9.

Brümmer F, Bräuner T, Brenner J, Hülser DF. Effects of lithotriptor-generated shock waves on L1210 mouse leukemia cells detected by flow cytometry. Eur J Cell Biol 1988;46:12.

Brümmer F, Brenner J, Bräuner T, Hülser DF. Effect of shock waves on suspended and immobilized L1210 cells. Ultrasound Med Biol 1989;15:229–39.

Bundesverband der Ortskrankenkassen. Statistik der Ortskrankenkassen. Krankheitsarten-, Krankheitsursachen- und Sterblichkeitsstatistik 1975–1979.

Burchhardt P. Über konservativ behandelte Ausgusssteine und Restkonkremente. Urologe (A) 1982;21:45–48.

Burns JR, Shoemaker BE, Finlayson B. The effect of irrigation agents on in vitro dissolution of magnesium ammonium phosphate hexahydrate. World J Urol 1983;1:159–62.

Bush W, Gibbons RP, Lewis GP, Brannen GE. Impact of extracorporeal shock wave lithotripsy on percutaneous stone procedures. Am J Radiol 1986;147:89–93.

Carini M, Selli C, Fiorelli, C. Elective treatment of ureteral stones with extracorporeal shock wave lithotripsy. Eur Urol 1987;13:289.

Chang R, Marshall FF. Management of ureteroscopic injuries. J Urol 1987;139:1132.

Charig CR, Webb DR, Payne SR, Wickham JE. Comparison of treatment of renal calculi by open surgery, percutaneous nephrolithotomy, and extracorporeal shock wave lithotripsy. Br Med J 1986;292:879–82.

Chaussy C. ESWL: past, present, and future. J Endourol 1988;2:97–105.

Chaussy C, Fuchs G. Erfahrungen mit der extrakorporalen Stosswellenlithotripsie nach 5 Jahren klinischer Anwendung. Urologe (A) 1985;24:305–10.

Chaussy C, Schmiedt E. Shock wave treatment for stones in the upper urinary tract. Urol Clin North Am 1983;10:743–50.

Chaussy C, Schmiedt E. Extracorporeal shock wave lithotripsy (ESWL) for kidney stones: an alternative to surgery? Urol Radiol 1984;6:80–7.

Chaussy C, Staehler G. Berührungsfreie Nierensteinzertrümmerung durch extrakorporal erzeugte, fokussierte Stosswellen. In: Schmiedt E, Bauer HW, eds. Beiträge zur Urologie. Basle: Karger, 1980.

Chaussy C, Eisenberger F, Wanner K, Forssmann B, Hepp W, Schmiedt E, Brendel W. The use of shock waves for the destruction of calculi without direct contact. Urol Res 1976;4:175.

Chaussy C, Eisenberger F, Wanner K. Die Implantation humaner Nierensteine. Ein einfaches experimentelles Steinmodell. Urologe (A) 1977;16:35–8.

Chaussy C, Eisenberger F, Wanner K, Forssmann B. Extrakorporale Anwendung von hochenergetischen Stosswellen. Ein neuer Aspekt in der Behandlung des Harnsteinleidens, Teil 2. Aktuel Urol 1978;9:95–102.

Chaussy C, Schmiedt E, Forssmann B, Brendel W. Contact-free renal stone destruction by means of shock waves. Eur Surg Res 1979;11:36.

Chaussy C, Brendel W, Schmiedt E. Extracorporeally induced destruction of kidney stones by shock waves. Lancet 1980;13:1265–68.

Chaussy C, Schmiedt E, Jocham D, Brendel W, Forssmann B, Moser E. Berührungsfreie Nierensteinzertrümmerung durch Stosswellen. Dtsch Ärztebl 1981;78:881–6.

Chaussy C, Schmiedt E, Jocham D, Brendel W, Forssmann B, Walther W. First clinical experience with extracorporeally induced destruction of kidney stones by shock waves. J Urol 1982;127:417–20.

Chaussy C, Schmiedt E, Jocham D, Walther V, Brendel W. Stosswellentherapie zur Behandlung von Nierensteinen. Münchn Med Wochenschr 1983;125:151–5.

Chaussy C, Schmiedt E, Jocham D, Schüller J, Brandl H. Extrakorporale Stosswellenlithotripsie. Beginn einer Umstrukturierung in der Behandlung des Harnsteinleidens. Urologe (A) 1984a;23:25–9.

Chaussy C, Schmiedt E, Jocham D, Schüller J, Brandl J, Liedl B. Extracorporeal shock wave lithotripsy (ESWL) for treatment of urolithiasis. Urology 1984b;23:59–66.

Chaussy C, Schmiedt E, Jocham D, et al. Extracorporeal shock wave lithotripsy. Basle: Karger, 1986.

Chaussy C, Randazzo RF, Fuchs GJ. The effects of extracorporeal shock waves on human renal carcinoma cells and normal human embryonic kidney cells. J Urol 1988a;139:320A.

Chaussy C, Randazzo RF, Fuchs GJ. The effects of extracorporeal shock waves on FANFT bladder tumors in C3H/He mice. J Urol 1988b;139:289a.

Chinn SKB, Michaels EK, Fowler JE, Behnia R, Linde HW, Ray V. Hemodynamic and adrenal response to shock wave energy. J Urol 1988;139:324A.

Chuong CJ, Zhong MS, Preminger GM. Pressure measurements in a Wolf Piezolith 2200 lithotriptor. In: Lingeman JE, Newman DM, eds. Shock wave lithotripsy: state of the art. New York: Plenum Press, 1988:395–8.

Clayman RV. Techniques in percutaneous removal of renal calculi. Urol 1984;23(suppl)11–19.

Clayman RV, Castaneda-Zuniga W. Nephrolithotomy: percutaneous removal of renal calculi. Urol Radiol 1984;6:95–112.

Clayman RV, Surya V, Miller RP, Castaneda-Zuniga W, Amplatz K, Lange PH. Percutaneous nephrolithotomy: an approach to branched and staghorn renal calculi. J Am Med Assoc 1983;250:73–5.

Clayman RV, Surya V, Miller RP, et al. Percutaneous nephrolithotomy: extraction of renal and ureteral calculi from 100 patients. J Urol 1984;131:868–71.

Cole RS, Shuttleworth KE. Is extracorporeal shockwave lithotripsy suitable treatment for lower ureteric stones? Brit J Urol 1988;62:525.

Coleman AJ, Saunders JE. Comparison of extracorporeal shock wave lithotriptors based on measurements in the acoustic field. In: Coptcoat MJ, Miller RA, Wickham JEA, eds. Lithotripsy, vol 2. London: BDI, 1987:121–31.

Coleman AJ, Saunders JE. A comparison of PVDF hydrophone measurements in the acoustic field of a shock wave source. In: Ell C, Marberger M, Berlien P, eds. Extra- und intrakorporale Lithotripsie bei Harn-, Gallen-, Pankreas- und Speichelsteinen. Stuttgart: Thieme, 1990: 14–22..

Coleman AJ, Saunders JE. A survey of the acoustic input of commercial extracorporeal shock wave lithotriptors. Ultrasound Med Biol 1989;15:213–27.

Coptcoat MJ. The Steinstrasse: classification and management. In: Coptcoat MJ, Miller RA, Wickham JEA, eds. Lithotripsy, vol 2. London: BDI, 1987:133–8.

Coptcoat MJ, Webb DR, Kellett MJ, et al. The complications of extracorporeal shock wave lithotripsy: management and prevention. Br J Urol 1986;58:578–80.

Das G, Birch B, Samuel C, Whitfield HN, Wickham JEA. Enzymuria as a marker of tubular recovery following extracorporeal shock wave lithotripsy. In: Lingeman JE, Newman DE, eds. Shock wave lithotripsy: state of the art. New York: Plenum Press, 1988:369–70.

Delius M, Enders G, Heine G, Stark J, Remberger K, Brendel W. Biological effects of shock waves: lung hemorrhage by shock waves in dogs – pressure dependence. Ultrasound Med Biol 1987;13:61–7.

Delius M, Enders G, Xuan Z, Liebich HG, Brendel W. Biological effects of shock waves: kidney damage by shock waves in dogs – dose dependence. Ultrasound Med Biol 1988;14:117–22.

Delius M, Jordan M, Eizenhofer H, et al. Biological effects of shock waves: kidney hemorrhage by shock waves in dogs – adminstration rate dependence. Ultrasound Med Biol 1988;689–94.

DiSilverio F, Gallucci M, Gambardella P, et al. Blood cellular and biochemical changes after extracorporeal shock wave lithotripsy. Urol Res 1990;18:49–51.

Drach GW, Dretler SP, Fair WR. Report of the United States cooperative study of extracorporeal shock wave lithotripsy. J Urol 1986;135:1127.

Dreikorn K, Horsch R. Aktueller Stand renoprotektiver Massnahmen bei Operationen an der insuffizienten Niere. Urologe (A) 1984;23:3–8.

Dretler SP. An evaluation of ureteral laser lithotripsy: 225 consecutive patients. J Urol 1990;43:267–72.

Dretler SP, Keating MA, Riley J. An algorithm for the management of ureteral calculi. J Urol 1986;136:1190.

Dretler SP, Pfister RC, Newhouse JH, Prien EL Jr. Percutaneous catheter dissolution of cystine calculi. J Urol 1984;131:216–19.

Dretler SP, Watson G, Parrish JA, Murray S. Pulsed dye laser fragmentation of ureteral calculi: Initial clinical experience. J Urol 1986;137:386.

Dretler SP, Weinstein A. A modified algorithm for the management of ureteral calculi: 100 consecutive cases. J Urol 1988;140:732.

Dretler SP. Techniques of Laser Lithotripsy. J Endourol 1988;2:123.

Dretler SP. Stone fragility: an new therapeutic distinction. J Urol 1988;139:290.

Eisenberger F. [Editorial.] Z Allgemeine Med 1985; 61:961–2.

Eisenberger F, Rassweiler J. Extrakorporale Stosswellen-lithotripsie im Wandel. Aktuel Urol 1986;17:229–33.

Eisenberger F, Schmidt A. ESWL: What is proven and what remains controversial? In: Proceedings of the Seventh World Congress on Endourology and ESWL, November 27–30, 1989, Kyoto, Japan (abstract L7).

Eisenberger F, Chaussy C, Klein U, Pfeifer KJ, Rothe R, Schellong H. In-situ Perfusion und Unterkühlung der Niere. Verh Dtsch Ges Urol 1973;29:225.

Eisenberger F, Chaussy C, Wanner K. Entwicklung eines steintragenden Hundemodells zur in-vivo Untersuchung der Wirkung fokussierter Stosswellen auf Nierensteine. Biophysikalische Verfahren zur Diagnose und Therapie von Steinleiden der Harnwege. Meersburg, West Germany: Dornier, 1976. (Wissenschaftliche Berichte der Firma Dornier.)

Eisenberger F, Chaussy C, Hofstetter A, Marx FJ. Langzeituntersuchungen nach hypothermer Perfusion der Niere. Aktuel Urol 1977a;8:239–42.

Eisenberger F, Chaussy C, Wanner K. Extrakorporale Anwendung von hochenergetischen Stosswellen. Ein neuer Aspekt in der Behandlung des Harnsteinleidens. Aktuel Urol 1977b;8:3–15.

Eisenberger F, Schmiedt E, Chaussy C, et al. Berührungsfreie Harnsteinzertrümmerung. Stand der Forschung. Dtsch Ärztebl 1977c;74:1145–50.

Eisenberger F, Fuchs G, Miller K. Nierensteintherapie: Erste klinische Erfahrungen mit der berührungsfreien Nierensteintherapie. ESWL am Katharinenhospital Stuttgart. Ärztebl Baden-Württemberg 1983;12:504–6.

Eisenberger F, Fuchs G, Miller K, Rassweiler J. Extracorporeal shock wave lithotripsy and endourology: an ideal combination for the treatment of kidney stones. World J Urol 1985a;3:41–8.

Eisenberger F, Fuchs G, Miller K, Rassweiler J. Noninvasive renal stone therapy with extracorporeal shock wave lithotripsy (ESWL). In: Donner W, Heuck FH. Radiology today, vol 3. Berlin: Springer, 1985b:161–7.

Eisenberger F, Gumpinger R, Miller K, Horbaschek H, Sklebitz H. Stereo-Röntgen in der Endourologie. Urologe (A) 1985c;24:342–5.

Eisenberger F, Rassweiler J, Bab P, Kallert B, Miller K. Differentiated approach to staghorn calculi using extracorporal shock wave lithotripsy and percutaneous nephrolithotomy: an analysis of 131 cases. World J Urol 1987; 5: 248–54.

Eisenberger F, Rassweiler J, Kallert B, Bub P. Die Behandlung des Ausgusssteines. Strategien und Ergebnisse des kombinierten Einsatzes neuer Techniken. Urologe (A) 1989;138–44.

Eisenmenger W. Eine elekromagnetische Impulsschallquelle zur Erzeugung von Druckstössen in Flüssigkeiten und Festkörpern. In: Cremer L, ed. Proceedings of the Third International Congress on Acoustics, July 1961. Amsterdam: Elsevier, 1962:326–9.

Eisenmenger W. Elektromagnetische Erzeugung von ebenen Druckstössen in Flüssigkeiten. Acustica 1962; 12:185–202.

Eisenmenger W. Physikalisch-medizinische Aspekte selbstfokussierter elektromagnetisch erzeugter Stosswellen. Verh Ber Dtsch Ges Urol 1988;39:69–70.

El-Faqih SR, Husain I, Ekman PE, Sharma ND, Chakrabary A, Talic R. Primary choice of intervention for distal ureteric stone: Ureteroscopy or ESWL? Brit J Urol 1988;62:13.

Erlich N, Lobel B, Guille F, et al. Influence of high energy shock waves on benign prostatic hypertrophy. In: Proceedings of the Seventh World Congress on Endourology and ESWL, November 27–30, 1989, Kyoto, Japan. (abstract P13–13).

Erturk E, Streem S, Stower NT. The effects of ESWL on renal function and systemic blood pressure: preliminary report of an experimental study. In: Lingeman JE, Newman DE, eds. Shock wave lithotripsy: state of the art. New York: Plenum Press, 1988:383–6.

Eshghi M. Pressure-controlled hydraulic dilation of the ureter: "one-step" ureteroscopy. J Urol 1988;140:950.

Fair HD. In vitro destruction of urinary calculi by laser-induced stress waves. Med Instrum 1978;12:100–5.

Fernstroem I, Johannson B. Percutaneous pyelolithotomy: a new extraction technique. Scand J Urol Nephrol 1976;4:257.

Fetner CD, Preminger GM, Kettelhut MC, Elkins SL. Morbidity of ureteral stenting during ESWL. J Urol 1989;141:270A (abstract 402).

Fischer N, Rübben H, Hofsäss S, et al. Alternative Stosswellenerzeugungsverfahren mit dem Dornier Lithoripter HM3. Urologe (A) 1987;26:29–32.

Fischer N, Müller HM, Gulhan A, et al. Cavitation effects: possible cause of tissue injury during extracorporeal shock wave lithotripsy. J Endourol 1988;2:215–20.

Fitzpatrick JM, Sleight MW, Braack A, Marberger M, Wickham JEA. Intrarenal access: effects on renal function and morphology. Br J Urol 1980;52:409–14.

Folbert W. Pressure-optimized lithotripsy with the Siemens Lithostar: successful and tissue-protecting treatment of urinary stones. Eur Urol 1990; 17:51–7.

Folbert W, Hassler D. Die Wertigkeit von "in-line" und "out-line" Ultraschall-Lokalisation in der extrakorporalen Stoßwellen-Lithotripsie. Z Urol 1990; 2:46−7.

Ford TF, Watson G, Wickham JE. Transurethral ureteroscopic retrieval of ureteric stones. Br J Urol 1983;55:626−8.

Ford TF, Payne SR, Wickham JE. The impact of transurethral ureteroscopy on the management of ureteric calculi. Br J Urol 1984;56:602−3.

Forssmann B, Hepp W. Stosswellen in der Medizin. Med unserer Zeit 1980;4:10−14.

Forssmann B, Hepp W, Hoff G, Eisenberger F, Chaussy C, Wanner K. Entwicklung eines Verfahrens zur berührungsfreien Zerkleinerung von Nierensteinen durch Stosswellen. Biophysikalisches Verfahren zur Diagnose und Therapie von Steinleiden der Harnwege. Meersburg, West Germany: Dornier, 1976. (Wissenschaftliche Berichte der Firma Dornier.)

Forssmann B, Hepp W, Chaussy C, Eisenberger F, Wanner K. Eine Methode zur berührungsfreie Zertrümmerung von Nierensteinen durch Stosswellen. Biomed Tech 1977;22:164.

Forssmann B, Hepp W, Chaussy C, Jocham D, Schmiedt E, Brendel W. Prototyp für die klinische Anwendung der berührungsfreien Nierensteinzertrümmerung durch Stosswellenimpulse. Biomed Tech 1980; 9 (suppl): 414−16.

Fritz KW, Seitz W, Aeikens B. Der Einsatz von Prilocain zur lumbalen Periduralanästhesie bei extracorporaler Stosswellenlithotripsie (ESWL). Aktuel Urol 1985; 16:317−19.

Fritz KW, Reimann P, Schröder D, Allhoff E, Spangehl-Meridjen P, Jonas U. Extrakorporale Stosswellenlithotripsie (ESWL) mit dem modifizierten HM3-Lithotripter. Eine klinische Untersuchung zum Anästhesiemanagement. Klinikarzt 1989;18:363−5.

Fuchs AM, Coulson W, Fuchs GJ. Effect of extracorporeally induced high-energy shock waves on the rabbit kidney and ureter: a morphologic and functional study. J Endourol 1988;2:341−4.

Fuchs G, Fuchs A. Intrarenal surgery − indications and results. J Endourol 1990;4:5−142 (Suppl.)

Fuchs G, Miller K, Rassweiler J. Alternatives to open surgery for renal calculi: percutaneous nephrolithotomy and extracorporeal shock wave lithotripsy. In: Schilling A, ed. Klinische und experimentelle Urologie, vol 8. Munich: Zuckschwerdt, 1984b:153−77.

Fuchs G, Miller K, Rassweiler J, Eisenberger F. Extracorporeal shock wave lithotripsy: one-year experience with the Dornier lithotripter. Eur Urol 1985;11:145−9.

Fuchs GJ, Chaussy CG. Extracorporeal shock wave lithotripsy for staghorn stones: reassessment of our treatment strategy. Wld J Urol 1987;5:237.

Fuchs GJ, Chaussy CG, Stenzl A. Current management concepts in the treatment of ureteral stones. J Endourol 1988;2:117.

Fuchs GJ, Fuchs AM, Royce Pl, Stenzl A, Chaussy CG. Staghorn stone treatment with extracorporeal shock wave lithotripsy: the fate of residual stones. In: Lingeman JE, Newman DE, eds. Shock wave lithotripsy: state of the art. New York: Plenum Press, 1988a:101−6.

Fuchs GJ, Randazzo RF, Fuchs AM, Stenzl A, Chaussy CG. The in vitro and in vivo effects of extracorporeal shock waves on tumor cells. In: Lingeman JE, Newman DE, eds. Shock wave lithotripsy: state of the art. New York: Plenum Press, 1988:351−6.

Fuchs GJ, David RM, Wolfson B, Barbaric Z. Comparative morphological and functional study of the bioeffects of open surgery, percutaneous surgery and ESWL on renal morphology and function: creation of an animal model. In: Proceedings of the Seventh World Congress on Endourology and ESWL, November 27−30, 1989, Kyoto, Japan (abstract 04−7).

Gilbert BR, Riehle RA, Vaughan ED Jr. Extracorporeal shock wave lithotripsy and its effect on renal function. J Urol 1988;139:482−5.

Gil-Vernet J. New surgical concepts in removing renal calculi. Urol Int 1985;20:255−88.

Gil-Vernet JM. Minimum nephrostomy. Urology 1977;6:620.

Gleeson MJ, Griffith DP. Extracorporeal shock wave lithotripsy monotherapy for large renal calculi. Br J Urol 1989;64:329−32.

Goetz AE, Königsberger R, Feyh J, Conzen PF, Lumper W. Breakdown of tumor microcirculation induced by shock waves or photodynamic therapy. In: Baethmann F, Messmer G, eds. Surgical research: recent concepts and results. Berlin: Springer, 1987:82−93.

Goodwin WE, Casey WC. Percutaneous trocar nephrostomy in hydronephrosis. J Am Med Assoc 1955;157:891.

Graff J, Pastor J, Herberhold D, et al. Technical modifications of the Dornier HM3 lithotriptor with an improved anesthesia technique. World J Urol 1987;5:202−7.

Graff J, Pastor J, Funke PJ, Mach P, Senge T. Extracorporeal shock wave lithotripsy for ureteral stones: a retrospective analysis of 417 cases. J Urol 1988a;139:513−16.

Graff J, Richter KO, Pastor J. Wirkung von hochenergetischen Stosswellen auf Knochengewebe. Verh Ber Dtsch Ges Urol 1988b;39:76.

Griffith DP, Moskowith PA, Carlton CE. Adjunctive chemotherapy of infection-induced staghorn calculi. J Urol 1979;121:711.

Griffith DP, McCue P, Lee H, Benson J, Carlton CE Jr. Stone cancer: palliative treatment with acetohydroxamide acid. World J Urol 1983;1:170−5.

Grote R, Döhring W, Aeikens B. Computertomographischer und sonographischer Nachweis von renalen und perirenalen Veränderungen nach einer extrakorporalen Stosswellenlithotripsie. RöFo 1986;144:434−9.

Grunberger I, Laungani GB, Armel H, et al. Initial experience with the therasonic lithotripor. In: Proceedings of the Seventh World Congress on Endourology and ESWL, November 27−30, 1989, Kyoto, Japan (abstract 02−3).

Gumpinger R, Miller K, Fuchs G, Eisenberger F. Antegrade ureteroscopy for stone removal. Eur Urol 1985;11:199−202.

Gupta NP, Kochar GS, Wadhwa SN, Singh SM. Management of patients with renal and ureteric calculi presenting with chronic renal insufficiency. Br J Urol 1985;57:130−2.

Habermehl A, Hackelöer BJ. Physikalische und technische Grundlagen der Sonographie. Dtsch Ärztebl 1983;80:41−57.

Habersetzer R, Schneider B, Schleiuer S, Illner W. Aktueller Stand der Nierentransplantation und ihre Ergebnisse. Lebensversicherungsmedizin 1985;3:72−4.

Haupt G, Haupt A, Gerety B, Chvapil M. Enhancement of fracture healing with extracorporeal shock waves. J Urol 1990;143(2):2311.

Häusler E, Kiefer W. Anregung von Stosswellen in Flüssigkeiten durch Hochgeschwindigkeitswassertropfen. Verh Dtsch Physik Ges 1971;10:36.

Häusler E, Kiefer W. Nierensteinzertrümmerung mit geführten Stosswellen. Ann Univ Saraviensis Med 1974;11:150–9.

Häusler E, Kiefer W. Zerstörung von spröden Einschlüssen in flüssiger Umgebung durch autofokussierte Stosswellen. Verh Dtsch Physik Ges 1975;10:35.

Hautmann R. Cystine stone therapy with alpha-mercaptopropionylglycine. World J Urol 1983;1:186–91.

Hautmann R. Urolithiasis. Epidemiologie und Pathogenese. Dtsch Ärztebl 1985a;82:27.

Hautmann R. Urolithiasis. Prophylaxe und Metaphylaxe. Dtsch Ärztebl 1985b;82:401.

Hautmann R, Lutzeyer W (Eds.). Harnsteinfibel. Deutscher Ärzte Verlag, Köln. 1986.

Hautmann R, Mauermeyer W. Möglichkeiten und Grenzen der intraoperativen Pyeloskopie beim Nierenbeckenausgussstein. In: Porpaczy P, ed. Internationales Symposium über Ausgusssteine. Vienna: Egermann, 1979:71.

Hepp W. Survey of the development of shock wave lithotripsy. Meersburg, West Germany: Dornier Medical Systems, 1984.

Hepp W, Heine G, Schneider W, et al. The Dornier lithotripter (Dornier GmbH): HM3, HM4, HM5. In: Coptcoat MJ, Miller RA, Wickham JEA, eds. Lithotripsy, vol 2. London: BDI, 1987:15–56.

Higashihara E, Horie S, Takeuchi T, et al. Laser ureterolithotripsy with combined rigid and flexible ureterorenoscopy. J Urol 1990;143:273–4.

Hoffmann R, Hartung R, Geissdörfer K, et al. Laser-induced shock wave lithotripsy: biologic effects of nanosecond pulses. J Urol 1988;139:1077–9.

Hoffmann R, Hartung R, Schmidt–Kloiber H, Reichel E. Laser-induced shock wave lithotripsy. Urol Res 1990;18:45–8.

Holl R. Wellenfokussierung in Fluiden [dissertation]. Aachen, West Germany: Rheinisch-Westfälische Technische Hochschule, 1982.

Holm HH, Hald T, Kristensen J, Holm-Bentzen M, Schultz A. The Danish extracorporeal lithotriptor. In: Lingeman JE, Newman DE, eds. Shock wave lithotripsy: state of the art. New York: Plenum Press, 1988:301–2.

Holmes RP. Tumor growth suppression by shock waves and cisplatin. AUA Today 1990;3:12.

Holmes RP, Yeaman LD, Taylor RG, Lewis JC, McCullough DL. Enhanced adriamycin uptake by neutrophils exposed to shock waves. J Urol 1988;139:304A.

Huffman JL, Bagley DH. Balloon dilation of the ureter for ureteroscopy. J Urol 1988;140:954.

Huffmann J, Bagley DH, Schoenberg HW, Lyon ES. Transurethral removal of large ureteral and renal pelvic calculi using ureteroscopic ultrasonic lithotripsy. J Urol 1983;130:31–4.

Huffmann JL, Bagley DH, Lyon ES. Treatment of distal ureteral calculi using a rigid ureteroscope. Urology 1982;20:574.

Hulbert JC, Lange PH. The percutaneous control of difficult upper urinary tract calculi. World J Urol 1985;3:19–23.

Hunter DW, Castaneda-Zuniga WR, Young AT, et al. Percutaneous removal of ureteral calculi: clinical and experimental results. Radiology 1985;156:341–8.

Hunter P, Newman R, Finlayson B, Drylie D, Leal J, Hawkins FF. Retrograde nephrostomy in 100 patients. World J Urol 1985;3:2–6.

Iro H, Wessel B, Benzel W, et al. Gewebereaktionen unter Applikation von piezoelektrischen Stosswellen zur Lithotripsie von Speichelsteinen. Laryngol Rhinol Otol 1990;69:102–7.

Ison K. Physical and technical introduction to lithotripsy. In: Coptcoat MJ, Miller RA, Wickham JEA, eds. Lithotripsy, vol 2. London: BDI, 1987:7–14.

Jaeger P, Redha F, Uhlschmid G, Hauri D. Morphologic changes in canine kidneys following extracorporeal shock wave treatment. J Endourol 1988;2:205–13.

Jaeger P, Redha F, Alund G, Uhlschmid G. Schadet die Stosswelle der Niere? Schweiz Med Wochenschr 1989;119:944–9.

Janetschek G, Kunzel KH. Percutaneous nephrolithotomy in horseshoe kidneys applied anatomy and clinical experience. Brit J Urol 1988;62:117.

Janetschek G. Intrarenale perkutane Chirurgie bei Kelchsteinen, Kelchhalsstenose, Kelchdivertikeln und Ureterabgangsstenosen. Urologe (A) 1988;27:256.

Jenkins A. ESWL: alternative technologies. Paper presented at the 44th Annual Meeting of the Mid-Atlantic Section of the AUA, Bermuda, September 28 to October 2, 1986.

Jenner R, Rassweiler J, Bub P, Eisenberger F. Ureter-katheter-Dilatationsset. Eine wertvolle Ergänzung des endurologischen Instrumentariums. Urologe (B) 1989;29:112–13.

Jocham D. Die extrakorporale Stosswellenlithtripsie: Indikationen, Grenzen, Resultate. Medwelt 1987;38:766–71.

Jocham D, Chaussy C, Schmiedt E. Extracorporeal shock wave lithotripsy. Urol Int 1986;41:357–68.

Jocham D, Liedl B, Chaussy CG, et al. Preliminary clinical experience with the HM4 bath-free Dornier lithrotripter. World J Urol 1987;5:208–12.

Jocham D, Liedl B, Ludwig W, Jaenicke U, Hofstetter A. Clinical experience with a Dornier lithotripter using electomagnetic shock wave generation. In: Proceedings of the Seventh World Congress on Endourology and ESWL, November 27–30, 1989, Kyoto, Japan. (abstract 2–5).

Jocham D, Liedl B, Lunz C, Schuster C, Chaussy C. Langzeiterfahrungen nach ESWL von Harnsteinpatienten. Urologe (A) 1989b;28:134–7.

Jones BJ, Ryan PC, Fenton D, Nowlan P, Voorheis HP, Butler MR. Targeting of drug carriers using piezoelectric shock waves. In: Proceedings of the Seventh World Congress on Endourology and ESWL, November 27–30, 1989, Kyoto, Japan. (abstract P13–11).

Kahn RJ. Percutaneous flexible fiberoptic nephroscopy. World J Urol 1985;3:11–18.

Karlin GS, Badlani GH, Smith AD. Endopyelotomy versus open pyeloplasty: Comparison in 88 patients. J Urol 1988;140:476.

Kaude JV, Williams CM, Millner MR, Scott KN, Finlayson B. Renal morphology and function immediately after extracorporeal shock wave lithotripsy. Am J Radiol 1985;145:305–13.

Kellett MJ, Wickham JE, Payne SR. Combined retrograde and antegrade manipulations for percutaneous nephrolithotomy of ureteric calculi: "push-pull" technique. Urology 1985;25:391–2.

Kishimoto T, Yamamoto K, Sugimoto T, Yoshihara H, Maekawa M. Side-effects of extracorporeal shock wave exposure in patients treated by extracorporeal shock wave lithotripsy for upper urinary tract stones. Eur Urol 1986;12:308–13.

Kitada S, Kuramoto H, Kumazawa J, Yamaguchi A, Nakasu H, Hara S. Effects of extracorporeal shock wave lithotripsy on urinary excretion of N-acetylbeta-D-glucosamides. Urol Int 1989;44:35–7.

Knoll LD, Segura JW, Patterson DE, LeRoy AJ, Smith LH. Long-term follow-up in patients with cystine urinary calculi treated by percutaneous ultrasonic lithotripsy. J Urol 1988;140:246.

Korth K. Perkutane Lithotripsie mit einem neuen Dauerspül-Pyeloskop. Urologe (A) 1983;22:219–21.

Korth K. Percutaneous renal stone surgery. Berlin: Springer, 1984.

Kramolowsky EV. Ureteral perforation during ureterorenoscopy: Treatment and management. J Urol 1987;138:36.

Kramolowsky EV, Kratz C. Extracorporeal shock wave lithotripsy for the treatment of bulbous urethral stones. J Urol 1988;139:362–3.

Krongrad A, Saltzman B, Tannenbaum M, Droler MJ. Enzymuria following extracorporeal shock wave lithotripsy (ESWL). J Urol 1988;139:324A.

Kroovand RL, Harrison LH, McCullough DL. Extracorporeal shock wave lithotripsy in childhood. J Urol 1987;138:1106–9.

Kurth KH, Hohenfellner R, Altwein JE. Ultrasound litholapaxy of a staghorn calculus. J Urol 1977;117:242–3.

Kurzweil SJ, Smith JE, Arsdalen K van. Effects of extracorporeal shock waves on skeletal and renal growth in the infant rabbit. J Urol 1988;139:325A.

Kuwahara M, Kambe K, Kurosu S, et al. Extracorporeal stone disintegration using chemical explosive pellets as an energy source of underwater shock waves. J Urol 1986a;135:133A.

Kuwahara M, Kurosu S, Kambe K, Kageyama S, Orikasa S, Tahayama S. Extracorporeal microexplosive lithotripsy: experience with 40 clinical cases. J Urol 1986b;135(2):182A abstract no. 313.

Kuwahara M, Kambe K, Kurosu S, et al. Clinical application of extracorporeal shock wave lithotripsy using microexplosions. J Urol 1987;137:837–40.

Kuwahara M, Ioritani N, Kambe K, et al. A new overhead-–type ESWL machine with an anti-miss shot control device. In: Proceedings of the Seventh World Congress on Endourology and ESWL, November 27–30, 1989, Kyoto, Japan (abstract 1–6).

Kuwahara M, Ioritani N, Kambe K, et al. Hyperechoic region induced by focused shock waves in vitro and in vivo: possibility of acoustic cavitation bubbles. J Lithotripsy Stone Dis 1989;1:282–8.

Lazare JN, Saltzman B, Sotolongo J. Extracorporeal shock wave lithotripsy treatment of spinal cord injury patients. J Urol 1988;140:266.

Lensch G. Ein neues Röntgenverfahren in der Nierensteinchirurgie. Urologe (A) 1970;9:182–8.

Libby JM, Meacham RB, Griffith DP. The role of silicone ureteral stents in extracorporeal shock wave lithotripsy of large renal calculi. J Urol 1988;139:15–17.

Liedl B, Jocham D, Lunz C, Schuster C, Chaussy C. Prävalenz und Inzidenz der arteriellen Hypertonie bei ESWL–behandelten Nierensteinpatienten. Urologe (A) 1989;28:130–3.

Lin PJ, Hrejsa AF. Patient exposure and radiation environment of an extracorporeal shock wave lithotriptor system. J Urol 1987;138:712–15.

Lingeman JE, Shirrel WI, Newman DM, Mosbaugh PG, Steele RE, Woods JR. Management of upper ureteral calculi with extracorporeal shock wave lithotripsy. J Urol 1987;138:720.

Lingeman JE. Current concepts in the relative efficacy of percutaneous nephrostolithotomy and extracorporeal shock wave lithotripsy. Wld J Urol 1987;5:229.

Lingeman JE, Newman D, Mertz J, et al. Extracorporeal shock wave lithotripsy: the Methodist Hospital of Indiana experience. J Urol 1986a;135:1134–7.

Lingeman JE, Sonda LP, Kahnoski RJ, et al. Ureteral stone management: emerging concepts. J Urol 1986b;135:1172–4.

Lingeman JE, McAteer JA, Kempson SA, Evan AP. Bioeffects of extracorporeal shock wave lithotripsy. J Endourol 1987;1:89–98.

Loening SA, Mardan AH, Holmes J, Lubaraoff DM. In vivo and in vitro effects of shock waves on Dunning prostate tumors. J Urol 1988;139:303A.

Lupu AN, Fuchs GJ, Chaussy CG. Calcification of ureteral stent treated by extracorporeal shock wave lithotripsy. J Urol 1986;136:1297–8.

Lustenberger FX, Zingg EJ. Die operative Behandlung von Nierenausgusskonkrementen. Schweiz Med Wochenschr 1981;111:2005–11.

Lyon ES. Editorial comment. J Urol 1988;140:952.

Lyon ES, Kyker JS, Schoenberg HW. Transurethral ureteroscopy in women: a ready addition to the urological armamentarium. J Urol 1978;119:35–6.

Lyon ES, Huffmann JL, Bagley DH. Ureteroscopy and ureteropyeloscopy. Urology 1984;23:29–36.

Lytton B, Weiss RM, Green DF. Complications of ureteral endoscopy. J Urol 1986; 137:649.

McCullough DL, Yeaman LD, Bo WJ, et al. Do extracorporeal shock waves affect fertility and fetal development? A study of shock wave effects on the rat ovary and fetus. J Urol 1988a;139:325A.

McCullough DL, Yeaman LD, Bo WJ, Kroovand RL, Assimos DG, Griffin AS. Experimental effects of extracorporeal shock waves on the rat ovary and fetus. In: Lingeman JE, Newman DE, eds. Shock wave lithotripsy: state of the art. New York: Plenum Press, 1988b:327–8.

McMurty JM, Clayman RV, Sicord GA, Anderson CB. Pulmonary embolism and deep venous thrombosis following extracorporeal shock wave lithotripsy. In: Lingeman JE, Newman DE, eds. Shock wave lithotripsy: state of the art. New York: Plenum Press, 1988:177–80.

McNicholas TA, Ramsay JWA, Crocker PR, Webb DR, Wickham JEA. The effects of extracorporeal shock wave lithotripsy on urological prostheses and endoprostheses. Urol Res 1986;14:309–13.

Manzone DJ, Chiang B. Extracorporeal shock wave lithotripsy of stones in the upper, mid and lower ureter. J Endourol 1988;2:107.

Marberger M. Regionale Kühlung der Niere bei Nierensteinoperationen: wann und weshalb? Aktuel Urol 1979;10:313–20.

Marberger M. Die endoskopische Behandlung des Uretersteins. Urologe (A) 1984;23:308–16.

Marberger M, Eisenberger F. Regional hypothermia of the kidney: surface or transarterial perfusion cooling? J Urol 1980;124:179–83.

Marberger M, Stackl W. New developments in endoscopic surgery for ureteric calculi. Br J Urol 1983;54(suppl):34–7.

Marberger M, Stackl W. Surgical treatment of renal calculi. In: Schneider HJ, ed. Urolithiasis: therapy, prevention. Berlin: Springer, 1986:85.

Marberger M, Stackl W, Hruby W. Percutaneous litholapaxy of renal calculi with ultrasound. Eur Urol 1982;8:236–42.

Marberger M, Hruby W, Stackl W, Kroiss A. Late sequelae of ultrasonic lithotripsy of renal calculi. J Urol 1985a;133:170–3.

Marberger M, Stackl W, Hruby W, Wurster H, Schnedl W. Ultrasonic lithotripsy and soft tissue. World J Urol 1985b;3:27–32.

Marberger M, Türk C, Steinkogler I. Painless piezoelectric extracorporeal lithotripsy. J Urol 1988;139:695–9.

Marberger M, Türk C, Albrecht W, Steinkogler I, Hasun R. Aktueller Stand und Perspektiven in der Harnsteinbehandlung. In: Ell C, Marberger M, Berlien P, eds. Extra- und intrakorporale Lithotripsie von Harn-, Gallen-, Pankreas- und Speichelsteine. Stuttgart: Thieme, 1990:150–61.

Marshall F, Makofski R, Mark F, et al. Shock wave destruction of renal calculi: new technical modifications. J Urol 1984;131:133A.

Marshall F, Makofski R, Mark F, et al. Shock wave destruction of renal calculi: new technical modifications. J Urol 1985;133(2):118A.

Marshall F, Weiskopf F, Singh A, et al. A prototype device for nonimmersion shock wave lithotripsy using ultrasonography for calculus localization. J Urol 1988;249–53.

Martin X, Mestas DL, Cathignol D, Margohari I, Dubernard IM. Ultrasound stone localisation for extracorporeal shock wave lithotripsy. Br J Urol 1986;58:349–52.

Matouschek E. The lithotripsy of stones in the ureter under visual control. Eur Urol 1984;10:60–1.

May P. Nierenbeckenkelchausgussstein. Grenzen der Operabilität. Urologe (A) 1974;13:244–7.

Mayo ME, Krieger JN, Rudd TG. Effect of percutaneous nephrolithotomy on renal function. J Urol 1985;133:167–8.

Mayo ME, Chapman WH, Anwell JS. Progress report on the laser triptor. J Urol 1986;135:160A.

Mebel M, Brien G, Bick C, Gremske D, Fahlenkamp D, Eger E. Results of surgical and conservative therapy on patients with nephrolithiasis and chronic renal insufficiency. Eur Urol 1982;8:150–4.

Medstone International. Medstone 1000 shock wave lithotripter [product description]. Irvine, CA: Medstone International, 1985.

Meyer WH, Klosterhalfen H, Becker H, Schulte am Esch J, Kochs E. Effektivitätssteigerung der extrakorporealen Stosswellenlithotripsie (ESWL) durch highfrequency jet ventilation (HFJV). Aktuel Urol 1985;16:250–4.

Meyer WW, Jonas D. First experiences with the Storz Modulith lithotripter. In: Proceedings of the Seventh World Congress on Endourology and ESWL, November 27–30, 1989b, Kyoto, Japan (abstract 2–1).

Meyer WW, Michels-Maisch B, Jonas D. The effect of shock waves on MDCK cells. In: Proceedings of the Seventh World Congress on Endourology and ESWL, November 27–30, 1989a, Kyoto, Japan (abstract P13–4).

Michaelis EK, Fowler JE, Mariano M. Bacteriuria following extracorporeal shock wave lithotripsy of infection stones. J Urol 1988;140:254.

Miller K, Bachor R, Hautmann R. Extracorporeal shock wave lithotripsy of stones in the prone position: Technique, indications, results. J Endourol 1988;2:113.

Miller K, Bachor R, Hautmann R. Percutaneous nephrolithotomy/ESWL vs. ureteral stent/ESWL for the treatment of large renal calculi and staghorn stones: a prospective randomized study. J Endourol 1988;2:131.

Miller K, Bachor R, Sauter T, Hautmann R. PCNL/ESWL vs. ureteral stent/ESWL for the treatment of large renal stones and staghorn stone – what did we learn? J Endourol 1989;3:287–293.

Miller K, Bachor R, Sauter T, Hautmann R. Management or ureteral calculi – the impact of anesthesia-free ESWL. J Endourol 1989;3:295–300.

Miller K, Hautmann R. Treatment of distal ureteral calculi with ESWL: experience with more than 100 consecutive cases. World J Urol 1987;5:259–65.

Miller K, Fuchs G, Bub P, Rassweiler J, Eisenberger F. Kombination von perkutaner Nephrolithotomie (PCN) und extrakorporaler Stosswellenlithotripsie (ESWL). Eine neue Möglichkeit zur Behandlung von Nierensteinen. Aktuel Urol 1984a;15:317–21.

Miller K, Fuchs G, Rassweiler J, Eisenberger F. Financial analysis, personnel planning and organizational requirements for the installation of a kidney lithotripter at an urologic department. Eur Urol 1984b;10:212–15.

Miller K, Fuchs G, Bub P, Rassweiler J, Eisenberger F. Stuttgart group experience after one year with extracorporeal shock wave lithotripsy (ESWL) and endourology: review of current stone treatment. J Urol 1985a;133(2):182.

Miller K, Fuchs G, Rassweiler J, Eisenberger F. Extrakorporal Stosswellenlithotripsie (ESWL). Z Allgemeinmed 1985b;61:963–7.

Miller K, Fuchs G, Rassweiler J, Eisenberger F. PCN als Möglichkeit zur Indikationserweiterung der berührungsfreien Nierensteinzertrümmerung bei komplizierter Nephrolithiasis. Urologe (B) 1985c;25:11–16.

Miller K, Fuchs G, Rassweiler J, Eisenberger F. Treatment of ureteral stone disease: the role of ESWL and endourology. World J Urol 1985d;3:53–7.

Miller K, Gumpinger R, Fuchs G, Rassweiler J. Perkutane Nierensteinchirurgie. Z Allgemeinmed 1985e;61:968–72.

Miller K, Gumpinger R, Fuchs G, Rassweiler J, Eisenberger F. Antegrade Ureteroskopie – das Ende der offenen Chirurgie beim hohen Harnleiterstein? Aktuel Urol 1985f;16:291–3.

Miller K, Gumpinger R, Fuchs G, Rassweiler J. Ureterorenoskopie (URS). Z Allgemeinmed 1985g;61:973–6.

Miller K, Bubeck J, Hautmann R. Extracorporeal shock wave lithotripsy of distal ureteral calculi. Eur Urol 1986;12:305–7.

Miller K, Bachor R, Hautmann R. Extracorporeal shock wave lithotripsy in the prone position: technique, indications, results. In: Lingeman JE, Newman DE, eds. Shock wave lithotripsy: state of the art. New York: Plenum Press, 1988a:43–6.

Miller K, Bachor R, Hautmann R. Percutaneous nephrolithotomy and ESWL versus ureteral stent and ESWL for the treatment of large renal calculi and staghorn calculi: preliminary results of a prospective randomized study. In: Lingeman JE, Newman DE, eds. Shock wave lithotripsy: state of the art. New York: Plenum Press, 1988b:89–94.

Miller K, Bachor R, Sauter T, Hautmann R. Aktuelle Therapie des Harnleitersteins. Urologe (A) 1989;28: 148–51.

Miller K, Weber HM, Hautmann RE. Laser lithotripsy with the pulsed alexandrite: in vitro results. In: Proceedings of the Seventh World Congress on Endourology and ESWL, November 27–30, 1989, Kyoto, Japan (abstract 5–13).

Miller RA. Endoscopic application of shock wave technology for the destruction of renal calculi. World J Urol 1985;3:36–40.

Miller RA, Wickham JE. Percutaneous nephrolithotomy: advances in equipment and endoscopic techniques. Urology 1984;23:2–6.

Miller RA, Wickham JE, Kellett MJ. Percutaneous destruction of renal calculi: clinical and laboratory experience. Br J Urol 1983;(suppl):51–4.

Miller RA, Payne S, Wickham JE. Electrohydraulic nephrolithotripsy: a preferable alternative to ultrasound. Br J Urol 1984a;56:589–3.

Miller RA, Wickham JE, Reynold S, Westcott A, Bailey A. Explosive nephrolitholapaxy: reality or fiction. Urology 1984b;23:67–71.

Mininberg Dt. Extracorporeal shock wave lithotripsy in children: an overview. J Endourol 1989;3:385–9.

Müller M. Stosswellenfokussierung in Wasser [dissertation]. Aachen: Rheinisch-Westfälische Technische Hochschule, 1987.

Müller SC, Havereke J von, El Seeifi A, Alken P. Der hohe Harnleiterstein. Ein Problem trotz extrakorporaler Stosswellenlithotripsie. Aktuel Urol 1985;16:294–8.

Müller SC, Wilbert D, Thüroff JW, Alken P. Extracorporeal shock wave lithotripsy of ureteral stones: clinical experience and experimental findings. J Urol 1986;135:831–4.

Müller-Klieser W. Multicellular spheroids: a review on cellular aggregates in cancer research. J Cancer Res Clin Oncol 1987;113:101–22.

Mulley AG Jr, Carlson KJ, Dretler SP. Extracorporeal shock wave lithotripsy: slam-bang effects, silent side-effects? Am J Radiol 1988;150:316–18.

Muschter R, Kutscher KR, Bohle A, et al. Die ESWL mit dem Dornier Lithotripter HM3 mit modifiziertem Stosswellengenerator. Urologe (A) 1987;26:33–7.

Muschter R, Schmeller NT, Kutscher KR, Reis M, Hofstetter AG, Löhrs U. Histological findings in renal parenchyma after extracorporeal shock wave lithotripsy. In: Lingeman JE, Newman DE, eds. Shock wave lithotripsy: state of the art. New York: Plenum Press, 1988a:405–6.

Muschter R, Schmeller NT, Scheu W, Hofstetter AG, Krech R, Löhrs U. Reduktion der ESWL-bedingten Nierenparenchymschädigung. Der modifizierte Dornier HM3 im Tierexperiment. Verh Ber Dtsch Ges Urol 1988b;39:72–3.

Muschter R, Thomas S, Knipper A, Engelhardt R, Brinkmann R, Maghraby H. The feasibility of blind application of the pulsed dye laser for lithotripsy. In: International Congress on Laser Lithotripsy and Conventional Therapy of Urinary and Biliary Stones, Lübeck/Travemünde, 1989.

Muschter R, Thomas S, Knipper A, Maghraby H. Intrakorporale laserinduzierte Lithotripsie. Lübecker Erfahrungen mit dem Telemit-System. In: Ell C, Marberger M, Berlien P, eds. Extra- und intrakorporale Lithotripsie von Harn-, Gallen-, Pankreas- und Speichelsteinen. Stuttgart: Thieme, 1990:128–31.

Nakatsuka S, Kinoshita H, Ueda H, Araki T, Tanaka H. Combined treatment of medullary sponge kidney by EDTA, potassium citrate, and extracorporeal shock wave lithotripsy. Eur Urol 1988;14:339–42.

Neisius D. extrakorporale piezoelektrische Lithotripsie von Harnsteinen. Homburger Erfahrungen und Perspektiven. In: Ell C, Marberger M, Berlien P, eds. Extra- und intrakorporale Lithotripsie von Harn-, Gallen-, Pankreas- und Speichelsteinen. Stuttgart: Thieme, 1990:93–100.

Neisius D, Gebhardt T, Seitz G, Ziegler M. Histological examination of the liver and gallbladder after application of extracorporeal shock waves to the gallbladder with the Piezolith 2200. J Lithotripsy Stone Dis 1989a;1:26–33.

Neisius D, Zwergel U, Becht E, Ziegler M. Extracorporeal piezoelectric lithotripsy (EPL) of urinary calculi in children. J Urol 1989b;141(2):270A (abstract 401).

Neisius D, Zwergel U, Moll V, Kanokogi M. Extracorporeal lithotripsy of ureteral stones in situ. In: Proceedings of the Seventh World Congress on Endourology and ESWL, November 27–30, 1989, Kyoto, Japan (abstract P2–20).

Nemoy NJ, Stemay TS. Use of hemiacridin in management of infected stones. J Urol 1977;117:159.

Newman DM, Coury T, Lingeman JE, et al. Extracorporeal shock wave lithotripsy: experience in children. J Urol 1987;138:238–40.

Newman R, Hackett R, Senior D, et al. Pathologic effects of ESWL on canine renal tissue. Urology 1987;29:194–200.

Newman RC, Hunter PT, Hawkins IF, Finlayson B. The ureteral access system: A review of the immediate results in 43 cases. J Urol 1986;137:380.

O'Brian WM, Maxted WC, Pahira JJ. Ureteral stricture: Experience with 31 cases. J Urol 1988;140:737.

Pak C. Medical management of nephrolithiasis. J Urol 1983;128:1157–60.

Pak CY, Nicar MJ, Britton F. Clinical experience with sodium cellulose phosphate. World J Urol 1983;1: 180–5.

Pastor J, Graff J, Senge T, et al. New development in ESWL without invasive anesthesia. Dornier User Letter 1987;2:10–14.

Patel V. Coagulum-Pyelolithotomie. Urologe (A) 1974;13:168–72.

Patterson D, Segura J, LeRoy A, Benson R, May G. The etiology and treatment of delayed bleeding following percutaneous lithotripsy. J Urol 1985;133:447–50.

Pensel J, Frank F, Rothenberger K, Hofstetter A, Unsöld E. Destruction of urinary stones by Nd:YAG laser irradiation. In: Proceedings of the Fourth Congress for Laser Surgery, Tokyo, 1981.

Perez-Castro Ellendt E, Martinez-Pineiro JA. Transurethral ureteroscopy: a current urological procedure. Arch Esp Urol 1980;33:445.

Perez-Castro Ellendt E, Martinez-Pineiro JA. Transurethral ureteropyeloscopy. Urologe (A) 1981;258–60.

Perez–Castro Ellendt E, Martinez-Pineiro JA. Ureteral and renal endoscopy. Eur Urol 1982;8:117–20.

Peschke P, Hahn EW, Lorenz WJ, et al. Pulsed highenergy ultrasound shock waves: biological effects on the Dunning prostate rat tumor. In: Proceedings of the Seventh World Congress on Endourology and ESWL, November 27–30, 1989, Kyoto, Japan (abstract P13–7).

Pfeifer KJ, Heinze HG, Eisenberger F, Chaussy C, Wirth H. Änderung der Durchblutung und Durchblutungsverteilung nach normo- und hypothermer Ischämie der Nieren. Nuklearmedizin 1976;15:161−7.

Pode D, Lenkovski Z, Shapiro A, Pfau A. Can extracorporeal shockwave lithotripsy eradicate persistent urinary infection associated with infected stones? J Urol 1988;140:257.

Pode D, Verstandig A, Shapiro A, Katz G, Caine M. Treatment of complete staghorn calculi by extracorporeal shock lithotrips monotherapy with special reference to internal stenting. J Urol 1988;140:260.

Pollack HM, Banner MP. Work in progress: percutaneous fiberoptic endoscopy of the upper urinary tract. Radiology 1982;145:651−4.

Politis G, Griffith DP. ESWL: stone-free efficacy based upon stone size and location. Wld J Urol 1987;5:255.

Preminger GM, Clayman R. The changing face of lithotripsy: impact of "second generation" machines. In: Proceedings of the Seventh World Congress on Endourology and ESWL, November 27−30, 1989, Kyoto, Japan (abstract P7−18).

Psihramis KE, Dretler SP. Extracorporeal shock wave lithotripsy of caliceal diverticula calculi. J Urol 1987;138:707−11.

Puppo P, Bottino P, Germinale F, Caviglia C, Ricciotti G. Extracorporeal shock wave lithotripsy using double-J stents: technique, pitfalls, results and complications. In: Lingeman JE, Newman DE, eds. Shock wave lithotripsy: state of the art. New York: Plenum Press, 1988:35−8.

Puppo P, Bottino P, Germinale F, Giuliani L. Lithoring multi one: experimental studies and clinical applications. In: Proceedings of the Seventh World Congress on Endourology and ESWL, November 27−30, 1989, Kyoto, Japan (abstract 1−7).

Puppo P, Bottino P, Germinale F, Giuliani L. First experience with the Lithoring in the management of irinary stones. Eur Urol 1990;18:1−5.

Rambow A, Staritz M, Klose P, Thelen M, Meyer zum Büschenfelde KH. Extrakorporale Stosswellenlithotripsie von Gallenblasensteinen: Wie viele Patienten sind geeignet? Dtsch Med Wochenschr 1989;114:895−8.

Rapado A, Mancha A, Castrillo JM, Traba ML, Santos M, Cifueales Delatte L. Ätiologische Klassifikation des Harnsteinleidens. In: Feldmann HU, Mewes D, eds. Urolithiasis. Erlangen: Perimed, 1976.

Rassweiler J, Buck J, Miller K, Fuchs G. Computertomographische Steindichtemessung zur Steinanalyse vor extrakorporaler Stosswellenlithotripsie (ESWL). Aktuel Urol 1985a;16:30−5.

Rassweiler J, Miller K, Fuchs G, Eisenberger F. Kosten und Nutzen der berührungsfreien Nierenlithotripsie. Lebensversicherungsmedizin 1985b;37:80−5.

Rassweiler J, Gumpinger R, Miller K, Hölzermann F, Eisenberger F. Multimodal treatment (extracorporeal shock wave lithotripsy and endourology) of complicated renal stone disease. Eur Urol 1986a;12:294−304.

Rassweiler J, Hath U, Lutz K, Eisenberger F. Insitu-ESWL beim distalen Harnleiterstein. Das Ende der Zeiss-Schlinge. Aktuel Urol 1986b;17:328−31.

Rassweiler J, Lutz K, Gumpinger R, Eisenberger F. Efficacy of in situ extracorporeal shock wave lithotripsy for upper ureteral calculi. Eur Urol 1986c;12:377−86.

Rassweiler J, Bub P, Eisenberger F. The role of ESWL for ureteric stones. In: Coptcoat MJ, Miller RA, Wickham JEA, eds. Lithotripsy, vol 2. London: BDI, 1987a:135−50.

Rassweiler J, Lutz K, Gumpinger R, Eisenberger F. The efficacy of in situ ESWL for upper ureteral calculi. Eur Urol 1987b;13:32−6.

Rassweiler J, Gumpinger R, Mayer R, Kohl H, Schmidt A, Eisenberger F. Extracorporeal piezoelectric lithotripsy with modified Dorner HM3: a cooperative study. World J Urol 1987c;5:218−24.

Rassweiler J, Schmidt A, Gumpinger R, et al. Experimental basis of ESWL using different principles of shock wave generation. J Urol 1987d;137(2):278.

Rassweiler J, Bub P, Seibold J, et al. Dornier MPL 9000: urologic use in an interdisciplinary stone center. J Endourol 1988a;2:375−9.

Rassweiler J, Westhauser A, Bub P, Eisenberg F. Second-generation lithotripters: a comparative study. J Endourol 1988b;2:192−203.

Rassweiler J, Köhrmann KU, Berle B, Pfenninger T, Marlinghaus EH, Alken P. Experimental classification of a newly designed electromagnetic shock wave source for lithotripsy. In: Proceedings of the Seventh World Congress on Endourology and ESWL, November 27−30, 1989a, Kyoto, Japan (abstract 1−2).

Rassweiler J, Köhrmann KU, Heine G, Wess O, Alken P. Modulith SL 10/20: first clinical experience with a new interdisciplinary lithotripter. In: Proceedings of the Seventh World Congress on Endourology and ESWL, November 27−30, 1989b, Kyoto, Japan (abstract P7−19).

Rassweiler J, Irion U, Strauss R, Bub P, Eisenberger F. Technical considerations using a pulsed neodymium-YAG laser for endoscopic shock wave lithotripsy. Eur Urol 1989c;16:374−7.

Rassweiler J, Löbelenz M, Köhrmann U, Eisenberger F, Alken P. In vitro comparison of second-generation lithotripters using two stone models. In: Vahlensieck W, Gasser G, Hesse A, Schöneich G, eds. Proceedings of the First European Symposium on Urolithiasis, Bonn 1989. Amsterdam: Excerpta Medica, 1990a:133−6.

Rassweiler J, Köhrmann U, Heine G, Potempa D, Wess O, Alken P. Modulith SL10/20: first clinical experience with a new interdisciplinary lithotripter. Z Urol 1990b;2:75−7.

Rassweiler J, Schmidt A, Eisenberger F. Operative technique for extracorporeal shock wave lithotripsy with the elektrohydraulic lithotripter Dornier HM3. In: Wickham JEA, Buck AC, eds. Renal tract stone: metabolic basis and clinical practice. Edinburgh: Churchill Livingstone, 1990:579−90.

Recker F, Hofstädter E, Daus HJ, et al. Morphological pathomechanism following extracorporeal shock wave lithotripsy in rat kidneys. In: Lingeman JE, Newman DE, eds. Shock wave lithotripsy: state of the art. New York: Plenum Press, 1988:357−62.

Recker F, Konstantinidis K, Jaeger P, Krönagel H, Alund G, Hauri D. Der Nierenbeckenausgussstein: Anatrophe Nephrolithotomie versus perkutane Litholapaxie und ESWL versus ESWL Monotherapie. Ein Bericht über 6 Jahre Erfahrung. Urologe (A) 1989;28:152−7.

Reddy PK, Lange PH, Hulbert JC, et al. Percutaneous removal of caliceal and other "inaccessible" stones: results. J Urol 1984;132:443−7.

Reddy PK, Hulbert JC, Lange PH, et al. Percutaneous removal of renal and ureteral calculi: experience with 400 cases. J Urol 1985;134:662−5.

Reichel E, Schmidt-Kloiber H. Die Anwendung laserinduzierter Stosswellen am Beispiel der Zerstörung von Harnwegskonkrementen. Med Phys 1983:197−201.

Resnick MJ, Boyce WH. Bilateral staghorn calculi: patient evaluation and management. J Urol 1980;123:338–41.

Reuter JH. Transurethrale Ultraschallithotripsie im Ureter. Aktuel Urol 1984;15:28–31.

Reuter MJ, Reuter HJ. Diagnostische und operative transurethrale Ureterorenoskopie. Erste Erfahrungen an 69 Patienten. Erprobung des neueren rigiden Kompaktendoskops von 9.5 Ch. Z Urol Nephrol 1983;76:7–14.

Riedlinger R, Überle F, Wurster H, et al. Die Zertrümmerung von Nierensteinen durch piezoelektrisch erzeugte Hochenergie-Schallpulse. Physikalische Grundlagen und experimentelle Untersuchungen. Urologe (A) 1986;25:188–92.

Riedlinger R, Überle F. Berührungsfreie piezoelektrische Nierensteinzertrümmerung. In: Proceedings of the 12. Gemeinschaftstagung mit Kolloquien der Deutsche Arbeitsgemeinschaft für Akustik, 10.–13. März, 1986.

Riedmiller J, Thüroff J, Alken P, Hutschenreiter G, Hohenfellner R. Gefäß- und Steinlokalisation durch Ultraschall – das Ende von Ischämie Kühlung in der Nierensteinchirurgie? Aktuel Urol 1981;12:210–15.

Riedmiller H, Thüroff J, Alken P, Hohenfellner R. Doppler and B-mode ultrasound for avascular nephrotomy. J Urol 1983;130:224–7.

Rigatti P, Colombo R, Centemero A, et al. Histological and ultrastructural evaluation of extracorporeal shock wave lithotripsy-induced acute renal lesions: preliminary report. Eur Urol 1989;16:207–11.

Rittenberg MH, Koolpe H, Keeler L, McNamara T, Baley DH. Pain control: comparison of percutaneous and operative nephrolithotomy. Urology 1985;25:468–71.

Robertson WG. Physikalisch-chemische Aspekte der Kalziumsteinbildung in den harnableitenden Wegen. In: Feldmann HU, Mewes D, eds. Urolithiasis. Erlangen: Perimed, 1976.

Rocco F, Mandressi A, Larcher P. Classfication of renal calculi. Eur Urol 1984;10:121–3.

Roth RA, Beckmann CF. Complications of extracorporeal shock wave lithotripsy and percutaneous nephrolithotomy. Urol Clin North Am 1988;15:155–66.

Rous SN, Turner WR. Retrospective study of 95 patients with staghorn calculus disease. J Urol 1977;118:902–4.

Royce PL, Fuchs GJ, Lupu AN, Chaussy CG. The treatment of uric acid calculi with extracorporeal shock wave lithotripsy. Br J Urol 1987;60:6–9.

Rubin JI, Argeer PH, Pollack HM, et al. Kidney changes after extracorporeal shock wave lithotripsy: CT evaluation. Radiology 1987;162:21–4.

Ruiz-Marcellán JR, Servio LI. Evaluation of renal damage in extracorporeal lithotripsy by shock waves. Eur Urol 1986;12:73–5.

Russo P, Stephenson RA, Mies C, et al. High energy shock waves suppress tumor growth in vitro and in vivo. J Urol 1986;135(2):626–8.

Russo P, Mies C, Huryk R, Heston WDW, Fair WR. Histopathologic and ultrastructural correlates of tumor growth suppression by high-energy shock waves. J Urol 1987;137:338–41.

Rutner AB. Ureteral balloon dilatation and stone basketing. Urology 1984;23:44–53.

Ryan Pc, Seery J, Colhoun E, et al. Functional, morphological and microbiological effects of piezoelectric shock wave lithotripsy (EDAP LT01): an experimental and clinical study. In: Lingeman JE, Newman DE, eds. Shock wave lithotripsy: state of the art. New York: Plenum Press, 1988:399–404.

Sackmann M, Delius M, Sauerbruch T, et al. Shock wave lithotripsy of gallbladder stones. N Engl J Med 1988;318:393–7.

Saltzman B. Ureteral stenting during extracorporeal shock wave lithotripsy: friend or foe? In: Proceedings of the Seventh World Congress on Endourology and ESWL, November 27–30, 1989, Kyoto, Japan (abstract L4).

Sant G, Blaivas J, Meaves E Jr. Hemiacridin irrigation in the management of struvite calculi: long-term results. J Urol 1983;130:1048–50.

Sauerbruch T, Delius M, Paumgartner G, et al. Fragmentation of gallstones by extracorporeal shock waves. N Engl J Med 1986;314:818–22.

Saunders JE, Coleman AJ. Physical characteristics of the Dornier extracorporeal shock wave lithotriptor. Urology 1987;29(5):506–9.

Schmeller N, Hofstetter AG, Frank F, Hessell S, Thomas S, Wondrazek F. Laser-induced shock wave lithotripsy (LISL). In: International Congress on Laser Lithotripsy and Conventional Therapy of Urinary and Biliary Stones, Lübeck/Travemünde, 1989.

Schmeller NT, Baumüller A, Hofstetter AG. Nicht-operative Behandlung von Harnleitersteinen mit Hilfe der Ureteroskopie. Fortschr Med 1984a;36:895–9.

Schmeller NT, Kersting H, Schüller J, Chaussy C, Schmidt E. Combination of chemolysis and shock wave lithotripsy in the treatment of cystine renal calculi. J Urol 1984b;13:434–8.

Schmiedt E, Chaussy C. Extrakorporale Stosswellenlithotripsie von Harnleitersteinen. Therapiewoche 1984a:6567–73.

Schmiedt E, Chaussy C. Extracorporeal shock wave lithotripsy (ESWL) of kidney and ureteric stones. Int Urol Nephrol 1984b;16:273–83.

Schmiedt E, Chaussy C. Extracorporeal shock wave lithotripsy of kidney and ureteric stones. Urol Int 1984c;39:193–8.

Schmiedt E, Chaussy C. Die extrakorporale Stosswellenlithotripsie von Nieren– und Harnleitersteinen. Dtsch Ärztebl 1985;82:247–51.

Schneider HJ. Urolithiasis: etiology, diagnosis. In: Handbook of urology, vol. 17/1. Berlin: Springer, 1985.

Schneider HJ. Urolithiasis: therapy, prevention. In: Handbook of urology, vol. 17/2. Berlin: Springer, 1986.

Schneider HJ, Berg C. Epidemiologische Aussagen zum Harnsteinleiden auf der Grundlage von 100 000 Harnsteinanalysen unter besonderer Berücksichtigung der Rezidive. In: Vahlensieck W, Gasser G, eds. Pathogenese und Klinik der Harnsteine, vol 8. Darmstadt: Steinkopff, 1983:38–42.

Schneider HJ, Hienzsch E. Welche Bedeutung hat die operative Therapie der Urolithiasis heute? Z Urol Nephrol 1975;68:574–6.

Schneider HJ, Rugendorff EW. Bedeutung der Nachsorge Harnsteinkranker im Zeitalter von extrakorporaler Stosswellentherapie, perkutane Litholapaxie und Ureterorenoskopie. Urologe (B) 1986;26:23–7.

Schüller J, Chaussy C, Johann D, Brandl H, Liedl B, Schmiedt E. Erweiterung der ESWL durch auxiläre Methoden. Urologe (A) 1984;23:317–32.

Schüller J, Schuldes H, Berendsen G, Nagel R. Perkutane und transurethro-uretale Harnleiterschlitzung. Aktuel Urol 1986;17:203–7.

Schuldes H, Boehle A, Berendsen G, Schüller J, Nagel R. Die Bedeutung des Harnleitersteins mit der ESWL. Aktuel Urol 1985;16:299–303.

Schulze H, Falkenberg F, Mondorf AW, Engelmann U, Senge T. Enhanced secretion of kidney-derived antigens in the urine of patients after ESWL treatment. J Urol 1988;139:323A.

Segura JW. Endourology. J Urol 1984;132:1079–84.

Segura JW. Percutaneous endourology: vascular complications. World J Urol 1985;3:24–6.

Seibold J, Rassweiler J, Schmidt A, et al. Advanced technology in extracorporeal shock wave lithotripsy: the Dornier MPL 9000 versus the upgraded Dornier HM3. J Endourol 1988;2:173–5.

Servadio C, Livne P, Winkler H. Extracorporeal shock wave lithotripsy using a new compact and portable unit. J Urol 1988;139:685–8.

Shore N, Somers W, Riehle RA Jr. Evolution of pretreatment stenting and local anesthesia for extracorporeal shock wave lithotripsy at a single university center. J Urol 1990;143:257–60.

Sigman M, Laudone VP, Jenkins AD, et al. Initial experience with extracorporeal shock wave lithotripsy in children. J Urol 1987;138:839–41.

Singh M, Tresidder GC, Blandy J. The long-term results of removal of staghorn calculi by extended pyelolithotomy without cooling or renal artery occlusion. Br J Urol 1971;43:658–64.

Singh SM, Yadar R, Gupta NP, Wadhwa SN. The treatment of renal and ureteric calculi in renal failure. Br J Urol 1982;54:445–7.

Smith MJ, Boyce H. Anatrophic nephrotomy and plastic calyrrhapy. J Urol 1968;99:521–7.

Snyder JA, Rosenblum JL, Smith AD. Endourological removal of staghorn calculi in the elderly: analysis of 42 cases. J Endourol 1987;1:123.

Sonda LP, Lipson S, Ross L, Hammond G, Drake D, Bowers G. Report on safety and efficacy of the Medstone 1050 lithotripter. In: Lingeman JE, Newman DE, eds. Shock wave lithotripsy: state of the art. New York: Plenum Press, 1988:255–60.

Sonda LP, Wang S, Ellis J, Kielczewski P, Fleenor S. Resolution of bacteriuria in patients with infection stones: Comparison of results employing treatment modalities. J Endourol 1988;2:151.

Stackl W, Marberger M. Late sequelae of the management of ureteral calculi with the ureterorenoscope. J Urol 1986;136: 386.

Stephenson TP, Banner S, Hargreave TB, Turner-Warwick RT. The technique and results of pyelocalycotomy for staghorn calculi. Br J Urol 1976;47:751–8.

Streem SB, Pontes JE, Novick AC, Montie JE. Ureteropyeloscopy in the evalutation of upper tract filling defects. J Urol 1986;136:383.

Sturm W, Marx FJ, Chaussy C, Eisenberger F. Zum Stellenwert der Unterkühlungsmethode zur operativen Steinentfernung. Urologe (A) 1984;23:9–12.

Sutherland RM. Cell and environment interactions in tumor microregions: the multicell spheroid model. Science 1988;240:177–84.

Tanaka M, Matsumoto T, Kitada S, Kumazawa J, Hara S, Yamaguchi A. Endotoxemia in patients who underwent ultrasonic lithotripsy and extracorporeal shock wave lithotripsy. Eur Urol 1988;14:173–7.

Terhorst B, Cichos M, Versin F, Buss H. Der Einfluss von elektrohydraulischer Schlagwelle und Ultraschall auf das Uroepithel. Urologe (A) 1975;14:41–5.

Thibault P, Dory J, Cotard JP, Moraillon JY, Vallancien G, André-Bougaren J. Lithotripsie à impulsions ultracourtes: étude expérimentale sur une lithiase rénale du chien. Ann Urol 1986;20:20–5.

Thomas R, Harmon E, Sloane B, Hurwitz G, Figueroa TE. Effect of extracorporeal shock wave lithotripsy in children. J Urol 1989;141(2):272A (abstract 412).

Thomas R, Sloane B, Roberts J. Effect of extracorporeal shock wave lithotripsy on renal function. J Urol 1988;139:323A.

Thüroff JW, Alken P, Riedmüller H, Hohenfellner R. Doppler and real-time ultrasound in renal stone surgery. Eur Urol 1982;8:298–303.

Tiselius HG, Hellgren E, Wall I. Infected staghorn stones treated with extracorporeal shock wave lithotripsy and hemiacidrin. J Endourol 1988;2:137.

Tomera KM, Benson RC, Martin X. Sonolith 2000. In: Coptcoat MJ, Miller RA, Wickham JEA, eds. Lithotripsy, vol 2. London: BDI, 1987:65–90.

Tshada R, Miekisch G, Knebel L, Alken P. Ureteral stenting or percutaneous nephrostomy for palliative long-term urinary diversion? In: Proceeding of the sixth World Congress on Endourology and ESWL, September 1–3, 1988, Paris (abstract 211).

Überle f. Ein Konzept für Ultraschall-Ortung und Erkennung von Zielen für Schallpulse hoher Amplitude [dissertation]. University of Karlsruhe, 1988.

Ueda T, Momose S. Modified inferior pyelocalycotomy for staghorn calculi and multiple stones: the use of renal pedicle clamp and fibrin coagulum. Urol Int 1982;37:49–56.

Vahlensieck W, Hesse A, Bach D. Zur Prävalenz des Harnsteinleidens in der Bundesrepublik Deutschland. Urologe (B) 1980;273–6.

Vahlensieck W, Bach D, Hesse A. Inzidenz, Prävalenz und Mortalität des Harnsteinleidens in der BRD. Helv Clin Acta 1982;49:445.

Vahlensieck W Jr, Kürz JJ, Steinhauer H, Friedburg H, Sommerkamp H. Side–effects of extracorporeal piezoelectric shock wave lithotripsy (EPL). Urol Res 1990;18:53–6.

Valchanov V, Michailov P, Patrashkov T. New possibilities of the HM3 lithotripter for treatment of disturbed bone union. In: Proceedings of the Seventh World Congress on Endourology and ESWL, November 27–30, 1989, Kyoto, Japan (abstract P13–14).

Valensic M, Sökeland J. Endoskopische Harnsteinentfernung mit dem Ureterorenoskop. Dtsch Ärztebl 1985;82:268–9.

Vallancien G, Brisset JM, Veillon B, et al. Clinical results with piezoelectric second-generation LT01 lithotripter. J Urol 1987;137:144–9.

Vallancien G, Aviles J, Munoz R, Veillon B, Charton M, Brisset JM. Piezoelectric extracorporeal lithotripsy by ultrashort waves with the EDAP LT01 device. J Urol 1988;139:689–94.

Vandeursen H, Baert L. Extracorporeal shock wave lithotripsy monotherapy for bladder stones with the second-generation lithotriptors. J Urol 1990;143:18–19.

Vandeursen H, Baert L. Extracorporeal shock wave lithotripsy monotherapy for staghorn stones with the second-generation lithotriptors. J Urol 1990;143:252–6.

Vargas AD, Bragin SD, Mendez R. Staghorn calculus: its clinical presentation, complication and management. J Urol 1982;127:860–2.

Vergunst H, Terpstra OT, Schröder FH, Matura E. Assessment of shock wave pressure profiles in vitro: clinical implications. J Lithotripsy Stone Dis 1989;1:289–98.

Vergunst H, Terpstra OT, Schröder FH, Matura E. Assessment of shock wave pressure profiles in vivo. In: Proceedings of the Seventh World Congress on Endourology and ESWL, November 27–30, 1989, Kyoto, Japan (abstract 1–4).

Vögeli T, Mellin HE, Ackermann R. Narkosefreie Ureteroskopie. Urologe A, 28 (Supplement): A 46, 1989

Watson GM, Wickham JE. The pulsed dye laser for stone fragmentation. In: Fourth World Congress on Endourology and ESWL. Madrid 1986.

Watson GM, Wickham JE, Mills TN, Brown P, Salmon PR. Laser fragmentation of renal calculi. Br J Urol 1983;55R613–16.

Watson G, Murray S, Dretler SP, Parrish JA. An assessment of the pulsed dye laser for fragmenting calculi in the pig ureter. J Urol 1987;138:199–202.

Watson G, Murray S, Dretler SP, Parrish JA. The pulsed dye laser for fragmenting urinary calculi. J Urol 1987;138:195.

Webb R, McNicholas TA, Whitfield HN, Wickham JEA. Extracorporeal shock wave lithotripsy, endourology and open surgery: the management and follow-up of 200 patients with urinary calculi. J R Coll Surg Lond 1985;67:337–40.

Webb DR, Fitzpatrick JM. Experimental ureterolithotomy. World J Urol 1985;3:33–5.

Weber HM, Miller K, Hautmann RE. Laser lithotripsy with the pulsed alexandrite: biological side-effects. In: Proceedings of the Seventh World Congress on Endourology and ESWL, November 27–30, 1989, Kyoto, Japan (abstract P5–12).

Weirich W, Ackermann D, Riedmüller H, Alken P. Die Auflösung von Cystinsteinen mit N-Acetylcystein nach perkutaner Nephrostomie. Aktuel Urol 1981;12:224–6.

Weirich W, Haas H, Alken P. Perkutane Chemolyse von Struvitsteinen bei Nierenbecken- und Kelchhalsobstruktion. Aktuel Urol 1982;13:256–8.

Weirich W, Frohnenberg D, Ackermann D, Alken P. Praktische Erfahrungen mit der antegraden lokalen Chemolyse von Struvit/Apatit-, Harnsäure- und Cystinsteinen der Niere. Urologe (A) 1984;23:95–8.

Wess OJ, Marlinghaus Eh, Katona J. A new design of an optimal acoustic source for extracorporeal lithotripsy. In: Second Interdisciplinary International Symposium on Biliary Lithotripsy, Vancouver, April 24–26, 1989.

Whitfield HN. Percutaneous nephrolithotomy. Br J Urol 1983;55:609–12.

Wickham JE. Clinical experience in renal hypothermia. Br J Urol 1963;35:416.

Wickham JE. Urinary calculus disease. Edinburgh: Churchill Livingstone, 1979.

Wickham JE, Kellett MJ. Percutaneous nephrolithotomy. Br J Urol 1981;53:297–9.

Wickham JE, Miller R. Percutaneous surgery of renal calculi. Edinburgh: Churchill Livingstone, 1983.

Wickham JE, Coe N, Ward JP. One hundred cases of nephrolithotomy under hypothermia. J Urol 1974; 112:702–5.

Wickham JE, Fernando AR, Hendry WF, Whitfield HN, Fitzpatrick JM. Intravenous inosine for ischaemic renal surgery. Br J Urol 1979;51:437.

Wickham JE, Kellett MJ, Miller RA. Elective percutaneous nephrolithotomy in 50 patients: an analysis of the technique, results and complications. J Urol 1983;129:904–6.

Wickham JE, Miller RA, Kellett MJ, Payne SR. Percutaneous nephrolithotomy: one stage or two? Br J Urol 1984;56:582–5.

Wickham JE, Webb DR, Payne SR, Kellett MJ, Watkinson G, Whitfield HN. Extracorporeal shock wave lithotripsy: the first 50 patients treated in Britain. Br Med J 1985;290:1188–9.

Wilbert DM, Jungbluth A, Rosenkranz T. et al. Experimental evaluation of a new electromagnetic shock wave source. In: Jacobi GH, et al., eds. Investigative urology, vol 2. Berlin: Springer, 1987a:98–102.

Wilbert DM, Reichenberger H, Hutschenreiter G, et al. Second-generation shock wave lithotripsy: experience with the Lithostar. World J Urol 1987;5:255–9.

Wilbert DM, Hutschenreiter G, Schärfe T, Riedmiller H, Alken P, Hohenfellner R. Zweite Generation der berührungslosen Nierensteinzertrümmerung. Klinische Ergebnisse der lokalen Stosswellenlithotripsie. Aktuel Urol 1988;19:93–6.

Williams CM, Kaude JV, Newman RC, Peterson JC, Thomas WC. Extracorporeal shock wave lithotripsy: long-term complications. Am J Radiol 1988; 150:311–15.

Willscher MK, Conway JF, Babayan RK, Morrisseau P, Sant GR, Bertagnoll A. Safety and efficacy of electrohydraulic lithotripsy by ureteroscopy. J Urol 1988;140:957.

Wilmer A, Gambihler S, Delius M, Brendel W. Shock waves enhance the cytotoxicity of cisplatin but not of adriamycin. Eur Surg Res 1988;20:89–90.

Woodhouse CR, Farrell CR, Paris AM, Blandy JP. The place of extended pyelolithotomy in the management of renal staghorn calculi. Br J Urol 1981;53:520–3.

Wu W, Wu H, Zhou XM. "Dry lithotripsy" by a simple modification of the Chinese lithotripter KDE-1. Urol Res 1990;18:57–8.

Wurster H, Ziegler M, Marberger M. Piezolith 2200 (Richard Wolf GmbH). In: Coptcoat MJ, Miller RA, Wickham JEA, eds. Lithotripsy, vol 2. London: BDI, 1987:91–108.

Yeaman LD, McCullough DL, Jerome CP. Effects of extracorporeal shock waves on immature bone growth of the rat. J Urol 1988;139:324A.

Yendt ER, Chohanin M. Experience with thiazide diuretics in calcium oxalate urolithiasis. World J Urol 1983;1:176–9.

Yokoyama M, Kitahara K, Yanagizawa R, Shoji F, Osaka M. Tissue damage by extracorporeal shock wave lithotripsy treatment in patients with urolithiasis: clinical evaluation. In: Lingeman JE, Newman DE, eds. Shock wave lithotripsy: state of the art. New York: Plenum Press, 1988:377–82.

Zechner O, Köller A. Die superselektive anatrophe Nephrotomie. Aktuel Urol 1983;14:132–5.

Zeiss L. Über eine neue Methode der konservativen Harnsteinbehandlung. Z Urol 1939;33:121.

Ziegler M, Kopper B, Riedlinger R, et al. Die Zertrümmerung von Nierensteinen mi einem piezoelektrischen Gerätesystem. Urologe (A) 1986;25:193–7.

Ziegler M, Mast G, Neisius D, et al. Results in the use of extracorporeal piezoelectric lithotripsy (EPL) for treatment of urinary calculi. Urol Int 1988;43:35–41.

Zwergel U, Neisius D, Zwergel T, et al. Results and clinical management of extracorporeal piezoceramic lithotripsy (EPL) in 1,321 consecutive treatments. World J Urol 1987;5:213–19.

Index